Advances in Experimental Medicine and Biology

Volume 890

More information about this series at http://www.springer.com/series/5584

Aamir Ahmad • Shirish M. Gadgeel
Editors

Lung Cancer and Personalized Medicine: Novel Therapies and Clinical Management

Springer

Editors
Aamir Ahmad
Karmanos Cancer Institute
Wayne State University
Detroit, MI, USA

Shirish M. Gadgeel
Karmanos Cancer Institute
Wayne State University
Detroit, MI, USA

ISSN 0065-2598 ISSN 2214-8019 (electronic)
Advances in Experimental Medicine and Biology
ISBN 978-3-319-79702-1 ISBN 978-3-319-24932-2 (eBook)
DOI 10.1007/978-3-319-24932-2

Springer Cham Heidelberg New York Dordrecht London

Softcover reprint of the hardcover 1st edition 2016

Printed on acid-free paper

Springer International Publishing AG Switzerland is part of Springer Science+Business Media (www.springer.com)

Preface

This is the second part of volume *Lung Cancer and Personalized Medicine*. Part I of this volume, available as a separate book, discussed lung cancer as a disease, the available therapies and the associated challenges. In this edition, we focus on the upcoming and novel strategies to better understand and target lung cancer. As discussed in the chapters presented here, our understanding of lung cancer and the various factors associated with its onset and progression has vastly improved in last several years. All this information is critical to developing personalized therapies tailored for the benefit of individual patients.

A major component of personalized therapy is the ability to profile an individual lung cancer patient. The molecular and genomic profiling of lung cancers are steps in this direction. *Chapter 1* focuses on the advancements in these areas of lung cancer research. *Chapter 2* summarizes all of the emerging biomarkers, relevant to personalized care of lung cancer patients. This chapter discusses the many potential biomarkers, such as ROS1, RET, MET, HER2 and BRAF that are under investigation. This is in addition to EGFR and ALK, the more established biomarkers covered in more detailed chapters in part I of this volume. For a successful personalized profiling of lung cancer patients, a comprehensive signature, with relative status of multiple biomarkers, is very critical. *Chapter 3* focuses on the process of epithelial to mesenchymal transition (EMT), a phenomenon that is particularly relevant to metastasis of lung cancers. The important role that EMT plays in acquisition of stem cell-like properties and resistance to targeted therapies is now well accepted, and all these topics are covered in this chapter.

Chapter 4 continues on the topic of cancer stem cells (CSCs) and provides a more detailed overview of our knowledge on the topic. The existence of CSCs has been a hotly debated topic for last several years. In addition to the various markers and a role of CSCs in the recurrence and drug resistance mechanisms of lung cancers, this chapter also describes the emerging evidence of natural agents and their synthetic derivatives as compounds that can effectively target CSCs. *Chapter 5* details the current knowledge of lung cancer cells' niche—the microenvironment—which feeds and sustains lung cancer cells, providing them the perfect environment to acquire an aggressive phenotype. A better understanding of tumor microenvironment is critical to the development of future personalized therapies for lung cancer patients. The next chapter, *Chapter 6*, examines the epigenetic changes associated with lung cancer progression and their possible validation as therapeutic targets. This chapter discusses the epigenetic changes that are now known to influence the expression of oncogenes as well as the tumor suppressors, and the various epigenetic events that can potentially be targeted as part of personalized management of lung cancer patients.

Chapter 7 provides a detailed overview of next-generation sequencing and the associated promise of early detection and molecular profiling of lung cancers. The importance of early detection and complete profiling cannot be over-stated, and, moving forward, such methodologies will be very handy at the time of making decisions for personalized treatment plans. *Chapter 8* discusses the promising field of 'cancer nanomedicine'. The nanoparticle-based systems, discussed in this chapter, can be an invaluable tool in the delivery of novel therapeutic agents in an attempt to enhance their effectiveness. According to the American Cancer Society, lung cancers are three distinct types: non-small cell lung cancers; small cell lung cancers; and lung carcinoid tumors. While non-small cell lung cancers represent a major subtype with up to 85% of all lung cancers, small cell lung cancers are known to be particularly aggressive. *Chapter 9* describes the recent updates towards personalized therapy of small cell lung cancers.

The foregoing chapters address the various characteristics of lung cancers and the putative targets of therapy, knowledge of which is essential to the development of personalized clinical management. The manner in which the personalized approach is actually applied in clinical management of lung cancers is discussed in the last two chapters of this section. Radiation therapy is a major treatment option for lung cancers, and *Chapter 10* discusses the concept of personalized radiation therapy that promises to improve treatment outcomes with substantially reduced toxicity. Finally, *Chapter 11* details the approaches to making a decision for personalized treatment of lung cancer patients, based on the individual clinical characteristics, biomarkers and other parameters that an individual lung cancer patient presents.

Between the two parts, this volume comprehensively covers many aspects of modern day lung cancer research, with special focus on personalized therapy. We are so excited to have a panel of experts and leading lung cancer scientists contribute to this volume, and it is our distinct pleasure to present this volume to the scientific community.

Detroit, USA

Aamir Ahmad, PhD
Shirish M. Gadgeel, MD

Contents

Contributors

Aamir Ahmad Karmanos Cancer Institute, Wayne State University, Detroit, MI, USA

Shadan Ali Department of Oncology, Karmanos Cancer Institute, Wayne State University School of Medicine, Detroit, MI, USA

Nasser K. Altorki Department of Cardiothoracic Surgery, Weill Medical College of Cornell University, New York, NY, USA

Neuberger Berman Lung Cancer Research Center, Weill Medical College of Cornell University, New York, NY, USA

Aliccia Bollig-Fischer Department of Oncology, Barbara Ann Karmanos Cancer Institute, Wayne State University, Detroit, MI, USA

Philip T. Cagle Houston Methodist Hospital, Weill Medical College of Cornell University, Houston, TX, USA

Shirish M. Gadgeel Karmanos Cancer Institute, Wayne State University, Detroit, MI, USA

Mary Helen Barcellos-Hoff Department of Radiation Oncology, New York University School of Medicine, New York, NY, USA

Sajid Hussain NCI-designated Cancer Center, Sanford Burnham Prebys Medical Discovery Institute, La Jolla, CA, USA

Jian-Yue Jin Cancer Center, Georgia Regents University, Augusta, GA, USA

Gregory P. Kalemkerian Division of Hematology/Oncology, University of Michigan, Ann Arbor, MI, USA

Feng-Ming (Spring) Kong Cancer Center, Georgia Regents University, Augusta, GA, USA

Kristina M. Kruglyak Oncology, Illumina, Inc., San Diego, CA, USA

Erick Lin Medical Affairs, Ambry Genetics, Inc., Aliso Viejo, CA, USA

Timothy E. McGraw Department of Cardiothoracic Surgery, Weill Medical College of Cornell University, New York, NY, USA

Neuberger Berman Lung Cancer Research Center, Weill Medical College of Cornell University, New York, NY, USA

Department of Biochemistry, Weill Medical College of Cornell University, New York, NY, USA

Vivek Mittal Department of Cardiothoracic Surgery, Neuberger Berman Foundation Lung Cancer Center, New York, NY, USA

Department of Cell and Developmental Biology, Weill Medical College of Cornell University, New York, NY, USA

Navneet Narula Department of Pathology, Weill Medical College of Cornell University, New York, NY, USA

Frank S. Ong Medical Affairs and Clinical Development, NantHealth, LLC, Culver City, CA, USA

Philip A. Philip Department of Oncology, Karmanos Cancer Institute, Wayne State University School of Medicine, Detroit, MI, USA

Bryce P. Portier Houston Methodist Hospital, Houston, TX, USA

Kirtee Raparia Department of Pathology, Northwestern University, Feinberg School of Medicine, Chicago, IL, USA

Tina El Rayes Department of Cardiothoracic Surgery, Weill Medical College of Cornell University, New York, NY, USA

Neuberger Berman Lung Cancer Research Center, Weill Medical College of Cornell University, New York, NY, USA

Department of Cell and Developmental Biology, Weill Medical College of Cornell University, New York, NY, USA

Weill Cornell Graduate School of Medical Sciences, Weill Medical College of Cornell University, New York, NY, USA

Fazlul H. Sarkar Department of Pathology, Karmanos Cancer Institute, Wayne State University School of Medicine, Detroit, MI, USA

Department of Oncology, Karmanos Cancer Institute, Wayne State University School of Medicine, Detroit, MI, USA

Bryan J. Schneider Division of Hematology/Oncology, University of Michigan, Ann Arbor, MI, USA

Raagini Suresh Department of Pathology, Karmanos Cancer Institute, Wayne State University School of Medicine, Detroit, MI, USA

Priyanga Wijesinghe Department of Oncology, Barbara Ann Karmanos Cancer Institute, Wayne State University, Detroit, MI, USA

Lung Cancer Genomics in the Era of Accelerated Targeted Drug Development

Priyanga Wijesinghe and Aliccia Bollig-Fischer

Abstract Lung cancer is the leading cause of cancer-related deaths in the United States and the 5-year overall survival outlook for a patient has not improved in several decades. Recently, however, molecular and genomic profiling of the lung tumors has revealed recurring somatic mutations. As a result the therapeutic landscape of lung cancer is undergoing a paradigm shift from a purely histology-based understanding of the disease to subtype distinctions based on tumor genetics, which has launched cancer-specific, mechanism-based targeted therapies with clear benefit to patients. While targeted therapy advancements are being made at an ever increasing rate, a new challenge in the form of drug resistance has also emerged. This review summarizes the current literature for these issues.

Keywords Lung cancer • Targeted therapy • Genomics • Tyrosine-kinase inhibitors • Molecular biomarkers • Fusion genes • Drug resistance • EGFR • ALK

1 Oncogenes, Tumor Suppressors and Targeted Therapeutics

Carcinogenesis and the course of the disease for each patient are influenced by many factors including ancestral genetics or germ-line polymorphisms and behavioral or life-style issues. But ultimately cancer is a disease dictated by somatic mutations. Decades of research has contributed to the understanding that cancer initiation and progression are governed by the activation of cancer driver genes, termed oncogenes, and inactivation of key tumor suppressor genes. The importance of oncogenes is underscored by the progress made in developing molecularly targeted drugs to block the function of oncogenes, often proteins with kinase function such as the epidermal growth factor receptors *EGFR* and *HER2* [1].

P. Wijesinghe, Ph.D. • A. Bollig-Fischer, Ph.D. (✉)
Department of Oncology, Barbara Ann Karmanos Cancer Institute,
Wayne State University, 4100 John R, Detroit, MI 48201, USA
e-mail: wijesinp@karmanos.org; bollig@karmanos.org

A. Ahmad, S.M. Gadgeel (eds.), *Lung Cancer and Personalized Medicine: Novel Therapies and Clinical Management*, Advances in Experimental Medicine and Biology 890, DOI 10.1007/978-3-319-24932-2_1

There is a fundamental distinction for activating mutations arising in oncogenes compared to other mutations that are termed passenger mutations. If the mutations confer a selective growth advantage to the cancer cells they are considered to be driver oncogene mutations. Molecularly targeted therapy exploits tumor dependence on activation of driver oncogenes. Although tumor suppressors are not as directly amenable to targeted therapy, other therapeutic avenues are being explored. There are occasions where tumor suppressor gene inactivation by mutation results in the activation of kinases downstream the signaling pathway [2]. For example, the inactivation of the tumor suppressor gene *PTEN* activates the *AKT* kinase thus giving the hope in targeted therapy [3, 4]. Also, an active line of research explores mechanisms and drugs with potential to re-activate tumor suppressor pathways [5, 6].

Recently, the therapeutic landscape of Non-Small Cell Lung Cancer (NSCLC) underwent a paradigm shift from a purely histology based approach to a treatment of molecular subtypes driven by distinct genetic alterations. The evolution of this new direction started with the discovery that gain-of-function somatic mutations in epidermal growth factor receptor (*EGFR*) recurring in NSCLC are sensitive to EGFR tyrosine kinase inhibitors like gefitinib [7–9]. This led to the finding of a number of other genes with driver mutations in lung cancer such as *HER2, KRAS, BRAF, NRAS, PIK3CA, AKT* [10]. In 2007, Soda et al. discovered an *EML4-ALK* fusion gene, a product of a chromosomal rearrangement and a transforming agent of NSCLC [11]. After this pioneering work, the list of tumorigenic fusion genes in lung cancer is ever increasing. Therefore, this cause and effect based genomic research now links specific oncogenes and recurring mutations to the disease and provides rationale for biomarkers and molecularly targeted treatments that are improving lung cancer patient outcomes [12].

With in-depth mechanistic understanding it is appreciated that there are various ways to aberrantly or constitutively activate a proto-oncogene, but fundamentally and chief among them are genomic aberrations in the form of somatic coding mutations, copy number changes and genomic rearrangements leading to tumorigenic gene fusions. It is often straightforward to appreciate how genome aberrations in the form of coding mutations or somatic copy number alterations (SCNAs) contribute to cancer. DNA coding mutations can activate an oncogene directly or disrupt protein regulatory domains, and disruption of tumor suppressor function occurs when mutations translate to missense or truncated protein sequence. In SCNA, the operative effect of DNA imbalance disrupts the gene expression levels and thus the proper availability of the protein to function normally.

Knowledge of lung cancer molecular biology and mutation drivers has rapidly increased in recent years largely due to advancements made in high-throughput technologies that allow for genomic and transcriptomic-scale analyses. This review captures the present state of molecular genomics research of lung cancer. The diversity of oncogenic somatic mutations in lung cancer subtypes, the heightened status of fusion genes in lung cancer, and how the information is translating to the clinic are major topics.

2 Somatic Copy Number Alterations and Coding Mutation Frequencies According to Lung Cancer Subtype

Lung cancers are a heterogeneous group of tumors that are traditionally categorized by histology. By far the majority of lung cancers are categorized as non-small cell lung cancer (NSCLC) and about 15 % minority are small cell lung cancer. NSCLCs are further subdivided into adenocarcinomas (~45 %), squamous cell lung cancer (~23 %), and large cell lung cancer (~3 %), with other subtypes representing the remaining approximate 28 % [13]. During the last decade there has been a shift in classification of lung cancer based on tumor genetics. This attempt not only provided the actionable targets for the effective therapy but highlighted the importance of reconsidering the tumor reclassification, from histology based to molecular based. For example, in a recent genomic study of lung cancer classification, existence of the large cell lung cancer subtype was brought into question when these specimens were discovered to fit with adenocarcinomas or squamous cell lung cancer [12]. Moreover, the genomics approach used in this study recognized adenocarcinoma and squamous cell lung cancer cases that were not classifiable by histology.

2.1 Lung Adenocarcinoma

Of the three major subtypes of lung cancers, patients with adenocarcinoma benefit the most from molecular genomic based cancer therapeutics today. While 25–30 % of patients receive targeted therapies like gefitinib and erlotinib, another 25–30 % can enroll in clinical trials targeting other known oncogenic drivers [14]. The major oncogenic drivers in lung adenocarcinoma include activating mutations in *EGFR, KRAS, BRAF, HER2, MET* or translocations of *ALK, ROS1* and *RET* [15, 16]; and all of these targets have drugs that are approved or in clinical trials. Tumor suppressor loss-of-function mutations occurring in lung adenocarcinoma include *TP53, CDKN2A, PTEN, STK11, RB1, NF1, KEAP1* and *SMARCA4* [16–18]. Targeting these tumor suppressor alterations is therapeutically challenging at the moment [16], but their presence may be highly informative such as in the case of *TP53* mutation association with lack of response to EGFR inhibitors and recurrence [12, 19]. The key genes that are targets for treatment or that hold therapeutic potential for adenocarcinoma are discussed in greater detail below; focusing on *EGFR* as the model gene for lung cancer targeted therapy.

2.1.1 *EGFR*

The epidermal growth factor receptor is a transmembrane tyrosine kinase that has an extracellular ligand-binding domain and an intracellular tyrosine kinase domain (Fig. 1a). EGFR belongs to the ErbB/HER family of growth factors and these

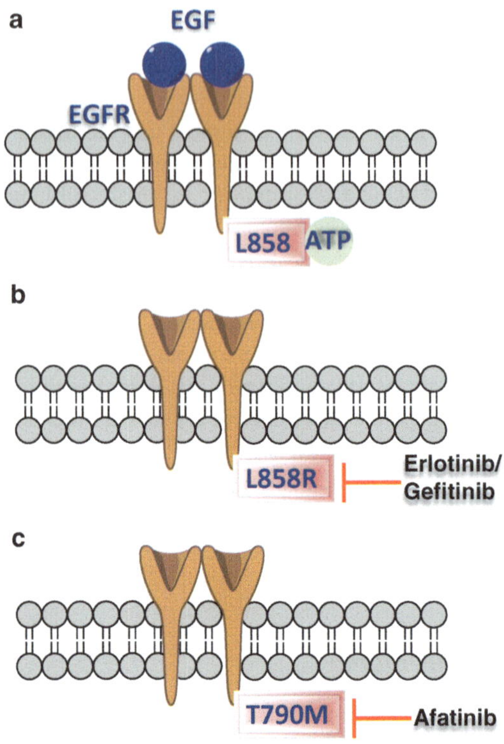

Fig. 1 Oncogenic EGFR, targeted therapy and drug resistance. (**a**) The *EGFR* proto-oncogene encodes a tansmembrane protein (EGFR) containing an extracellular ligand-binding domain and an intracellular component with a catalytic tyrosine kinase domain. Under normal physiology, binding of a ligand (e.g. EGF) causes homodimerization of EGFR or heterodimerization with other ERBB family members to activate kinase function and induce phosphorylation. (**b**) With the transversion (T>G) point mutation at nucleotide position 2573, *EGFR* becomes oncogenic and this genetic change substitutes an arginine (R) for leucine (L) at codon 858 in exon 21. This L858R amino acid change leads to ligand-independent, constitutive activation of EGFR signaling. While this alteration disrupts the autoinhibitory interactions it also sensitizes the protein to inhibition by tyrosine kinase inhibitors like erlotinib and gefitinib. (**c**) More than half of the patients acquire resistance to reversible tyrosine kinase inhibitors erlotinib or gefitinib through a second mutation at T790M. This threonine to methionine amino acid change markedly decreased drug binding affinity. Afatinib is an irreversible ERBB family blocker shown to inhibit the effects of T790M mutation

proteins play a pivotal role in cell proliferation, adhesion, migration and invasion [20]. When the reversible tyrosine kinase inhibitors erlotinib and gefitinib were first used in early clinical trials in an unselected patient cohort, it showed only a modest efficacy (a response rate of about 10 %) over placebo [21]. Then in 2004 an underlying connection between *EGFR* activating mutations and improved lung cancer response to tyrosine kinase inhibitors laid the groundwork for molecularly informed targeted therapy [7–9]. In lung cancer, the key *EGFR* mutations occur in exons 18 through 21 and alter the ATP binding pocket of the kinase domain. Most mutations detected are exon 19 deletions of which there are over 20 variants (most common delE746-A750). The next most common are missense mutations in exon 21—the most frequent point mutation is the L858R (Fig. 1b). Biochemical studies later showed how these *EGFR* mutants preferentially bind the tyrosine kinase inhibitors like erlotinib or gefitinib over ATP [22, 23]. Therefore, these mutations are the cause of ligand-independent activation of the EGFR signaling and confer sensitivity to tyrosine kinase inhibitors. A range of less frequent in-frame insertions and duplication mutations in exon 20 have also been reported [24, 25]. As research continues, less frequent novel *EGFR* mutations with biologically plausible activating function are likely to be discovered. For example, a recent high-throughput whole genome and exome sequencing study using 183 lung adenocarcinoma and matched normal pairs detected two novel exon 25 and 26 deletions truncating C-terminus of the *EGFR* [16].

Having understood the association between gain-of-function mutations of *EGFR* and sensitivity to EGFR tyrosine kinase inhibitors, studies demonstrated the superiority of EGFR tyrosine kinase inhibitors over chemotherapy in terms of progression-free survival, response and quality of life [26, 27]. Currently, gefitinib has been approved in Europe to treat NSCLC harboring *EGFR* mutations. Erlotinib was approved by the United States Food and Drug Administration (FDA) for the first line treatment of NSCLC with detected sensitizing mutations.

Although patients with *EGFR* mutations respond to tyrosine kinase inhibitor drugs initially, all eventually develop resistance due to the secondary mutations or other mechanisms. The most common secondary point mutation is the *EGFR* T790M activating mutation in exon 20 (Fig. 1c). This amino acid substitution introduces a bulky methionine at the wild-type threonine [28]. Presumably this gatekeeper mutation alters the ATP binding pocket of EGFR to reduce inhibitor binding capacity and increase affinity for ATP [23]. The second-generation irreversible EGFR tyrosine kinase inhibitor, afatinib was recently given FDA approval as a first-line therapy. When gefitinib, erlotinib or afatinib are administered as the first-line therapy for the patients with sensitization *EGFR* mutations, 60–80 % of the patients responded with median progression-free survival of 9–12 months and median survival in excess of 2 years [27].

Finally, it is of note that *EGFR* alterations are primarily in adenocarcinoma subtype and present in approximately 10 % of patients of European or African descent [29–31] though there is some dispute in the literature [32–34], while 40 % Asian patients harbor an *EGFR* mutation [35–37]. The majority of them are never smoker, younger, female patients [24, 36–38]. *EGFR* mutations are very rare in histologically pure squamous cell lung cancer [39, 40].

2.1.2 *KRAS*

KRAS belongs to the *RAS* family of proto-oncogenes and it plays a central role in downstream signal transduction induced by an array of growth factor receptors including EGFR [41]. The *KRAS* encoded G-protein acts as an on or off switch depending on whether the binding partner is GTP (guanosine triphosphate) or GDP (guanosine diphosphate). Mutated *KRAS* codes for a protein lacking GTPase activity; thus, binding of GTP locks in constitutive activation of downstream RAF/MEK/ERK and

PI3K/AKT/mTOR signaling pathways [42, 43]. The most common activating mutations for *KRAS* include those in codon 12 and less frequently in codons 13 and 61. *KRAS* mutation is the most frequent oncogenic alteration in lung adenocarcinoma representing between 25 and 40 % of cases [38, 44, 45]. In general *KRAS* mutations do not co-occur with *EGFR* mutations hence it can be used as a potential negative predictive marker for the efficacy of EGFR tyrosine kinase inhibitors [24, 38]. Moreover, if *KRAS* is mutated it is logical that such tumors are resistant to EGFR tyrosine kinase inhibitors since KRAS acts on molecules downstream in the EGFR signaling pathway [46]. MEK1/MEK2 inhibitor selumetinib (in combination with docetaxel) was recently used in a randomized phase II study using 87 patients with advanced NSCLC having *KRAS* mutations [47]. In this study the combination arm, selumetinib plus docetaxel compared to placebo plus docetaxel, showed superior overall survival, though results did not reach statistical significance. Therefore, a phase III trial with a larger group of patients is needed to confirm the above results [27]. Ongoing clinical trials to inhibit *KRAS* mutations by targeting downstream pathways in NSCLC are studying the effects of a variety of drugs and targets, including the MEK inhibitors trametinib; tivantinib with erlotinib; or the hsp90 inhibitor IPI504 plus the mTOR inhibitor everolimus [27].

2.1.3 *BRAF*

The proto-oncogene *BRAF* encodes a serine/threonine protein kinase. This is the downstream effector protein of KRAS that activates the MAPK pathway regulating cell proliferation and survival [48]. *BRAF* mutations are very common in melanomas (approximately 66 % [48]) and they represent about 3 % of NSCLC [49]. Of all *BRAF* mutations in lung adenocarcinoma the V600E codon mutation accounts for 50 % [50]. V600E is within exon 15 and is an activating point mutation resulting in increased kinase activity, while most other *BRAF* codon mutations identified in lung adenocarcinoma, including G469A in exon 11 and D594G in exon 15, show low or intermediate kinase activity [48–50]. A recent case report showed the clinical benefit of the drug vemurafenib in treating a NSCLC patient with a tumor V600E mutation [51]. The ongoing clinical trials targeting either BRAF or its downstream effectors are studying outcomes for BRAF inhibitor dabrafenib on NSCLC patients with *BRAF* V600E mutation, the MEK inhibitor, trametinib for patients with non-V600E mutations and the drug dasatinib for the NSCLC patients with uncharacterized *BRAF* mutations [27].

2.1.4 *HER2*

Like *EGFR, HER2* is also a member of the ErbB family of epidermal growth factor receptor tyrosine kinases. HER2 is activated in 25–30 % of breast cancers due to focal amplification of the chromosome region 17q12 comprising the *HER2* gene. The contribution of *HER2* amplification in lung adenocarcinoma has been estimated to be 35 % based on immunohistochemistry studies [52]. Although not found in breast cancer, *HER2* is also observed to be activated in approximately 2 % of lung adenocarcinomas due to an in-frame insertion [53]. These activating mutations occur in exon 20 as in-frame insertions of 3 to 12 base pairs [54]. A clinical trial investigating outcomes of monoclonal antibody trastuzumab targeting HER2 overexpression in NSCLC showed no benefit alone [55] or in combination with chemotherapy [56]. However, individual clinical case reports support the potential for patients with *HER2* amplification in lung cancer [57]. Moreover, studies of HER2 binding tyrosine kinase inhibitors including afatinib [58], dacomitinib and neratinib [59] have yielded promising preliminary results against *HER2* mutants in NSCLC.

2.1.5 *MET*

The proto-oncogene *MET* codes for the transmembrane receptor tyrosine kinase also known as hepatocyte growth factor receptor. The binding of hepatocyte growth factor (HGF ligand) to the MET receptor activates the downstream RAS/RAF/MEK/MAPK; PI3K/AKT and c-SRC kinase pathways [60]. Mutations in *MET* are rare and it is most often gene copy number increase that leads to overexpression of the MET protein [61, 62]. A key observation for this mutation is that the amplification of *MET* gene is associated with developing secondary resistance to EGFR tyrosine kinase inhibitors. Evidence suggests that 5 % of the patients with *EGFR* mutations who initially responded to gefitinib or erlotinib acquire resistance due to *MET* amplification [63–65]. Here, the increased MET kinase activity drives the PI3K/AKT pathway bypassing the EGFR-directed tyrosine kinase inhibition [65]. The findings indicate the importance of blocking both EGFR and MET as a means of treating patients with acquired resistance. A recent randomized double blind phase II study investigating the effect of the MET receptor-targeted monoclonal antibody onartuzumab plus erlotinib compared to placebo plus erlotinib showed significant improvements in clinical outcomes with respect to progression-free survival and overall survival [66]. Moreover, this study illustrated the importance of parallel diagnostic testing after seeing worse outcomes with *MET* amplification negative patients. Therefore, the MET immunohistochemisty assay developed in the phase II study was incorporated as a diagnostic test for use of onartuzumab in the randomized phase III trial investigating the effect of onartuzumab and erlotinib [67]. A number of MET inhibitors and neutralizing antibodies are drugs presently in development. Some of the examples are MET inhibitor cabozantinib [68], MET tyrosine kinase inhibitor crizotinib [69], and hepatocyte growth factor neutralizing antibody rilotumumab [70, 71]. It has been noted that *MET* amplifications and *KRAS* mutations are mutually exclusive, meaning they are not co-expressed in lung cancer specimens [72].

2.2 *Squamous Cell Lung Cancer*

Of the major subtypes of lung cancers, squamous cell lung cancer shows the strongest association with cigarette smoking [73]. Furthermore unlike lung adenocarcinoma, presently there are no targeted therapies used in treatment of squamous cell lung cancer patients. Past trials to treat squamous cell lung cancer with chemotherapy and EGFR tyrosine kinase inhibitors showed the ineffectiveness of such treatments [74, 75]. This puts increased emphasis on the need for genomic analyses to find potential oncogenes that may present druggable targets for this cancer subtype. The earliest genomic aberrations found in squamous cell lung cancer included allelic loses at chromosome 3p (3p21, 3p22–24, 3p25), 8p21–23, 9p21 [76]; followed by loses at 17p13 comprising the *TP53* tumor suppressor gene and 13q14 containing tumor suppressor *RB1* [77]. Using whole-exome sequencing to identify new somatic mutations in this lung cancer subtype, Zheng et al. reported *TP53*, *EP300*, *LPHN2*, C10orf137, *MYH2*, *TGM2* and *MS4A3* as mutated genes with oncogenic potential [78]. Comprehensive analyses by The Cancer Genome Atlas (TCGA) shed more light on squamous cell lung cancer in 2012. The project used 178 histopathologically reviewed samples to detect on average 323 SCNAs, 360 exonic mutations and 165 genomic rearrangements per tumor [3]. The study identified statistically significant, recurring mutations in 11 genes, including *TP53* mutations in nearly all the specimens. The mutation frequencies of the genes in TCGA data were compatible with the study carried out by Paik et al. that examined specimens from 52 patients [79]. In this study 60 % of the patients harbored functionally relevant mutations in druggable oncogene targets including *FGFR1*, *DDR2*, *PIK3CA* in addition to tumor suppressor *PTEN*. Research has continued and the evolving knowledge on the specifics of oncogenic drivers of squamous cell lung cancer is further discussed below. Moreover, results from clinical studies are necessary to appreciate if these findings will translate to improve the overall survival of squamous cell lung cancer patients.

2.2.1 Somatic Copy Number Alterations in Squamous Cell Lung Cancer

FGFR1 (Fibroblast growth factor receptor 1) is a transmembrane tyrosine kinase and is one of the promising drug targets in squamous cell lung cancer. The amplification of the chromosome region 8p12 was detected in 2010 and focal amplification of *FGFR1* was validated in 15 of 155 squamous cell tumors [80]. The amplification was confirmed in an independent cohort of squamous cell lung cancer samples with 22 % cases being positive by fluorescence in situ hybridization (FISH) analysis [80]. According to TCGA analysis amplification of *FGFR1* is observed in 7 % of squamous cell lung cancer [3]. Clinical trials employing small molecule inhibitors that block FGFR1 are on-going, these include molecules specific to FGFR1 kinase, multi-kinase inhibitors and pan-FGFR inhibitors [80–82]. *FGFR1* amplification and *MET* amplification frequency (reported at about 6 % in lung squamous cell lung cancer) are both considered to be more prevalent in lung squamous cell lung cancer than in adenocarcinoma [83].

SOX2 is a transcription factor that regulates pluripotency of embryonic stem cells as well as morphogenesis of trachea-bronchial epithelia [73]. This lineage-survival oncogene was discovered using comparative genomic hybridization with probes targeting the 3q26 region [84]. About 60–80 % of squamous cell lung cancers show amplifications in this region of chromosome 3 and approximately 20 % harbor a focal amplification that includes the *SOX2* gene [85, 86]. According to the TCGA study, *SOX2* was amplified in 21 % of the samples analyzed [3]. Although it was demonstrated that the inhibition of SOX2 suppresses cancer cell growth, research also suggests that *SOX2* amplification is not sufficient for carcinogenesis in the absence of other oncogenic mutations [84].

At a lower frequency than those estimated above, *PDGFRA* (platelet-derived growth factor receptor) tyrosine kinase, located in chromosomal region 4q12, is shown to be amplified in 4–8 % of squamous cell lung cancers [3, 87]. There are a number of multi-targeted tyrosine kinase inhibitors against *PDGFRA* that are in clinical development at this time; including sunitinib, pazopanib, cediranib and nintedanib [88]. *HER2* amplifications are also observed in about 4 % of squamous cell lung cancers [89]; evaluation of *HER2*-directed therapy needs to be done.

2.2.2 Somatic Coding Mutations in Squamous Cell Lung Cancer

Well-documented oncogene mutations recurring at significant frequency in squamous cell lung cancer include the *AKT1* codon E17K somatic mutation, which causes constitutive activation of the kinase [90]. Malanga et al. found this mutation in a subset of squamous cell lung cancer (2/36 lung squamous cell lung cancer and 0/53 lung adenocarcinoma) [91]. AKT kinase inhibitors such as MK2206 and GDC-0068 are in clinical trials [92]. *BRAF* mutations are present in about 4 % of squamous cell lung cancers [50]. A clinical trial is underway to test BRAF-specific kinase inhibitor GSK2118436 on patients with squamous cell lung cancer with BRAF mutations [82]; and other existing data point to MEK inhibition as potentially effective target for non-V600E *BRAF* mutations in this lung cancer subcategory [93]. *DDR2* (Discoidin domain receptor 2) tyrosine kinase is described as an oncogene that promotes cell proliferation and cell survival [94], and mutations in the *DDR2* gene render cells sensitive to the small molecule kinase inhibitor dasatinib [95]. A clinical trial is underway to find out the efficacy of dasatinib on the squamous cell lung cancer with activating *DDR2* mutations, which are observed at a rate of close to 4 %.

PIK3CA is one of the most common sequence mutated oncogenes in cancer and it is reported to present more frequently in squamous cell lung cancer than in lung adenocarcinoma [96]. In accordance with previous studies missense mutations at codon positions 545 and 1047 were found in 48 % of the samples in the TCGA study [3, 97]. *PIK3CA* encodes the catalytic subunit of the PI3K lipid kinases and a number of clinical trials are presently underway to examine the impact of targeted therapies and combination PI3K inhibitors and chemotherapy in lung cancer [98]. The PI3K inhibitors in clinical development include XL-147, XL-765, BEZ235, BKM120, GDC-0941, early evidence indicates the response rate to these single agents are low [10, 98, 99].

Other genes reported to show recurring mutations in squamous cell lung cancer include the *MLL2* gene encoding a histone methyltranferase that plays a key role in epigenetic programming and embryonic development. The therapeutic strategies to target epigenetic pathways; for example histone methyltransferase inhibitors are also emerging and mutation activated *MLL2* holds promise as a novel target [100, 101]. *PTEN* is a tumor suppressor gene often sequence mutated and inactivated in many types of cancer. The mutation frequency of *PTEN* reported at 15 % in squamous cell lung cancer is higher than compared to lung adenocarcinoma [3, 102]. Also, how loss of function mutations in the *HLA_A* class I Major Histocompatibility (MHC I) gene may help cancer cells avoid immune responses as has been proposed and raises the promise of immunotherapy [103, 104].

2.3 Small Cell Lung Cancer

Small cell lung cancer is the third most frequent subtype of lung cancer diagnosis representing around 200,000 cases worldwide annually. According to overall survival rates, patients with small cell lung cancer by far face the lowest probability of survival [105]. The 5-year overall survival outlook for these patients is about 5 % and this has not improved for the last four decades [106]. Efforts to study somatic mutations in small cell lung cancer, which is rarely treated by surgery, trail behind other histologic subtypes due to lack of specimens. However, very recent studies present the first results of comprehensive profiling of small cell lung cancer specimens. Rudin et al. characterized 80 small cell lung cancer specimens including cancer-derived cell lines and 36 primary tumors and paired normal tissue [107] A key finding was a significant *SOX2* amplification frequency ~27 % and the demonstration of decreased proliferation in a small cell lung cancer cell model using shRNA knockdown of *SOX2* [107]. Peifer et al., by accessing small cell lung tumor specimens from a global genome research consortium, were able to sequence 29 exomes, 2 genomes and 15 transcriptomes [108]. Their SCNA algorithm identified almost universal deletions at chromosome 3p and 13q (affecting *RB1*), 17p (containing *TP53*) and frequent gains of 3q and 5p as well as for the *FGFR1* gene.

Iwakawa et al. used genome-wide copy number analysis and whole-transcriptome sequencing to study the genome-wide amplifications and translocations in small cell lung cancer [109]. Their copy number analysis found 34 genes to be frequently amplified in small cell lung cancer. Among them three *MYC* family genes *MYCL1* (1p34.2), *MYCN* (2p24.3) and *MYC* (8q24.21) were frequently amplified in concordance with the previous small scale studies using [110–112]. This is an important finding in small cell lung cancer as inhibitors against *MYC* family protein products are gaining research traction [113–115]. In addition, the study identified the chromosomal region 9p24.1 as demonstrating mutual exclusivity with *MYC* amplifications. Furthermore, mRNA expression of the gene *KIAA1432* (from the 9p24.1 region) was strongly correlated with the *KIAA1432* amplification suggesting a novel cancer gene activated in small cell lung cancer. Compared to prevalence of kinase gene mutations in lung adenocarcinoma, targeting molecular markers of the small cell lung cancer (e.g. *SOX2*) may be therapeutically challenging. However, extensive basic and clinical research on the genomic aberrations of small cell lung cancer will enable efforts to understand and develop treatment options for this exceptionally aggressive disease. Since lack of small cell lung cancer patient specimens is a major problem, Sos et al. screened 267 compounds across 44 cell lines of this lung cancer subcategory to establish a genomic characterization framework [115]. By comparing SCNAs identified in 60 patient-derived small cell lung cancer cell lines with results from 63 primary tumor specimens described above, the authors demonstrated the comparable genomic landscape of small cell lung cancer between the two sample types. Then they showed the effectiveness of the Aurora kinase inhibitors against small cell lung cancer cell lines harboring *MYC* amplification.

3 Genomic Translocations and Expressed Fusion Genes

Compared to point mutations in oncogenes, a genomic translocation that gives rise to an oncogenic fusion gene can have more deleterious effects on protein function and on downstream cellular pathways (Fig. 2). Yet gene fusions are proving to be excellent cancer-specific drug targets and oncogenic tyrosine kinase gene fusions are the best examples. In 2007, Soda et al. discovered the first druggable

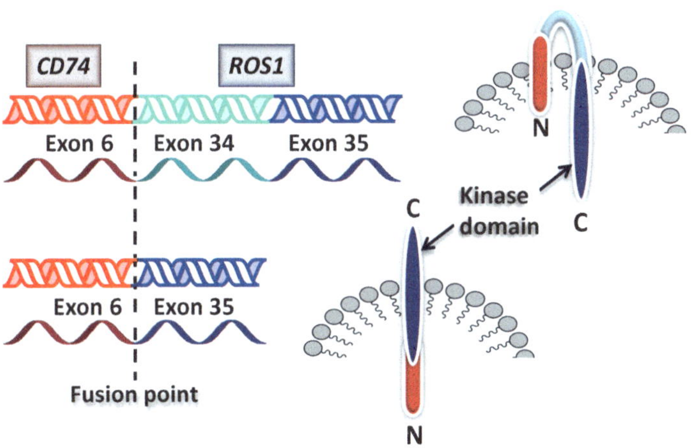

Fig. 2 *CD74-ROS1* translocation and expressed fusion genes. *CD74* and *ROS1* genomic rearrangements (double stranded DNA) results in the mRNA expression of two different fusion variants. *Left,* depiction of CD74 exon 6 (*red*) fusion with either ROS1 exon 34 (*light blue*) or exon 35 (*dark blue*). *Right,* the predicted protein configuration of the two spliced forms and their plasma membrane orientation are depicted. Of the two variants only the major spliced form CD74-ROS1 exon 34, which shows an additional transmembrane domain (*light blue*) that positions the ROS1 tyrosine kinase domain intracellularly, is considered to be oncogenic. The original patient with lung cancer expressing this mutation initially responded to crizotinib, later the drug resistance was developed due to the amino acid substitution G2032R

EML4-ALK fusion protein—an oncokinase—in NSCLC [11]. The marked response of patients with *ALK* positive NSCLC to the small-molecule tyrosine kinase inhibitor crizotinib [116, 117] catalyzed the field to search for expression of other novel oncogenic fusion genes. Application of high-throughput RNA sequencing analysis has greatly contributed to the identification of additional fusion genes in lung cancer involving kinases: *ROS1*[118], *RET* [119], *FGFR1*/2/3 [120, 121], *NTRK1*[122], *ERBB4* and *BRAF* [123], and AXL and PDGFRA [124]. Also, fusion genes involving the EGFR ligand NRG1 (*CD74-NRG1*, *SLC3A2-NRG1*) have been reported [123]. The particular importance of *ALK*, *ROS1* and *RET* fusion genes in lung cancer is expanded on below.

3.1 ALK

The inversion on chromosome 2p leads to the formation of the most commonly expressed ALK fusion, EML4-ALK. As the genomic inversion does not occur at the same location all the time, it results in expression of a number of EML4-ALK variants [11]. In all the variants, the intracellular tyrosine kinase domain of *ALK* starting at exon 20 is present while the *EML4* truncates at different points. The two most common variants E13:A20 (33 %) and E6a/b:A20 (29 %), which are also referred to as variant 1 and 3a/b respectively, represent approximately 60 % of detected EML4-ALK variants [125]. The NSCLC cell lines H3122 and DFC1031 contain the E13:A20 variant while H2228 harbors the E6a/b:A20 [126]. In NSCLC other *ALK* fusion partners have also been discovered, including *TFG* [118], *KIF5B* [127], *HIP1* [128], *KLC1* [129], *TPR* [130]. Each of these fusion partners mediates the ligand independent dimerization of *ALK* to constitutively activate ALK kinase function. The prevalence of the *ALK* rearrangements occurs in 3 to 7 % of unselected patients with NSCLC [11, 126]. This amounts to an estimated 65,000 new patients each year with *ALK* rearrangements [131] a number that is in the range of annual total number of Chronic Myeloid Leukemia cases [132, 133]. Like *EGFR* mutations, *ALK* rearrangements tend to occur in younger age patients with adenocarcinoma histology and never or light smoking history [117, 134]. Also, *ALK* rearrangements are the second genetic biomarker related to FDA-approved targeted therapy for NSCLC. Small molecule tyrosine kinase inhibitor crizotinib (originally developed for MET) was approved in 2011 along with the break apart FISH as the diagnostic test to detect the ALK positive advanced NSCLC patients [27, 125, 135]. In a recent phase 1 trial enrolling patients with *ALK* rearrangement positive lung cancer, the higher potency tyrosine kinase inhibitor ceritinib inhibited the resistance developed by the crizotinib treatment exemplifying the power of mechanism based rational drug design [136]. Mechanistically, the benefit of ceritinib over crizotinib is that it is uniquely effective at inhibiting secondary *ALK* mutation L1196M. For the first time in the history of targeted therapy, ceritinib received FDA approval just after the phase I clinical trial [137].

3.2 ROS1

The analysis of 41 cell lines and 150 NSCLC tumors led Rikova et al. to characterize the first *ROS1* rearrangement in NSCLC [118]. In one of the cell lines (HCC78) the authors identified the *ROS1-SLC34A2* fusion and one of the tumor samples harbored the *CD74-ROS1* fusion. Follow-up studies discovered a number of *ROS1* fusion gene partners: *TPM3* [138], *SDC4* [138, 139], *EZR* [140], *LRIG3* [138], *FIG* [141], *KDELR2* [142], *CCDC6* [124]. *ROS1* is located on human chromosome 6 and with the exception of *FIG* and *EZR* all other fusion partners are coming from different chromosomes [143]. In all the different fusion proteins, the ROS1 tyrosine kinase domain remains intact [138]. For *ROS1* fusion genes the mechanism remains unknown [119], but the likely oncogenic consequence is constitutive activation of ROS1 tyrosine kinase function. Furthermore, the expression of ROS1 fusion genes both in vitro and in vivo leads to oncogenic transformation [138]. Emerging data indicates that, *ROS1* fusion genes may preferentially activate downstream PI3K/AKT/mTOR and MAPK/ERK pathways [144].

3.3 RET

In 2011, researchers discovered the first RET gene fusion partnered with the gene KIF5B in NSCLC [145]. In 2012, three studies each added more variants to the list of expressed KIF5B-RET fusion genes [138, 146, 147]. Although *KIF5B* is the most common fusion partner of *RET*, other partners have also been reported such as *CCDC6*, *TRIM33* and *NCOA4* [148, 149]. The RET tyrosine kinase domain is conserved in all the fusions. In contrast to *ROS1*, *RET* fusion partners like *ALK* fusion partners contain a coiled-coil domain. Positioned at the 5′ end of the fusion gene this domain promotes ligand independent dimerization and hence constitutive activation of RET kinase function.

Although the prevalence of *ROS1* and *RET* fusion genes are about 1–2 % in an unselected population of NSCLC [138, 150], there is great interest for these two fusions as novel targets due to three main reasons. First, *ROS1* and *RET* fusions tend to occur without the presence of other driver mutations and this knowledge of mutual exclusivity can be used to strategize screening and detection [147]. Second, NSCLC patients harboring *ROS1* or *RET* fusions show unique clinicopathologic features [138, 150] (e.g. relatively younger age, never smoker with adenocarcinoma histology) facilitating clinical enrollments [119]. Third, there are already inhibitor drugs targeting *ROS1* and *RET* in clinical trials [148; 150]. It took only 4 years from the first identification of an ALK fusion gene in NSCLC for the FDA to conditionally approve an ALK-targeted tyrosine kinase inhibitor [135]; and in less than 6 months of publication on RET fusion genes, Drilon et al. initiated a clinical trial with cabozantinib [148]. Again underscoring how the transition from genomic research to molecularly-defined therapy in lung cancer can advance at an incredibly rapid rate.

With high-throughput sequencing of greater numbers of lung cancer transcriptomes across all histological subtypes, additional oncogenic variants of fusion genes may be discovered. However, it is important that complementary work be done to establish or refute if any one specific fusion gene event is tumorigenic and clinically actionable. For example, although the *ROS1* gene fusions *KDELR2-ROS1* and *CCDC6-ROS1* have been discovered in NSCLC, their tumorigenic potential has not been established [151]. In another example, a genomic translocation suggested to give rise to expression of a CCDC6-RET fusion gene has been detected in two forms: *CCDC6* exon 1 fused to *RET* exon 12 (C1; R12) and *CCDC6* intron 1 fused to *RET* exon 11 (C1; R11). However, only CCDC6-RET (C1; R12) is expressed and contributes to malignancy while *CCDC6-RET* (C1; R11) represents a benign breakpoint in the genome, therefore it is of no obvious clinical importance [152].

4 Challenges and Conclusions

The hallmarks of a cancer cell, distinct from normal cell biology, include the capacity for unlimited and unmitigated proliferation; resistance to anti-proliferative and apoptotic cues; and the ability to survive and proliferate in stressful conditions [103]. Underlying these malignant phenotypes is aberrant molecular biology in the form of deregulated signaling pathways or functional networks of genes that are ultimately governed by a mutated genome [153]. Much progress has been made to develop anti-cancer drugs that target the protein products of well-studied, recurrently mutated oncogenes. And to date the greatest clinical successes for molecularly targeted treatments in lung cancer have come from efforts to target EGFR and ALK kinases. Certainly more are on the horizon that will increasingly define and include all lung cancer subtypes, as stories of rapid discovery and drug development are unfolding in the literature.

Despite targeted treatment advances and marked improvements in patient outcomes over traditional chemotherapies, targeted therapies often fail for patients due to de novo or acquired drug resistance. A few examples of de novo resistance mechanisms in lung cancer stem from the observation that nearly 30 % of patients with tumors positive for *EGFR* mutations show no initial response [154–158]. *EGFR* mutations carrying exon 20 insertions are not sensitive to EGFR-tyrosine kinase inhibitor drugs. Unlike other *EGFR*-activating mutations, the exon 20 insertion D770_N771insNPG promotes EGFR function without increasing affinity for EGFR tyrosine kinase inhibitors [159, 160]. In another example, the *EGFR* T790M mutation, which confers EGFR-targeted drug resistance when it arises in a tumor, also exists as a heterozygous germ-line variant in 0.5 % of lung adenocarcinoma patients [161, 162].

The most frequent mechanism of acquired resistance is the gain of second-site *EGFR* mutations, which is estimated to occur in more than 50 % of the patients; among them the T790M mutation contributes more than 90 % [163]. In *EML4-ALK* fusion-gene positive patients, the gatekeeper mutation L1196M, analogous to *EGFR* T790M, requires the contribution from additional mutations within the *ALK* sequence and the net effect allows it to block crizotinib from its binding site [164, 165]. More recently, a second-site mutation was discovered within the *ROS1* fusion gene *CD74-ROS1*; it was causally linked to acquired resistance to crizotinib [166] (Fig. 2). The single G2032R amino acid change provides sufficient steric bulk to block inhibitor drug binding.

To better appreciate how acquired resistance arises, bear in mind that targeted therapies can promote minority populations of tumor cells harboring another driver oncogene, or cause reversible growth inhibition or autophagy allowing subpopulations of cancer cells the opportunity to evolve mechanisms for drug resistance leading to recurrence. Moreover, current targeted therapies inhibit the oncogene directly, and by default the proto-oncogene, thereby causing dose-limiting side effects. To overcome drug resistance, an array of new drugs including second and third generation EGFR and other tyrosine kinase inhibitors are being utilized and developed, as single and combination agents. The recent success of ceritinib in overcoming crizotinib drug resistance in *ALK* rearranged NSCLC is a milestone example [136].

A major challenge for research efforts to catalog the driver mutations in lung cancer is the high mutation frequency in lung cancer compared to other cancers. For example squamous cell lung carcinoma shows a median mutation frequency of 8.15 per megabase (Mb) while that of AML is only 0.28 mutations /Mb [167]. This poses the difficulty of detecting oncogenic drivers among the vast majority of passive mutations. Even the most comprehensive sequencing endeavors like the study of 183 lung adenocarcinomas raises gaps in our understanding [16]. In this study 15 % of the patients did not show a single mutation in known oncogenes or genes with known cancer function [103]. A recent saturation analysis across 21 tumor types estimated the requirement of 600–5000 samples per lung tumor type to achieve near-saturation [168]. The number of lung cancer samples necessary to detect a mutation at 3 % frequency extrapolates to about 2000 samples.

To conclude, the end-goal of research is transfer of the accumulated knowledge and evolution of knowledge of tumor biology to the clinic; here genomic technologies and cancer type-specific, single-pass comprehensive mutation panels are poised to transform clinical testing. The many complexities accompanying this paradigm shift should not be underestimated and difficulties remain for even the most forward thinking institutes, but they are foreseeably overcome by expert collaborative teams made up of health care professionals; basic and translational scientists; and regulatory agencies.

References

1. Sharma SV, Settleman J (2007) Oncogene addiction: setting the stage for molecularly targeted cancer therapy. Genes Dev 21:3214–3231
2. Vogelstein B, Papadopoulos N, Velculescu VE, Zhou S, Diaz LA Jr et al (2013) Cancer genome landscapes. Science 339:1546–1558
3. (2012) Comprehensive genomic characterization of squamous cell lung cancers. Nature 489:519–525

4. Vivanco I, Sawyers CL (2002) The phosphatidylinositol 3-kinase AKT pathway in human cancer. Nat Rev Cancer 2:489–501
5. Beltran AS, Blancafort P (2011) Reactivation of MASPIN in non-small cell lung carcinoma (NSCLC) cells by artificial transcription factors (ATFs). Epigenetics 6:224–235
6. Lee SH, Park BJ (2011) p53 activation by blocking Snail: a novel pharmacological strategy for cancer. Curr Pharm Des 17:610–617
7. Paez JG, Janne PA, Lee JC, Tracy S, Greulich H et al (2004) EGFR mutations in lung cancer: correlation with clinical response to gefitinib therapy. Science 304:1497–1500
8. Lynch TJ, Bell DW, Sordella R, Gurubhagavatula S, Okimoto RA et al (2004) Activating mutations in the epidermal growth factor receptor underlying responsiveness of non-small-cell lung cancer to gefitinib. N Engl J Med 350:2129–2139
9. Pao W, Miller V, Zakowski M, Doherty J, Politi K et al (2004) EGF receptor gene mutations are common in lung cancers from "never smokers" and are associated with sensitivity of tumors to gefitinib and erlotinib. Proc Natl Acad Sci U S A 101:13306–13311
10. Pao W, Girard N (2011) New driver mutations in non-small-cell lung cancer. Lancet Oncol 12:175–180
11. Soda M, Choi YL, Enomoto M, Takada S, Yamashita Y et al (2007) Identification of the transforming EML4-ALK fusion gene in non-small-cell lung cancer. Nature 448:561–566
12. (2013) A genomics-based classification of human lung tumors. Sci Transl Med 5:209ra153
13. Howlander N, Noone AM, Krapcho M, Neyman N, Aminou R, Waldron W, Altekruse SF, Kosary CL, Rulhl J, Tatalovich Z, Cho H, Mariotto A, Eisner MP, Lewis DR, Chen HS, Feuer EJ, Cronin KA, Edwards BK (2011) SEER cancer statistics review, 1975-2008. National Cancer Institute, Bethesda
14. Pao W, Iafrate AJ, Su Z (2011) Genetically informed lung cancer medicine. J Pathol 223:230–240
15. Pao W, Hutchinson KE (2012) Chipping away at the lung cancer genome. Nat Med 18:349–351
16. Imielinski M, Berger AH, Hammerman PS, Hernandez B, Pugh TJ et al (2012) Mapping the hallmarks of lung adenocarcinoma with massively parallel sequencing. Cell 150:1107–1120
17. Kan Z, Jaiswal BS, Stinson J, Janakiraman V, Bhatt D et al (2010) Diverse somatic mutation patterns and pathway alterations in human cancers. Nature 466:869–873
18. Sanchez-Cespedes M, Parrella P, Esteller M, Nomoto S, Trink B et al (2002) Inactivation of LKB1/STK11 is a common event in adenocarcinomas of the lung. Cancer Res 62:3659–3662
19. Huang S, Benavente S, Armstrong EA, Li C, Wheeler DL et al (2011) p53 modulates acquired resistance to EGFR inhibitors and radiation. Cancer Res 71:7071–7079
20. Prenzel N, Fischer OM, Streit S, Hart S, Ullrich A (2001) The epidermal growth factor receptor family as a central element for cellular signal transduction and diversification. Endocr Relat Cancer 8:11–31
21. Shepherd FA, Rodrigues Pereira J, Ciuleanu T, Tan EH, Hirsh V et al (2005) Erlotinib in previously treated non-small-cell lung cancer. N Engl J Med 353:123–132
22. Yun CH, Boggon TJ, Li Y, Woo MS, Greulich H et al (2007) Structures of lung cancer-derived EGFR mutants and inhibitor complexes: mechanism of activation and insights into differential inhibitor sensitivity. Cancer Cell 11:217–227
23. Yun CH, Mengwasser KE, Toms AV, Woo MS, Greulich H et al (2008) The T790M mutation in EGFR kinase causes drug resistance by increasing the affinity for ATP. Proc Natl Acad Sci U S A 105:2070–2075
24. Tam IY, Chung LP, Suen WS, Wang E, Wong MC et al (2006) Distinct epidermal growth factor receptor and KRAS mutation patterns in non-small cell lung cancer patients with different tobacco exposure and clinicopathologic features. Clin Cancer Res 12:1647–1653
25. Yamamoto H, Toyooka S, Mitsudomi T (2009) Impact of EGFR mutation analysis in non-small cell lung cancer. Lung Cancer 63:315–321
26. Hirsch FR, Janne PA, Eberhardt WE, Cappuzzo F, Thatcher N et al (2013) Epidermal growth factor receptor inhibition in lung cancer: status 2012. J Thorac Oncol 8:373–384

27. Cardarella S, Johnson BE (2013) The impact of genomic changes on treatment of lung cancer. Am J Respir Crit Care Med 188:770–775
28. Balak MN, Gong Y, Riely GJ, Somwar R, Li AR et al (2006) Novel D761Y and common secondary T790M mutations in epidermal growth factor receptor-mutant lung adenocarcinomas with acquired resistance to kinase inhibitors. Clin Cancer Res 12:6494–6501
29. Shigematsu H, Lin L, Takahashi T, Nomura M, Suzuki M et al (2005) Clinical and biological features associated with epidermal growth factor receptor gene mutations in lung cancers. J Natl Cancer Inst 97:339–346
30. Eberhard DA, Giaccone G, Johnson BE (2008) Biomarkers of response to epidermal growth factor receptor inhibitors in Non-Small-Cell Lung Cancer Working Group: standardization for use in the clinical trial setting. J Clin Oncol 26:983–994
31. Russell PA, Barnett SA, Walkiewicz M, Wainer Z, Conron M et al (2013) Correlation of mutation status and survival with predominant histologic subtype according to the new IASLC/ATS/ERS lung adenocarcinoma classification in stage III (N2) patients. J Thorac Oncol 8:461–468
32. Bauml J, Mick R, Zhang Y, Watt CD, Vachani A et al (2013) Frequency of EGFR and KRAS mutations in patients with non small cell lung cancer by racial background: do disparities exist? Lung Cancer 81:347–353
33. Yang SH, Mechanic LE, Yang P, Landi MT, Bowman ED et al (2005) Mutations in the tyrosine kinase domain of the epidermal growth factor receptor in non-small cell lung cancer. Clin Cancer Res 11:2106–2110
34. Reinersman JM, Johnson ML, Riely GJ, Chitale DA, Nicastri AD et al (2011) Frequency of EGFR and KRAS mutations in lung adenocarcinomas in African Americans. J Thorac Oncol 6:28–31
35. Sos ML, Koker M, Weir BA, Heynck S, Rabinovsky R et al (2009) PTEN loss contributes to erlotinib resistance in EGFR-mutant lung cancer by activation of Akt and EGFR. Cancer Res 69:3256–3261
36. Kosaka T, Yatabe Y, Endoh H, Kuwano H, Takahashi T et al (2004) Mutations of the epidermal growth factor receptor gene in lung cancer: biological and clinical implications. Cancer Res 64:8919–8923
37. Tokumo M, Toyooka S, Kiura K, Shigematsu H, Tomii K et al (2005) The relationship between epidermal growth factor receptor mutations and clinicopathologic features in non-small cell lung cancers. Clin Cancer Res 11:1167–1173
38. Ding L, Getz G, Wheeler DA, Mardis ER, McLellan MD et al (2008) Somatic mutations affect key pathways in lung adenocarcinoma. Nature 455:1069–1075
39. Rekhtman N, Paik PK, Arcila ME, Tafe LJ, Oxnard GR et al (2012) Clarifying the spectrum of driver oncogene mutations in biomarker-verified squamous carcinoma of lung: lack of EGFR/KRAS and presence of PIK3CA/AKT1 mutations. Clin Cancer Res 18:1167–1176
40. Ohtsuka K, Ohnishi H, Fujiwara M, Kishino T, Matsushima S et al (2007) Abnormalities of epidermal growth factor receptor in lung squamous-cell carcinomas, adenosquamous carcinomas, and large-cell carcinomas: tyrosine kinase domain mutations are not rare in tumors with an adenocarcinoma component. Cancer 109:741–750
41. Karnoub AE, Weinberg RA (2008) Ras oncogenes: split personalities. Nat Rev Mol Cell Biol 9:517–531
42. Downward J (2003) Targeting RAS signalling pathways in cancer therapy. Nat Rev Cancer 3:11–22
43. Rodenhuis S, Slebos RJ (1992) Clinical significance of ras oncogene activation in human lung cancer. Cancer Res 52:2665s–2669s
44. Sequist LV, Heist RS, Shaw AT, Fidias P, Rosovsky R et al (2011) Implementing multiplexed genotyping of non-small-cell lung cancers into routine clinical practice. Ann Oncol 22:2616–2624
45. Riely GJ, Kris MG, Rosenbaum D, Marks J, Li A et al (2008) Frequency and distinctive spectrum of KRAS mutations in never smokers with lung adenocarcinoma. Clin Cancer Res 14:5731–5734

46. Linardou H, Dahabreh IJ, Kanaloupiti D, Siannis F, Bafaloukos D et al (2008) Assessment of somatic k-RAS mutations as a mechanism associated with resistance to EGFR-targeted agents: a systematic review and meta-analysis of studies in advanced non-small-cell lung cancer and metastatic colorectal cancer. Lancet Oncol 9:962–972
47. Janne PA, Shaw AT, Pereira JR, Jeannin G, Vansteenkiste J et al (2013) Selumetinib plus docetaxel for KRAS-mutant advanced non-small-cell lung cancer: a randomised, multicentre, placebo-controlled, phase 2 study. Lancet Oncol 14:38–47
48. Davies H, Bignell GR, Cox C, Stephens P, Edkins S et al (2002) Mutations of the BRAF gene in human cancer. Nature 417:949–954
49. Brose MS, Volpe P, Feldman M, Kumar M, Rishi I et al (2002) BRAF and RAS mutations in human lung cancer and melanoma. Cancer Res 62:6997–7000
50. Paik PK, Arcila ME, Fara M, Sima CS, Miller VA et al (2011) Clinical characteristics of patients with lung adenocarcinomas harboring BRAF mutations. J Clin Oncol 29:2046–2051
51. Gautschi O, Pauli C, Strobel K, Hirschmann A, Printzen G et al (2012) A patient with BRAF V600E lung adenocarcinoma responding to vemurafenib. J Thorac Oncol 7:e23–e24
52. Hirsch FR, Varella-Garcia M, Franklin WA, Veve R, Chen L et al (2002) Evaluation of HER-2/neu gene amplification and protein expression in non-small cell lung carcinomas. Br J Cancer 86:1449–1456
53. Shigematsu H, Takahashi T, Nomura M, Majmudar K, Suzuki M et al (2005) Somatic mutations of the HER2 kinase domain in lung adenocarcinomas. Cancer Res 65:1642–1646
54. Stephens P, Hunter C, Bignell G, Edkins S, Davies H et al (2004) Lung cancer: intragenic ERBB2 kinase mutations in tumours. Nature 431:525–526
55. Clamon G, Herndon J, Kern J, Govindan R, Garst J et al (2005) Lack of trastuzumab activity in nonsmall cell lung carcinoma with overexpression of erb-B2: 39810: a phase II trial of Cancer and Leukemia Group B. Cancer 103:1670–1675
56. Gatzemeier U, Groth G, Butts C, Van Zandwijk N, Shepherd F et al (2004) Randomized phase II trial of gemcitabine-cisplatin with or without trastuzumab in HER2-positive non-small-cell lung cancer. Ann Oncol 15:19–27
57. Kelly RJ, Carter CA, Giaccone G (2012) HER2 mutations in non-small-cell lung cancer can be continually targeted. J Clin Oncol 30:3318–3319
58. De Greve J, Teugels E, Geers C, Decoster L, Galdermans D et al (2012) Clinical activity of afatinib (BIBW 2992) in patients with lung adenocarcinoma with mutations in the kinase domain of HER2/neu. Lung Cancer 76:123–127
59. Gandhi L, Camidge DR, Ribeiro de Oliveira M, Bonomi P, Gandara D et al (2011) Phase I study of Navitoclax (ABT-263), a novel Bcl-2 family inhibitor, in patients with small-cell lung cancer and other solid tumors. J Clin Oncol 29:909–916
60. Sadiq AA, Salgia R (2013) MET as a possible target for non-small-cell lung cancer. J Clin Oncol 31:1089–1096
61. Cappuzzo F, Marchetti A, Skokan M, Rossi E, Gajapathy S et al (2009) Increased MET gene copy number negatively affects survival of surgically resected non-small-cell lung cancer patients. J Clin Oncol 27:1667–1674
62. Toschi L, Cappuzzo F (2010) Clinical implications of MET gene copy number in lung cancer. Future Oncol 6:239–247
63. Sequist LV, Waltman BA, Dias-Santagata D, Digumarthy S, Turke AB et al (2011) Genotypic and histological evolution of lung cancers acquiring resistance to EGFR inhibitors. Sci Transl Med 3:75ra26
64. Yu HA, Arcila ME, Rekhtman N, Sima CS, Zakowski MF et al (2013) Analysis of tumor specimens at the time of acquired resistance to EGFR-TKI therapy in 155 patients with EGFR-mutant lung cancers. Clin Cancer Res 19:2240–2247
65. Engelman JA, Zejnullahu K, Mitsudomi T, Song Y, Hyland C et al (2007) MET amplification leads to gefitinib resistance in lung cancer by activating ERBB3 signaling. Science 316:1039–1043

66. Spigel DR, Ervin TJ, Ramlau RA, Daniel DB, Goldschmidt JH Jr et al (2013) Randomized phase II trial of Onartuzumab in combination with erlotinib in patients with advanced non-small-cell lung cancer. J Clin Oncol 31:4105–4114
67. Spigel DR, Edelman MJ, Mok T, O'Byrne K, Paz-Ares L et al (2012) Treatment Rationale Study Design for the MetLung Trial: a randomized, double-blind phase III study of onartuzumab (MetMAb) in combination with erlotinib versus erlotinib alone in patients who have received standard chemotherapy for stage IIIB or IV met-positive non-small-cell lung cancer. Clin Lung Cancer 13:500–504
68. Yakes FM, Chen J, Tan J, Yamaguchi K, Shi Y et al (2011) Cabozantinib (XL184), a novel MET and VEGFR2 inhibitor, simultaneously suppresses metastasis, angiogenesis, and tumor growth. Mol Cancer Ther 10:2298–2308
69. Cui JJ, Tran-Dube M, Shen H, Nambu M, Kung PP et al (2011) Structure based drug design of crizotinib (PF-02341066), a potent and selective dual inhibitor of mesenchymal-epithelial transition factor (c-MET) kinase and anaplastic lymphoma kinase (ALK). J Med Chem 54:6342–6363
70. Burgess TL, Sun J, Meyer S, Tsuruda TS, Elliott G et al (2010) Biochemical characterization of AMG 102: a neutralizing, fully human monoclonal antibody to human and nonhuman primate hepatocyte growth factor. Mol Cancer Ther 9:400–409
71. Gordon MS, Sweeney CS, Mendelson DS, Eckhardt SG, Anderson A et al (2010) Safety, pharmacokinetics, and pharmacodynamics of AMG 102, a fully human hepatocyte growth factor-neutralizing monoclonal antibody, in a first-in-human study of patients with advanced solid tumors. Clin Cancer Res 16:699–710
72. Beau-Faller M, Ruppert AM, Voegeli AC, Neuville A, Meyer N et al (2008) MET gene copy number in non-small cell lung cancer: molecular analysis in a targeted tyrosine kinase inhibitor naive cohort. J Thorac Oncol 3:331–339
73. Drilon A, Rekhtman N, Ladanyi M, Paik P (2012) Squamous-cell carcinomas of the lung: emerging biology, controversies, and the promise of targeted therapy. Lancet Oncol 13:e418–e426
74. Johnson DH, Fehrenbacher L, Novotny WF, Herbst RS, Nemunaitis JJ et al (2004) Randomized phase II trial comparing bevacizumab plus carboplatin and paclitaxel with carboplatin and paclitaxel alone in previously untreated locally advanced or metastatic non-small-cell lung cancer. J Clin Oncol 22:2184–2191
75. Scagliotti GV, Parikh P, von Pawel J, Biesma B, Vansteenkiste J et al (2008) Phase III study comparing cisplatin plus gemcitabine with cisplatin plus pemetrexed in chemotherapy-naive patients with advanced-stage non-small-cell lung cancer. J Clin Oncol 26:3543–3551
76. Wistuba II, Behrens C, Virmani AK, Mele G, Milchgrub S et al (2000) High resolution chromosome 3p allelotyping of human lung cancer and preneoplastic/preinvasive bronchial epithelium reveals multiple, discontinuous sites of 3p allele loss and three regions of frequent breakpoints. Cancer Res 60:1949–1960
77. Wistuba II, Behrens C, Milchgrub S, Bryant D, Hung J et al (1999) Sequential molecular abnormalities are involved in the multistage development of squamous cell lung carcinoma. Oncogene 18:643–650
78. Zheng CX, Gu ZH, Han B, Zhang RX, Pan CM et al (2013) Whole-exome sequencing to identify novel somatic mutations in squamous cell lung cancers. Int J Oncol 43:755–764
79. Roth BJ, Krilov L, Adams S, Aghajanian CA, Bach P et al (2013) Clinical cancer advances 2012: annual report on progress against cancer from the American Society of Clinical Oncology. J Clin Oncol 31:131–161
80. Weiss J, Sos ML, Seidel D, Peifer M, Zander T et al (2010) Frequent and focal FGFR1 amplification associates with therapeutically tractable FGFR1 dependency in squamous cell lung cancer. Sci Transl Med 2:62ra93
81. Perez-Moreno P, Brambilla E, Thomas R, Soria JC (2012) Squamous cell carcinoma of the lung: molecular subtypes and therapeutic opportunities. Clin Cancer Res 18:2443–2451

82. Kim CH (2013) Druggable targets of squamous cell lung cancer. Tuberc Respir Dis (Seoul) 75:231–235
83. Go H, Jeon YK, Park HJ, Sung SW, Seo JW et al (2010) High MET gene copy number leads to shorter survival in patients with non-small cell lung cancer. J Thorac Oncol 5:305–313
84. Bass AJ, Watanabe H, Mermel CH, Yu S, Perner S et al (2009) SOX2 is an amplified lineage-survival oncogene in lung and esophageal squamous cell carcinomas. Nat Genet 41:1238–1242
85. Hussenet T, du Manoir S (2010) SOX2 in squamous cell carcinoma: amplifying a pleiotropic oncogene along carcinogenesis. Cell Cycle 9:1480–1486
86. Hussenet T, Dali S, Exinger J, Monga B, Jost B et al (2010) SOX2 is an oncogene activated by recurrent 3q26.3 amplifications in human lung squamous cell carcinomas. PLoS One 5, e8960
87. Ramos AH, Dutt A, Mermel C, Perner S, Cho J et al (2009) Amplification of chromosomal segment 4q12 in non-small cell lung cancer. Cancer Biol Ther 8:2042–2050
88. Rooney M, Devarakonda S, Govindan R (2013) Genomics of squamous cell lung cancer. Oncologist 18:707–716
89. Grob TJ, Kannengiesser I, Tsourlakis MC, Atanackovic D, Koenig AM et al (2012) Heterogeneity of ERBB2 amplification in adenocarcinoma, squamous cell carcinoma and large cell undifferentiated carcinoma of the lung. Mod Pathol 25:1566–1573
90. Carpten JD, Faber AL, Horn C, Donoho GP, Briggs SL et al (2007) A transforming mutation in the pleckstrin homology domain of AKT1 in cancer. Nature 448:439–444
91. Malanga D, Scrima M, De Marco C, Fabiani F, De Rosa N et al (2008) Activating E17K mutation in the gene encoding the protein kinase AKT1 in a subset of squamous cell carcinoma of the lung. Cell Cycle 7:665–669
92. Heist RS, Sequist LV, Engelman JA (2012) Genetic changes in squamous cell lung cancer: a review. J Thorac Oncol 7:924–933
93. Solit DB, Garraway LA, Pratilas CA, Sawai A, Getz G et al (2006) BRAF mutation predicts sensitivity to MEK inhibition. Nature 439:358–362
94. Day E, Waters B, Spiegel K, Alnadaf T, Manley PW et al (2008) Inhibition of collagen-induced discoidin domain receptor 1 and 2 activation by imatinib, nilotinib and dasatinib. Eur J Pharmacol 599:44–53
95. Hammerman PS, Sos ML, Ramos AH, Xu C, Dutt A et al (2011) Mutations in the DDR2 kinase gene identify a novel therapeutic target in squamous cell lung cancer. Cancer Discov 1:78–89
96. Yamamoto H, Shigematsu H, Nomura M, Lockwood WW, Sato M et al (2008) PIK3CA mutations and copy number gains in human lung cancers. Cancer Res 68:6913–6921
97. Samuels Y, Diaz LA Jr, Schmidt-Kittler O, Cummins JM, Delong L et al (2005) Mutant PIK3CA promotes cell growth and invasion of human cancer cells. Cancer Cell 7:561–573
98. Shames DS, Wistuba II (2014) The evolving genomic classification of lung cancer. J Pathol 232:121–133
99. Thomas A, Rajan A, Lopez-Chavez A, Wang Y, Giaccone G (2013) From targets to targeted therapies and molecular profiling in non-small cell lung carcinoma. Ann Oncol 24:577–585
100. Popovic R, Licht JD (2012) Emerging epigenetic targets and therapies in cancer medicine. Cancer Discov 2:405–413
101. Zagni C, Chiacchio U, Rescifina A (2013) Histone methyltransferase inhibitors: novel epigenetic agents for cancer treatment. Curr Med Chem 20:167–185
102. Jin G, Kim MJ, Jeon HS, Choi JE, Kim DS et al (2010) PTEN mutations and relationship to EGFR, ERBB2, KRAS, and TP53 mutations in non-small cell lung cancers. Lung Cancer 69:279–283
103. Hanahan D, Weinberg RA (2011) Hallmarks of cancer: the next generation. Cell 144: 646–674
104. Brahmer JR, Tykodi SS, Chow LQ, Hwu WJ, Topalian SL et al (2012) Safety and activity of anti-PD-L1 antibody in patients with advanced cancer. N Engl J Med 366:2455–2465

105. van Meerbeeck JP, Fennell DA, De Ruysscher DK (2011) Small-cell lung cancer. Lancet 378:1741–1755
106. Chute JP, Chen T, Feigal E, Simon R, Johnson BE (1999) Twenty years of phase III trials for patients with extensive-stage small-cell lung cancer: perceptible progress. J Clin Oncol 17:1794–1801
107. Rudin CM, Durinck S, Stawiski EW, Poirier JT, Modrusan Z et al (2012) Comprehensive genomic analysis identifies SOX2 as a frequently amplified gene in small-cell lung cancer. Nat Genet 44:1111–1116
108. Peifer M, Fernandez-Cuesta L, Sos ML, George J, Seidel D et al (2012) Integrative genome analyses identify key somatic driver mutations of small-cell lung cancer. Nat Genet 44:1104–1110
109. Iwakawa R, Takenaka M, Kohno T, Shimada Y, Totoki Y et al (2013) Genome-wide identification of genes with amplification and/or fusion in small cell lung cancer. Genes Chromosomes Cancer 52:802–816
110. Kim YH, Girard L, Giacomini CP, Wang P, Hernandez-Boussard T et al (2006) Combined microarray analysis of small cell lung cancer reveals altered apoptotic balance and distinct expression signatures of MYC family gene amplification. Oncogene 25:130–138
111. Wistuba II, Gazdar AF, Minna JD (2001) Molecular genetics of small cell lung carcinoma. Semin Oncol 28:3–13
112. Larsen JE, Minna JD (2011) Molecular biology of lung cancer: clinical implications. Clin Chest Med 32:703–740
113. Soucek L, Whitfield J, Martins CP, Finch AJ, Murphy DJ et al (2008) Modelling Myc inhibition as a cancer therapy. Nature 455:679–683
114. Delmore JE, Issa GC, Lemieux ME, Rahl PB, Shi J et al (2011) BET bromodomain inhibition as a therapeutic strategy to target c-Myc. Cell 146:904–917
115. Sos ML, Dietlein F, Peifer M, Schottle J, Balke-Want H et al (2012) A framework for identification of actionable cancer genome dependencies in small cell lung cancer. Proc Natl Acad Sci U S A 109:17034–17039
116. Kwak EL, Bang YJ, Camidge DR, Shaw AT, Solomon B et al (2010) Anaplastic lymphoma kinase inhibition in non-small-cell lung cancer. N Engl J Med 363:1693–1703
117. Shaw AT, Yeap BY, Mino-Kenudson M, Digumarthy SR, Costa DB et al (2009) Clinical features and outcome of patients with non-small-cell lung cancer who harbor EML4-ALK. J Clin Oncol 27:4247–4253
118. Rikova K, Guo A, Zeng Q, Possemato A, Yu J et al (2007) Global survey of phosphotyrosine signaling identifies oncogenic kinases in lung cancer. Cell 131:1190–1203
119. Gainor JF, Shaw AT (2013) Novel targets in non-small cell lung cancer: ROS1 and RET fusions. Oncologist 18:865–875
120. Wu YM, Su F, Kalyana-Sundaram S, Khazanov N, Ateeq B et al (2013) Identification of targetable FGFR gene fusions in diverse cancers. Cancer Discov 3:636–647
121. Shaw AT, Hsu PP, Awad MM, Engelman JA (2013) Tyrosine kinase gene rearrangements in epithelial malignancies. Nat Rev Cancer 13:772–787
122. Vaishnavi A, Capelletti M, Le AT, Kako S, Butaney M et al (2013) Oncogenic and drug-sensitive NTRK1 rearrangements in lung cancer. Nat Med 19:1469–1472
123. Nakaoku T, Tsuta K, Ichikawa H, Shiraishi K, Sakamoto H et al (2014) Druggable oncogene fusions in invasive mucinous lung adenocarcinoma. Clin Cancer Res 20:3087–3093
124. Seo JS, Ju YS, Lee WC, Shin JY, Lee JK et al (2012) The transcriptional landscape and mutational profile of lung adenocarcinoma. Genome Res 22:2109–2119
125. Sasaki T, Rodig SJ, Chirieac LR, Janne PA (2010) The biology and treatment of EML4-ALK non-small cell lung cancer. Eur J Cancer 46:1773–1780
126. Koivunen JP, Mermel C, Zejnullahu K, Murphy C, Lifshits E et al (2008) EML4-ALK fusion gene and efficacy of an ALK kinase inhibitor in lung cancer. Clin Cancer Res 14:4275–4283
127. Takeuchi K, Choi YL, Togashi Y, Soda M, Hatano S et al (2009) KIF5B-ALK, a novel fusion oncokinase identified by an immunohistochemistry-based diagnostic system for ALK-positive lung cancer. Clin Cancer Res 15:3143–3149

128. Fang DD, Zhang B, Gu Q, Lira M, Xu Q et al (2014) HIP1-ALK, a novel ALK fusion variant that responds to crizotinib. J Thorac Oncol 9:285–294
129. Togashi Y, Soda M, Sakata S, Sugawara E, Hatano S et al (2012) KLC1-ALK: a novel fusion in lung cancer identified using a formalin-fixed paraffin-embedded tissue only. PLoS One 7, e31323
130. Choi YL, Lira ME, Hong M, Kim RN, Choi SJ et al (2014) A novel fusion of TPR and ALK in lung adenocarcinoma. J Thorac Oncol 9:563–566
131. Bray F, Ren JS, Masuyer E, Ferlay J (2013) Global estimates of cancer prevalence for 27 sites in the adult population in 2008. Int J Cancer 132:1133–1145
132. Ferlay J, Shin HR, Bray F, Forman D, Mathers C et al (2010) Estimates of worldwide burden of cancer in 2008: GLOBOCAN 2008. Int J Cancer 127:2893–2917
133. Jabbour E, Cortes JE, Ghanem H, O'Brien S, Kantarjian HM (2008) Targeted therapy in chronic myeloid leukemia. Expert Rev Anticancer Ther 8:99–110
134. Wong DW, Leung EL, So KK, Tam IY, Sihoe AD et al (2009) The EML4-ALK fusion gene is involved in various histologic types of lung cancers from nonsmokers with wild-type EGFR and KRAS. Cancer 115:1723–1733
135. Ou SH (2011) Crizotinib: a novel and first-in-class multitargeted tyrosine kinase inhibitor for the treatment of anaplastic lymphoma kinase rearranged non-small cell lung cancer and beyond. Drug Des Devel Ther 5:471–485
136. Shaw AT, Kim DW, Mehra R, Tan DS, Felip E et al (2014) Ceritinib in ALK-rearranged non-small-cell lung cancer. N Engl J Med 370:1189–1197
137. Chabner BA (2014) Approval after phase I: ceritinib runs the three-minute mile. Oncologist 19:577–578
138. Takeuchi K, Soda M, Togashi Y, Suzuki R, Sakata S et al (2012) RET, ROS1 and ALK fusions in lung cancer. Nat Med 18:378–381
139. Davies KD, Le AT, Theodoro MF, Skokan MC, Aisner DL et al (2012) Identifying and targeting ROS1 gene fusions in non-small cell lung cancer. Clin Cancer Res 18:4570–4579
140. Yoshida A, Kohno T, Tsuta K, Wakai S, Arai Y et al (2013) ROS1-rearranged lung cancer: a clinicopathologic and molecular study of 15 surgical cases. Am J Surg Pathol 37:554–562
141. Rimkunas VM, Crosby KE, Li D, Hu Y, Kelly ME et al (2012) Analysis of receptor tyrosine kinase ROS1-positive tumors in non-small cell lung cancer: identification of a FIG-ROS1 fusion. Clin Cancer Res 18:4449–4457
142. Govindan R, Ding L, Griffith M, Subramanian J, Dees ND et al (2012) Genomic landscape of non-small cell lung cancer in smokers and never-smokers. Cell 150:1121–1134
143. Suehara Y, Arcila M, Wang L, Hasanovic A, Ang D et al (2012) Identification of KIF5B-RET and GOPC-ROS1 fusions in lung adenocarcinomas through a comprehensive mRNA-based screen for tyrosine kinase fusions. Clin Cancer Res 18:6599–6608
144. Acquaviva J, Wong R, Charest A (2009) The multifaceted roles of the receptor tyrosine kinase ROS in development and cancer. Biochim Biophys Acta 1795:37–52
145. Ju YS, Lee WC, Shin JY, Lee S, Bleazard T et al (2012) A transforming KIF5B and RET gene fusion in lung adenocarcinoma revealed from whole-genome and transcriptome sequencing. Genome Res 22:436–445
146. Kohno T, Ichikawa H, Totoki Y, Yasuda K, Hiramoto M et al (2012) KIF5B-RET fusions in lung adenocarcinoma. Nat Med 18:375–377
147. Lipson D, Capelletti M, Yelensky R, Otto G, Parker A et al (2012) Identification of new ALK and RET gene fusions from colorectal and lung cancer biopsies. Nat Med 18:382–384
148. Drilon A, Wang L, Hasanovic A, Suehara Y, Lipson D et al (2013) Response to Cabozantinib in patients with RET fusion-positive lung adenocarcinomas. Cancer Discov 3:630–635
149. Chao BH, Briesewitz R, Villalona-Calero MA (2012) RET fusion genes in non-small-cell lung cancer. J Clin Oncol 30:4439–4441
150. Bergethon K, Shaw AT, Ou SH, Katayama R, Lovly CM et al (2012) ROS1 rearrangements define a unique molecular class of lung cancers. J Clin Oncol 30:863–870
151. Davies KD, Doebele RC (2013) Molecular pathways: ROS1 fusion proteins in cancer. Clin Cancer Res 19:4040–4045

152. Suzuki M, Makinoshima H, Matsumoto S, Suzuki A, Mimaki S et al (2013) Identification of a lung adenocarcinoma cell line with CCDC6-RET fusion gene and the effect of RET inhibitors in vitro and in vivo. Cancer Sci 104:896–903
153. Luo J, Solimini NL, Elledge SJ (2009) Principles of cancer therapy: oncogene and non-oncogene addiction. Cell 136:823–837
154. Rosell R, Carcereny E, Gervais R, Vergnenegre A, Massuti B et al (2012) Erlotinib versus standard chemotherapy as first-line treatment for European patients with advanced EGFR mutation-positive non-small-cell lung cancer (EURTAC): a multicentre, open-label, randomised phase 3 trial. Lancet Oncol 13:239–246
155. Zhou C, Wu YL, Chen G, Feng J, Liu XQ et al (2011) Erlotinib versus chemotherapy as first-line treatment for patients with advanced EGFR mutation-positive non-small-cell lung cancer (OPTIMAL, CTONG-0802): a multicentre, open-label, randomised, phase 3 study. Lancet Oncol 12:735–742
156. Maemondo M, Inoue A, Kobayashi K, Sugawara S, Oizumi S et al (2010) Gefitinib or chemotherapy for non-small-cell lung cancer with mutated EGFR. N Engl J Med 362:2380–2388
157. Mitsudomi T, Morita S, Yatabe Y, Negoro S, Okamoto I et al (2010) Gefitinib versus cisplatin plus docetaxel in patients with non-small-cell lung cancer harbouring mutations of the epidermal growth factor receptor (WJTOG3405): an open label, randomised phase 3 trial. Lancet Oncol 11:121–128
158. Mok TS, Wu YL, Thongprasert S, Yang CH, Chu DT et al (2009) Gefitinib or carboplatin-paclitaxel in pulmonary adenocarcinoma. N Engl J Med 361:947–957
159. Yasuda H, Kobayashi S, Costa DB (2012) EGFR exon 20 insertion mutations in non-small-cell lung cancer: preclinical data and clinical implications. Lancet Oncol 13:e23–e31
160. Yasuda H, Park E, Yun CH, Sng NJ, Lucena-Araujo AR et al (2013) Structural, biochemical, and clinical characterization of epidermal growth factor receptor (EGFR) exon 20 insertion mutations in lung cancer. Sci Transl Med 5:216ra177
161. Girard N, Lou E, Azzoli CG, Reddy R, Robson M et al (2010) Analysis of genetic variants in never-smokers with lung cancer facilitated by an Internet-based blood collection protocol: a preliminary report. Clin Cancer Res 16:755–763
162. Ohashi K, Maruvka YE, Michor F, Pao W (2013) Epidermal growth factor receptor tyrosine kinase inhibitor-resistant disease. J Clin Oncol 31:1070–1080
163. Arcila ME, Oxnard GR, Nafa K, Riely GJ, Solomon SB et al (2011) Rebiopsy of lung cancer patients with acquired resistance to EGFR inhibitors and enhanced detection of the T790M mutation using a locked nucleic acid-based assay. Clin Cancer Res 17:1169–1180
164. Heuckmann JM, Holzel M, Sos ML, Heynck S, Balke-Want H et al (2011) ALK mutations conferring differential resistance to structurally diverse ALK inhibitors. Clin Cancer Res 17:7394–7401
165. Sasaki T, Okuda K, Zheng W, Butrynski J, Capelletti M et al (2010) The neuroblastoma-associated F1174L ALK mutation causes resistance to an ALK kinase inhibitor in ALK-translocated cancers. Cancer Res 70:10038–10043
166. Awad MM, Katayama R, McTigue M, Liu W, Deng YL et al (2013) Acquired resistance to crizotinib from a mutation in CD74-ROS1. N Engl J Med 368:2395–2401
167. Kandoth C, McLellan MD, Vandin F, Ye K, Niu B et al (2013) Mutational landscape and significance across 12 major cancer types. Nature 502:333–339
168. Lawrence MS, Stojanov P, Mermel CH, Robinson JT, Garraway LA et al (2014) Discovery and saturation analysis of cancer genes across 21 tumour types. Nature 505:495–501

Emerging Biomarkers in Personalized Therapy of Lung Cancer

Philip T. Cagle, Kirtee Raparia, and Bryce P. Portier

Abstract The two clinically validated and Food and Drug Administration approved lung cancer predictive biomarkers (epidermal growth factor receptor mutations and anaplastic lymphoma kinase (*ALK*) translocations) occur in only about 20 % of lung adenocarcinomas and acquired resistance develops to first generation drugs. Several other oncogenic drivers for lung adenocarcinoma have emerged as potentially druggable targets with new predictive biomarkers. Oncologists are requesting testing for *ROS*1 translocations which predict susceptibility to crizotinib, already approved for *ALK* positive lung cancers. Other potential biomarkers which are currently undergoing clinical trials are RET, MET, HER2 and BRAF. Detection of these biomarkers includes fluorescent in situ hybridization and/or reverse transcriptase polymerase chain reaction (ROS1, RET, HER2), mutation analysis (*BRAF*) and immunohistochemistry (MET). Screening by immunohistochemistry may be useful for some biomarkers (ROS1, BRAF). Targeted next generation sequencing techniques may be useful as well. These five biomarkers are under consideration for inclusion in revised lung cancer biomarker guidelines by the College of American Pathologists, International Association for the Study of Lung Cancer and Association for Molecular Pathology.

Keywords ROS1 • RET • MET • HER2 • BRAF • Multikinase inhibitors • Fluorescent in situ hybridization • Crizotinib • Reverse transcriptase polymerase chain reaction • Immunohistochemistry

---

P.T. Cagle, M.D. (✉)
Houston Methodist Hospital, Weill Medical College of Cornell University, Houston, TX, USA
e-mail: pcagle@houstonmethodist.org

K. Raparia, M.D.
Department of Pathology, Northwestern University, Feinberg School of Medicine, Chicago, IL, USA
e-mail: kraparia@northwestern.edu

B.P. Portier, M.D., Ph.D.
Houston Methodist Hospital, Houston, TX, USA
e-mail: bpportier@houstonmethodist.org

A. Ahmad, S.M. Gadgeel (eds.), *Lung Cancer and Personalized Medicine: Novel Therapies and Clinical Management*, Advances in Experimental Medicine and Biology 890, DOI 10.1007/978-3-319-24932-2_2

1 Introduction

Two predictive biomarkers for personalized therapy of non-small cell lung cancers (NSCLC) have been well validated in clinical trials and approved by the Federal Drug Administration (FDA): epidermal growth factor receptor (EGFR) mutations and anaplastic lymphoma kinase (ALK) translocations [1]. These two biomarkers have been the subject of the first lung cancer biomarkers guidelines from the College of American Pathologists (CAP), International Association for the Study of Lung Cancer (IASLC) and Association for Molecular Pathology (AMP) [2] as well as the CAP Lung Cancer Biomarker Reporting Template [3].

The frequency of EGFR mutations found in non-small cell lung cancers (NSCLC), more specifically in adenocarcinomas, ranges from about 15 % of whites and Hispanics to about 19 % of African Americans to about 30 % of Asian patients [4–7]. ALK translocations creating fusion genes occur in about 4–5 % of adenocarcinomas [8–12]. Lung cancers that initially respond to first generation EGFR TKIs or to crizotinib eventually develop drug resistance and relapse, typically within a year [13–19]. Since about 80 % of adenocarcinomas lack *EGFR* mutations or *ALK* translocations and since lung cancers with these abnormalities develop acquired resistance to current therapies, there has been a robust search for additional oncogenic drivers in lung cancers that might be actionable. Investigations have not yet discovered drugs that target *KRAS*, the most frequent oncogenic driver in lung adenocarcinomas, occurring in about 30 % of cases [1, 2]. Oncogenic drivers have not yet been identified in a substantial number of lung adenocarcinomas and, of the additional drivers that have been identified, investigations of several are sufficiently advanced that they are being considered for revisions to the CAP/IASLC/AMP lung cancer biomarker guidelines and CAP lung cancer biomarker reporting template (See Fig. 1).

2 ROS1

Chromosomal rearrangements of the receptor tyrosine kinase gene c-ros oncogene 1 (*ROS1*) are found in approximately 1–2 % of lung cancers with adenocarcinoma histology, or about 2000–4000 new cases of ROS1 positive lung cancer each year in the United States [20–24]. ROS1 has considerable amino acid homology with ALK [25]. In 2012, Bergethon et al. [20] reported sensitivity of a *ROS*1 positive lung cancer cell line and *ROS*1 transfected cell lines to the small molecule multikinase inhibitor crizotinib. They also reported a near complete response of a *ROS*1 positive lung cancer to crizotinib in a single patient enrolled in an expansion cohort of an early phase study [20]. In an expansion of the PROFILE 1001 study, Shaw et al. [26] reported one complete response, six partial responses and four stable disease in thirteen patients with *ROS*1 positive lung cancers at 8 weeks of treatment with crizotinib. These observations indicating *ROS*1 positive lung adenocarcinomas might respond to crizotinib, a drug that already had FDA approval for treatment of

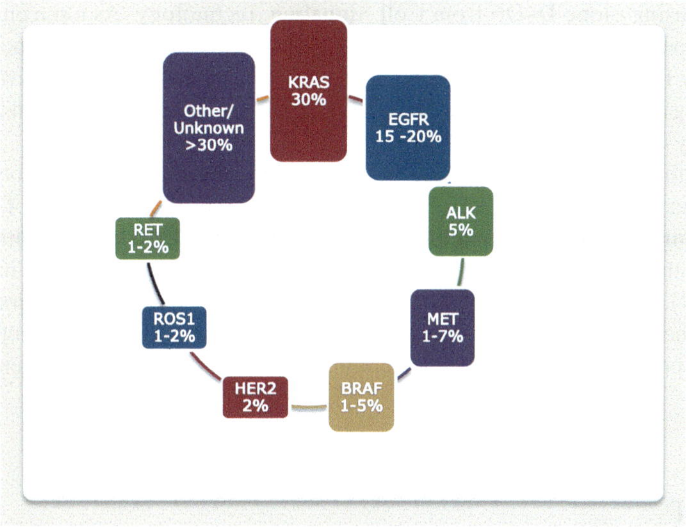

Fig. 1 Diagram showing the actionable and potentially actionable biomarkers in lung adenocarcinoma. *KRAS* mutation is the most common oncogenic driver, but no drugs specifically targeted to *KRAS* mutation are yet available. *EGFR* mutation and *ALK* translocation are clinically validated as predictive biomarkers for FDA approved TKI therapy. Emerging as biomarkers currently in clinical trials at this time are *ROS*1, *RET*, *MET*, *Her*2 and *BRAF*

ALK positive lung cancers, produced requests for ROS1 biomarker testing by medical oncologists for lung adenocarcinomas. Typically, this has been as part of an algorithm or after adenocarcinomas were reported negative for EGFR and ALK. As a result, ROS1 has moved to the forefront of new biomarkers for lung cancer.

Similar to *ALK* rearrangements, *ROS1* rearrangements with any of several fusion partners result in oncogenic kinase activation and the resultant oncogenic fusion kinase is susceptible to the multikinase inhibitor crizotinib [24, 27–31]. *ROS*1 positive adenocarcinomas share histologic and demographic features with *ALK* positive adenocarcinomas. *ROS*1 translocations tend to occur in adenocarcinomas with solid, papillary, cribriform or signet ring cell histologic patterns, tend to produce mucin and tend to arise in patients who are younger and never smokers. There are many exceptions to these general tendencies. As with other oncogenic drivers identified in lung adenocarcinomas, ROS1 translocation most often excludes the presence of other oncogenic drivers in the same tumor [20, 21, 28, 32–36].

Like *ALK* rearrangements, *ROS1* rearrangements can be detected by a break-apart fluorescent in situ hybridization (FISH) probe that is not dependent on the specific fusion partner [20, 22, 37, 38]. Specific fusion partners are detected by reverse transcriptase polymerase chain reaction (RT-PCR), including *CD74-ROS1, SDC4-ROS1, EZR-ROS1, SLC34A22-ROS1* and *FIG-ROS1* [20, 21, 29, 31, 34, 38–41]. Immunohistochemistry (IHC) can be used to screen for ROS1 positivity which can then be confirmed by FISH. IHC is performed on formalin-fixed, paraffin-embedded sections using clone D4D6 from Cell Signaling Technology. As a screening tool, IHC is reported to be highly sensitive (100 %) for ROS1 positive lung cancers confirmed by FISH and/or RT-PCR with strong diffuse staining. False positive immunostaining is reported to occur in some *ROS*1 negative lung cancers with considerable variability depending on the study [35, 37, 38, 42].

As with *ALK* positive adenocarcinomas, acquired resistance to crizotinib has been observed in *ROS*1 positive adenocarcinomas. Acquired resistance of a ROS1 positive lung cancer to crizotinib has been reported with a proposed mechanism of EGFR pathway activation [43] and, in another case, due to a mutation in *CD74-ROS*1 [44]. Therefore, similar to the situation with other oncogenic drivers of lung cancers, new drugs are under investigation for inhibiting ROS1. Davare et al. [45] reported preclinical studies which demonstrated that foretinib is a potent ROS1 inhibitor.

3 RET

The rearranged during transfection (*RET*) gene encodes for the RET receptor tyrosine kinase. Chromosomal rearrangements of the *RET* gene result in an oncogenic fusion kinase in about 1–2 % of lung cancers with adenocarcinoma histology. The majority are *KIF5B-RET* fusion genes with a lesser number of *CCDC6-RET, NCOA4* and *TRIM33* fusion genes reported [27, 34, 46–55]. Preclinical studies have reported that RET-positive lung cancer cell lines are sensitive to the multikinase inhibitors vandetanib, sunitinib, and sorafenib [56, 57]. One patient with *RET* positive advanced adenocarcinoma has been reported to respond to vandetanib [58]. Preliminary results from a phase II trial of the multikinase inhibitor cabozantinib were partial responses in two of three patients and stable disease in the third patient [54]. Therefore, oncologists may order *RET* tests for lung adenocarcinomas for possible enrollment of a patient in a clinical trial or RET may be detected in a lung cancer using next generation sequencing techniques.

Translocations of *RET* which result in oncogenic fusion kinases in lung adenocarcinomas have a tendency to occur in the same demographic and histologic groups as the reported tendencies for oncogenic fusion kinases from ROS1 and ALK translocations. Patients tend to be younger and never smokers and the adenocarcinomas tend to have solid, papillary and lepidic patterns and more often produce mucin. As with *ALK* and *ROS*1 positive adenocarcinomas, there are many exceptions to these general histologic and demographic tendencies for *RET* positive adenocarcinomas. Also, identification of a *RET* translocation usually excludes the presence of other oncogenic drivers such as *EGFR*, *ALK* and *ROS*1 in the same cancer [34, 48, 52, 54, 55].

RET translocations may be detected by FISH, by RT-PCR or by next generation sequencing [34, 48, 52, 54, 55, 59]. Immunohistochemistry for RET has had variable results and, currently, is not popular for identification of *RET* positive lung adenocarcinomas [52, 59].

4 MET

The MNNG-HOS transforming (*MET*) gene encodes a receptor tyrosine kinase and binding of its ligand hepatocyte growth factor (HGF) causes a conformational change in the MET receptor that facilitates receptor activation. *MET* can be activated in lung cancers by amplification and/or overexpression [60–67]. About 18 % of cases of acquired resistance to EGFR TKIs are associated with overexpression and/or amplification of *MET* or HGF, but prevalence of *MET* amplification in NSCLC patients who have not received treatment is 1–7 % [68].

Onartuzumab (MetMAb) is a recombinant, humanized, monovalent monoclonal antibody that targets MET [69]. In a phase II study patients with previously treated NSCLC were evaluated for therapy with onartuzumab plus erlotinib versus placebo plus erlotinib [70]. Patient lung cancer samples were classified as positive for MET expression or negative for MET expression by IHC using a cut-off of 50 % of malignant cells with moderate and/or strong staining intensity for classification as MET positive. The combination of onartuzumab and erlotinib resulted in improved progression free survival (PFS) and overall survival (OS) compared to placebo plus erlotinib in MET positive cases whereas the opposite was true in MET negative cases. Therefore, this IHC test provides the biomarker for MET treatment in this setting and is being considered as a companion diagnostic for onartuzumab in combination with erlotinib for treatment of lung cancer [71]. The phase II study is being followed by the MetLung phase III study [72].

ARQ 197 or tivantinib is a TKI that inhibits MET. The MARQUEE (**M**et Inhibitor **ARQ** 197 pl**u**s **E**rlotinib vs. **E**rlotinib plus placebo in NSCLC) phase III trial of tavantinib plus erlotinib in previously treated patients with locally advanced or metastatic non-squamous NSCLC was stopped not meet its primary endpoint of improved overall survival [73, 74]. Cabozantinib and ficlatuzumab, an anti-HGF monoclonal antibody, have undergone investigation in clinical trials for lung cancer combined with EGFR TKIs as well [75]. None of these drugs is currently approved for lung cancer therapy.

5 HER 2

HER2/ERBB2/NEU is a receptor tyrosine kinase of the epidermal growth factor family. Amplification or overexpression of HER2 is well known as a biomarker that predicts breast cancer response to targeted therapies. *HER*2 activation in lung cancer is associated with mutations, mostly insertions in exon 20, which are independent of *HER2* gene amplification. These mutations are not seen in breast cancer. *HER*2 mutations are found in 2 % of lung adenocarcinomas. *HER*2 mutations are more prevalent in lung adenocarcinomas from patients who are never smokers and perhaps are more common in Asians and women. Adenocarcinomas with *HER*2 mutations generally lack other oncogenic drivers such as *EGFR*, *ALK* and *KRAS* [76–83].

Clinical trials in patients with NSCLC that have *HER2* mutations have shown promising early results for therapy with afatinib [83, 84], trastuzumab [83], dacomitinib [85, 86] and neratinib plus temsirolimus [87, 88]. Therefore, detection of *HER2* mutations is a potential biomarker for a small subset of lung adenocarcinomas.

HER2 expression in lung cancers by IHC has not yet proven to be a successful biomarker for selecting patients for therapy [89]. *HER2* gene amplification is found in approximately 2 % of NSCLCs identified by FISH using the criteria for HER2 amplification in breast cancer [90]. Grob et al. [91] detected *HER2* amplification by FISH in 3 % of NSCLC, overwhelmingly adenocarcinomas, with high-level amplification in 2 %. They also reported that HER2 amplification in lung cancer may be heterogeneous, thus impacting the outcomes of trastuzumab or other HER2 therapies based on *HER2* amplification. *HER2* amplification also sometimes plays a role in acquired resistance to EGFR TKIs in lung cancer patients who initially respond to these therapies [92].

6 BRAF

The *BRAF* gene encodes for a nonreceptor serine/threonine kinase that is activated downstream of the Ras protein. About 50 % of melanomas have *BRAF* mutations which activate the BRAF kinase and increase phosphorylation of downstream targets, particularly MEK, and about 80–90 % are V600E mutations. The FDA has approved vemurafenib for the treatment of *BRAF V600E* mutation-positive, inoperable or metastatic melanoma [93, 94] and approved the cobas 4800 BRAF V600 Mutation Test as the companion diagnostic for the biomarker [95]. IHC using the primary mouse monoclonal antibody VE1, specific for BRAF p.V600E has been studied as a screening tool for the *BRAF V600E* mutation [96–98]. Dabrafenib, a mutant-*BRAF* kinase inhibitor [99], and trametinib, a MEK inhibitor [100], have also been approved for treatment of *BRAF V600E* positive unresectable or metastatic melanoma.

BRAF mutations occur in about 1–5 % of lung cancers. In contrast to melanomas, *V600E* mutations account for 50–60 % of these mutations and non-*V600E* mutations account for the remainder. With few exceptions, *BRAF* positive lung cancers are adenocarcinomas and, in some series, patients are more likely to be current or former smokers [101–105]. Marchetti et al. [103] reported that *V600E* mutations occurred more frequently in women and never smokers and were associated with micropapillary pattern whereas non-*V600E* mutations occurred in smokers.

Cases have been reported of *BRAF V600E* mutated lung adenocarcinomas which responded to vemurafenib [106–108], whereas a *BRAF* G469L mutated lung adenocarcinoma did not [109] which anecdotally suggests that *BRAF V600E* mutation is a predictive biomarker for therapy of lung adenocarcinoma with vemurafenib. Two patients with BRAF V600E mutated lung NSCLC, at least one an adenocarcinoma, are reported to have had a partial responses to dabrafenib [110, 111]. In these cases, patients have developed acquired resistance similar to what is observed with targeted therapies with the other biomarkers. Clinical trials with vemurafenib [94], dabrafenib [99] and trametinib [100] will hopefully validate these therapies for BRAF V600E mutated lung NSCLC.

Testing for *BRAF V600* mutations can be done by Sanger sequencing and various molecular techniques. As previously noted, the cobas 4800 BRAF V600 Mutation Test has been approved by the FDA as the companion diagnostic for *BRAF V600E* testing for vemurafenib therapy in melanoma [95]. *BRAF V600* mutations can be detected with targeted next generation sequencing [112, 113]. IHC using the aforementioned VE1 antibody has also been reported as a successful screening tool for BRAF V600E mutation in lung adenocarcinomas [114, 115].

References

1. Cagle PT, Allen TC (2012) Lung cancer genotype-based therapy and predictive biomarkers: present and future. Arch Pathol Lab Med 136(12):1482–1491
2. Lindeman NI, Cagle PT, Beasley MB et al (2013) Molecular testing guideline for selection of lung cancer patients for EGFR and ALK tyrosine kinase inhibitors: guideline from the college of american pathologists, international association for the study of lung cancer, and association for molecular pathology. Arch Pathol Lab Med 137(6):828–860
3. Cagle PT, Sholl LM, Lindeman NI et al (2014) Template for reporting results of biomarker testing of specimens from patients with non-small cell carcinoma of the lung. Arch Pathol Lab Med 138(2):171–174
4. Mitsudomi T, Yatabe Y (2007) Mutations of the epidermal growth factor receptor gene and related genes as determinants of epidermal growth factor receptor tyrosine kinase inhibitors sensitivity in lung cancer. Cancer Sci 98(12):1817–1824
5. Suda K, Tomizawa K, Mitsudomi T (2010) Biological and clinical significance of KRAS mutations in lung cancer: an oncogenic driver that contrasts with EGFR mutation. Cancer Metastasis Rev 29(1):49–60
6. Reinersman JM, Johnson ML, Riely GJ et al (2011) Frequency of EGFR and KRAS mutations in lung adenocarcinomas in African Americans. J Thorac Oncol 6(1):28–31
7. Zhang W, McQuitty EB, Olsen R et al (2014) EGFR mutations in US Hispanic versus non-Hispanic white patients with lung adenocarcinoma. Arch Pathol Lab Med 138(4): 543–545
8. Shaw AT, Yeap BY, Mino-Kenudson M et al (2009) Clinical features and outcome of patients with non-small-cell lung cancer who harbor EML4-ALK. J Clin Oncol 27(26): 4247–4253
9. Shaw AT, Yeap BY, Solomon BJ et al (2011) Effect of crizotinib on overall survival in patients with advanced non-small-cell lung cancer harbouring ALK gene rearrangement: a retrospective analysis. Lancet Oncol 12(11):1004–1012
10. Rodig SJ, Mino-Kenudson M, Dacic S et al (2009) Unique clinicopathologic features characterize ALK-rearranged lung adenocarcinoma in the western population. Clin Cancer Res 15(16):5216–5223
11. Atherly AJ, Camidge DR (2012) The cost-effectiveness of screening lung cancer patients for targeted drug sensitivity markers. Br J Cancer 106(6):1100–1106
12. Gaughan EM, Costa DB (2011) Genotype-driven therapies for non-small cell lung cancer: focus on EGFR, KRAS and ALK gene abnormalities. Ther Adv Med Oncol 3(3):113–125
13. Engelman JA, Janne PA (2008) Mechanisms of acquired resistance to epidermal growth factor receptor tyrosine kinase inhibitors in non-small cell lung cancer. Clin Cancer Res 14(10):2895–2899

14. Jackman D, Pao W, Riely GJ et al (2010) Clinical definition of acquired resistance to epidermal growth factor receptor tyrosine kinase inhibitors in non-small-cell lung cancer. J Clin Oncol 28(2):357–360
15. Yano S (2010) Studies for mechanism of drug resistance to EGFR-TKI. Gan To Kagaku Ryoho 37(8):1463–1466
16. Choi YL, Soda M, Yamashita Y et al (2010) EML4-ALK mutations in lung cancer that confer resistance to ALK inhibitors. N Engl J Med 363(18):1734–1739
17. Doebele RC, Pilling AB, Aisner DL et al (2012) Mechanisms of resistance to crizotinib in patients with ALK gene rearranged non-small cell lung cancer. Clin Cancer Res 18(5):1472–1482
18. Katayama R, Khan TM, Benes C et al (2011) Therapeutic strategies to overcome crizotinib resistance in non-small cell lung cancers harboring the fusion oncogene EML4-ALK. Proc Natl Acad Sci U S A 108(18):7535–7540
19. Katayama R, Shaw AT, Khan TM et al (2012) Mechanisms of acquired crizotinib resistance in ALK-rearranged lung cancers. Sci Transl Med 4(120):120ra17
20. Bergethon K, Shaw AT, Ou SH et al (2012) ROS1 rearrangements define a unique molecular class of lung cancers. J Clin Oncol 30(8):863–870
21. Janne PA, Meyerson M (2012) ROS1 rearrangements in lung cancer: a new genomic subset of lung adenocarcinoma. J Clin Oncol 30(8):878–879
22. Ou SH, Tan J, Yen Y, Soo RA (2012) ROS1 as a 'druggable' receptor tyrosine kinase: lessons learned from inhibiting the ALK pathway. Expert Rev Anticancer Ther 12(4):447–456
23. Rimkunas VM, Crosby K, Kelly M et al (2012) Analysis of receptor tyrosine kinase ROS1 positive tumors in non-small cell lung cancer: identification of a FIG-ROS1 fusion. Clin Cancer Res 18(16):4449–4457
24. Yasuda H, de Figueiredo-Pontes LL, Kobayashi S, Costa DB (2012) Preclinical rationale for use of the clinically available multitargeted tyrosine kinase inhibitor crizotinib in ROS1-translocated lung cancer. J Thorac Oncol 7(7):1086–1090
25. Chin LP, Soo RA, Soong R, Ou SH (2012) Targeting ROS1 with anaplastic lymphoma kinase inhibitors: a promising therapeutic strategy for a newly defined molecular subset of non-small-cell lung cancer. J Thorac Oncol 7(11):1625–1630
26. Shaw AT, Camidge DR, Engelman JA (2012) Clinical activity of crizotinib in advanced non-small cell lung cancer (NSCLC) harboring ROS1 gene rearrangement. J Clin Oncol 30(15 suppl):7508
27. Takeuchi K, Soda M, Togashi Y et al (2012) RET, ROS1 and ALK fusions in lung cancer. Nat Med 18(3):378–381
28. Forde PM, Rudin CM (2012) Crizotinib in the treatment of non-small-cell lung cancer. Expert Opin Pharmacother 13(8):1195–1201
29. Davies KD, Doebele RC (2013) Molecular pathways: ROS1 fusion proteins in cancer. Clin Cancer Res 19(15):4040–4045
30. Shaw AT, Hsu PP, Awad MM, Engelman JA (2013) Tyrosine kinase gene rearrangements in epithelial malignancies. Nat Rev Cancer 13(11):772–787
31. Heigener DF, Reck M (2014) Crizotinib. Recent Results Cancer Res 201:197–205
32. Go H, Kim DW, Kim D et al (2013) Clinicopathologic analysis of ROS1-rearranged non-small-cell lung cancer and proposal of a diagnostic algorithm. J Thorac Oncol 8(11):1445–1450
33. Kim HR, Lim SM, Kim HJ et al (2013) The frequency and impact of ROS1 rearrangement on clinical outcomes in never smokers with lung adenocarcinoma. Ann Oncol 24(9): 2364–2370
34. Pan Y, Zhang Y, Li Y et al (2014) ALK, ROS1 and RET fusions in 1139 lung adenocarcinomas: a comprehensive study of common and fusion pattern-specific clinicopathologic, histologic and cytologic features. Lung Cancer 84(2):121–126
35. Warth A, Muley T, Dienemann H et al (2014) ROS1 expression and translocations in non-small cell lung cancer: clinicopathological analysis of 1478 cases. Histopathology 65:187–194. doi:10.1111/his.12379

36. Yoshida A, Kohno T, Tsuta K et al (2013) ROS1-rearranged lung cancer: a clinicopathologic and molecular study of 15 surgical cases. Am J Surg Pathol 37(4):554–562
37. Sholl LM, Sun H, Butaney M et al (2013) ROS1 immunohistochemistry for detection of ROS1-rearranged lung adenocarcinomas. Am J Surg Pathol 37(9):1441–1449
38. Yoshida A, Tsuta K, Wakai S et al (2014) Immunohistochemical detection of ROS1 is useful for identifying ROS1 rearrangements in lung cancers. Mod Pathol 27(5):711–720
39. Matsuura S, Shinmura K, Kamo T et al (2013) CD74-ROS1 fusion transcripts in resected non-small cell lung carcinoma. Oncol Rep 30(4):1675–1680
40. Davies KD, Le AT, Theodoro MF et al (2012) Identifying and targeting ROS1 gene fusions in non-small cell lung cancer. Clin Cancer Res 18(17):4570–4579
41. Arai Y, Totoki Y, Takahashi H et al (2013) Mouse model for ROS1-rearranged lung cancer. PLoS One 8(2), e56010
42. Mescam-Mancini L, Lantuejoul S, Moro-Sibilot D et al (2014) On the relevance of a testing algorithm for the detection of ROS1-rearranged lung adenocarcinomas. Lung Cancer 83(2):168–173
43. Davies KD, Mahale S, Astling DP et al (2013) Resistance to ROS1 inhibition mediated by EGFR pathway activation in non-small cell lung cancer. PLoS One 8(12), e82236
44. Awad MM, Katayama R, McTigue M et al (2013) Acquired resistance to crizotinib from a mutation in CD74-ROS1. N Engl J Med 368(25):2395–2401
45. Davare MA, Saborowski A, Eide CA et al (2013) Foretinib is a potent inhibitor of oncogenic ROS1 fusion proteins. Proc Natl Acad Sci U S A 110(48):19519–19524
46. Gainor JF, Shaw AT (2013) Novel targets in non-small cell lung cancer: ROS1 and RET fusions. Oncologist 18(7):865–875
47. Ju YS, Lee WC, Shin JY et al (2012) A transforming KIF5B and RET gene fusion in lung adenocarcinoma revealed from whole-genome and transcriptome sequencing. Genome Res 22(3):436–445
48. Kohno T, Ichikawa H, Totoki Y et al (2012) KIF5B-RET fusions in lung adenocarcinoma. Nat Med 18(3):375–377
49. Li F, Feng Y, Fang R et al (2012) Identification of RET gene fusion by exon array analyses in "pan-negative" lung cancer from never smokers. Cell Res 22(5):928–931
50. Lipson D, Capelletti M, Yelensky R et al (2012) Identification of new ALK and RET gene fusions from colorectal and lung cancer biopsies. Nat Med 18(3):382–384
51. Suehara Y, Arcila M, Wang L et al (2012) Identification of KIF5B-RET and GOPC-ROS1 fusions in lung adenocarcinomas through a comprehensive mRNA-based screen for tyrosine kinase fusions. Clin Cancer Res 18(24):6599–6608
52. Tsuta K, Kohno T, Yoshida A et al (2014) RET-rearranged non-small-cell lung carcinoma: a clinicopathological and molecular analysis. Br J Cancer 110(6):1571–1578
53. Yokota K, Sasaki H, Okuda K et al (2012) KIF5B/RET fusion gene in surgically-treated adenocarcinoma of the lung. Oncol Rep 28(4):1187–1192
54. Drilon A, Wang L, Hasanovic A et al (2013) Response to cabozantinib in patients with RET fusion-positive lung adenocarcinomas. Cancer Discov 3(6):630–635
55. Wang R, Hu H, Pan Y et al (2012) RET fusions define a unique molecular and clinicopathologic subtype of non-small-cell lung cancer. J Clin Oncol 30(35):4352–4359
56. Chao BH, Briesewitz R, Villalona-Calero MA (2012) RET fusion genes in non-small-cell lung cancer. J Clin Oncol 30(35):4439–4441
57. Matsubara D, Kanai Y, Ishikawa S et al (2012) Identification of CCDC6-RET fusion in the human lung adenocarcinoma cell line, LC-2/ad. J Thorac Oncol 7(12):1872–1876
58. Gautschi O, Zander T, Keller FA et al (2013) A patient with lung adenocarcinoma and RET fusion treated with vandetanib. J Thorac Oncol 8(5):e43–e44
59. Sasaki H, Shimizu S, Tani Y et al (2012) RET expression and detection of KIF5B/RET gene rearrangements in Japanese lung cancer. Cancer Med 1(1):68–75
60. Bean J, Brennan C, Shih JY et al (2007) MET amplification occurs with or without T790M mutations in EGFR mutant lung tumors with acquired resistance to gefitinib or erlotinib. Proc Natl Acad Sci U S A 104(52):20932–20937

61. Cappuzzo F, Janne PA, Skokan M et al (2009) (2009) MET increased gene copy number and primary resistance to gefitinib therapy in non-small-cell lung cancer patients. Ann Oncol 20(2):298–304
62. Cappuzzo F, Marchetti A, Skokan M et al (2009) Increased MET gene copy number negatively affects survival of surgically resected non-small-cell lung cancer patients. J Clin Oncol 27(10):1667–1674
63. Chen HJ, Mok TS, Chen ZH et al (2009) Clinicopathologic and molecular features of epidermal growth factor receptor T790M mutation and c-MET amplification in tyrosine kinase inhibitor-resistant Chinese non-small cell lung cancer. Pathol Oncol Res 15(4):651–658
64. Engelman JA, Zejnullahu K, Mitsudomi T et al (2007) MET amplification leads to gefitinib resistance in lung cancer by activating ERBB3 signaling. Science 316(5827):1039–1043
65. Kong-Beltran M, Seshagiri S, Zha J et al (2006) Somatic mutations lead to an oncogenic deletion of met in lung cancer. Cancer Res 66(1):283–289
66. Kubo T, Yamamoto H, Lockwood WW et al (2009) MET gene amplification or EGFR mutation activate MET in lung cancers untreated with EGFR tyrosine kinase inhibitors. Int J Cancer 124(8):1778–1784
67. Onozato R, Kosaka T, Kuwano H, Sekido Y, Yatabe Y, Mitsudomi T (2009) Activation of MET by gene amplification or by splice mutations deleting the juxtamembrane domain in primary resected lung cancers. J Thorac Oncol 4(1):5–11
68. Sierra JR, Tsao MS (2011) c-MET as a potential therapeutic target and biomarker in cancer. Ther Adv Med Oncol 3(1 suppl):S21–S35
69. Surati M, Patel P, Peterson A, Salgia R (2011) Role of MetMAb (OA-5D5) in c-MET active lung malignancies. Expert Opin Biol Ther 11(12):1655–1662
70. Spigel DR, Ervin TJ, Ramlau RA et al (2013) Randomized phase II trial of onartuzumab in combination with erlotinib in patients with advanced non-small-cell lung cancer. J Clin Oncol 31(32):4105–4114
71. Koeppen H, Yu W, Zha J et al (2014) Biomarker analyses from a placebo-controlled phase II study evaluating erlotinib {+/-} onartuzumab in advanced non-small-cell lung cancer: MET expression levels are predictive of patient benefit. Clin Cancer Res. doi:10.1158/1078-0432.CCR-13-1836
72. Spigel DR, Edelman MJ, Mok T et al (2012) Treatment rationale study design for the MetLung trial: a randomized, double-blind phase III study of onartuzumab (MetMAb) in combination with erlotinib versus erlotinib alone in patients who have received standard chemotherapy for stage IIIB or IV met-positive non-small-cell lung cancer. Clin Lung Cancer 13(6):500–504
73. Scagliotti GV, Novello S, Schiller JH et al (2012) Rationale and design of MARQUEE: a phase III, randomized, double-blind study of tivantinib plus erlotinib versus placebo plus erlotinib in previously treated patients with locally advanced or metastatic, nonsquamous, non-small-cell lung cancer. Clin Lung Cancer 13(5):391–395
74. Sequist LV, von Pawel J, Garmey EG et al (2011) Randomized phase II study of erlotinib plus tivantinib versus erlotinib plus placebo in previously treated non-small-cell lung cancer. J Clin Oncol 29(24):3307–3315
75. Robinson KW, Sandler AB (2013) The role of MET receptor tyrosine kinase in non-small cell lung cancer and clinical development of targeted anti-MET agents. Oncologist 18(2):115–122
76. Buttitta F, Barassi F, Fresu G et al (2006) Mutational analysis of the HER2 gene in lung tumors from Caucasian patients: mutations are mainly present in adenocarcinomas with bronchioloalveolar features. Int J Cancer 119(11):2586–2591
77. Shigematsu H, Takahashi T, Nomura M et al (2005) Somatic mutations of the HER2 kinase domain in lung adenocarcinomas. Cancer Res 65(5):1642–1646
78. Stephens P, Hunter C, Bignell G et al (2004) Lung cancer: intragenic ERBB2 kinase mutations in tumours. Nature 431(7008):525–526
79. Arcila ME, Chaft JE, Nafa K et al (2012) Prevalence, clinicopathologic associations and molecular spectrum of ERBB2 (HER2) tyrosine kinase mutations in lung adenocarcinomas. Clin Cancer Res 18(18):4910–4918

80. Davies H, Hunter C, Smith R et al (2005) Somatic mutations of the protein kinase gene family in human lung cancer. Cancer Res 65(17):7591–7595
81. Sasaki H, Shimizu S, Endo K et al (2006) EGFR and erbB2 mutation status in Japanese lung cancer patients. Int J Cancer 118(1):180–184
82. Sonobe M, Manabe T, Wada H, Tanaka F (2006) Lung adenocarcinoma harboring mutations in the ERBB2 kinase domain. J Mol Diagn 8(3):351–356
83. Mazieres J, Peters S, Lepage B et al (2013) Lung cancer that harbors an HER2 mutation: epidemiologic characteristics and therapeutic perspectives. J Clin Oncol 31(16):1997–2003
84. De Greve J, Teugels E, Geers C et al (2012) Clinical activity of afatinib (BIBW 2992) in patients with lung adenocarcinoma with mutations in the kinase domain of HER2/neu. Lung Cancer 76(1):123–127
85. Kris M, Goldberg Z, Janne PA, Kim D, Martins R, Mok TSK (2012) Dacomitinib (PF-00299804), an irreversible pan-HER tyrosine kinase inhibitor (TKI), for first-line treatment of EGFR-mutant or HER2-mutant or -amplified lung cancers. Ann Oncol 23:1228
86. Reckamp KL, Giaccone G, Camidge DR et al (2014) A phase 2 trial of dacomitinib (PF-00299804), an oral, irreversible pan-HER (human epidermal growth factor receptor) inhibitor, in patients with advanced non-small cell lung cancer after failure of prior chemotherapy and erlotinib. Cancer 120(8):1145–1154
87. Gandhi L, Bahleda R, Cleary JM, Hollebecque A, Kwak EL, Pandya S (2011) Two dimensional phase I study of neratinib (NER) combined with temsirolimus (TEM) in patients (pts) with solid tumors. J Clin Oncol 29:3027
88. Gandhi L, Bahleda R, Tolaney SM et al (2014) Phase I study of neratinib in combination with temsirolimus in patients with human epidermal growth factor receptor 2-dependent and other solid tumors. J Clin Oncol 32(2):68–75
89. Clamon G, Herndon J, Kern J et al (2005) Lack of trastuzumab activity in nonsmall cell lung carcinoma with overexpression of erb-B2: 39810: a phase II trial of cancer and leukemia group B. Cancer 103(8):1670–1675
90. Heinmoller P, Gross C, Beyser K et al (2003) HER2 status in non-small cell lung cancer: results from patient screening for enrollment to a phase II study of herceptin. Clin Cancer Res 9(14):5238–5243
91. Grob TJ, Kannengiesser I, Tsourlakis MC et al (2012) Heterogeneity of ERBB2 amplification in adenocarcinoma, squamous cell carcinoma and large cell undifferentiated carcinoma of the lung. Mod Pathol 25(12):1566–1573
92. Takezawa K, Pirazzoli V, Arcila ME et al (2012) HER2 amplification: a potential mechanism of acquired resistance to EGFR inhibition in EGFR-mutant lung cancers that lack the second-site EGFRT790M mutation. Cancer Discov 2(10):922–933
93. Chapman PB, Hauschild A, Robert C et al (2011) Improved survival with vemurafenib in melanoma with BRAF V600E mutation. N Engl J Med 364(26):2507–2516
94. Garbe C, Abusaif S, Eigentler TK (2014) Vemurafenib. Recent Results Cancer Res 201:215–225
95. Anderson S, Bloom KJ, Vallera DU et al (2012) Multisite analytic performance studies of a real-time polymerase chain reaction assay for the detection of BRAF V600E mutations in formalin-fixed, paraffin-embedded tissue specimens of malignant melanoma. Arch Pathol Lab Med 136(11):1385–1391
96. Capper D, Berghoff AS, Magerle M et al (2012) Immunohistochemical testing of BRAF V600E status in 1,120 tumor tissue samples of patients with brain metastases. Acta Neuropathol 123(2):223–233
97. Capper D, Preusser M, Habel A et al (2011) Assessment of BRAF V600E mutation status by immunohistochemistry with a mutation-specific monoclonal antibody. Acta Neuropathol 122(1):11–19
98. Marin C, Beauchet A, Capper D et al (2014) Detection of BRAF p.V600E mutations in melanoma by immunohistochemistry has a good interobserver reproducibility. Arch Pathol Lab Med 138(1):71–75

99. Ballantyne AD, Garnock-Jones KP (2013) Dabrafenib: first global approval. Drugs 73(12): 1367–1376
100. Wright CJ, McCormack PL (2013) Trametinib: first global approval. Drugs 73(11):1245–1254
101. Brustugun OT, Khattak AM, Tromborg AK et al (2014) BRAF-mutations in non-small cell lung cancer. Lung Cancer 84(1):36–38
102. Kinno T, Tsuta K, Shiraishi K et al (2014) Clinicopathological features of nonsmall cell lung carcinomas with BRAF mutations. Ann Oncol 25(1):138–142
103. Marchetti A, Felicioni L, Malatesta S et al (2011) Clinical features and outcome of patients with non-small-cell lung cancer harboring BRAF mutations. J Clin Oncol 29(26):3574–3579
104. Paik PK, Arcila ME, Fara M et al (2011) Clinical characteristics of patients with lung adenocarcinomas harboring BRAF mutations. J Clin Oncol 29(15):2046–2051
105. Yousem SA, Nikiforova M, Nikiforov Y (2008) The histopathology of BRAF-V600E-mutated lung adenocarcinoma. Am J Surg Pathol 32(9):1317–1321
106. Gautschi O, Pauli C, Strobel K et al (2012) A patient with BRAF V600E lung adenocarcinoma responding to vemurafenib. J Thorac Oncol 7(10):e23–e24
107. Peters S, Michielin O, Zimmermann S (2013) Dramatic response induced by vemurafenib in a BRAF V600E-mutated lung adenocarcinoma. J Clin Oncol 31(20):e341–e344
108. Robinson SD, O'Shaughnessy JA, Lance Cowey C, Konduri K (2014) BRAF V600E-mutated lung adenocarcinoma with metastases to the brain responding to treatment with vemurafenib. Lung Cancer 85:326–330. doi:10.1016/j.lungcan.2014.05.009
109. Gautschi O, Peters S, Zoete V et al (2013) Lung adenocarcinoma with BRAF G469L mutation refractory to vemurafenib. Lung Cancer 82(2):365–367
110. Falchook GS, Long GV, Kurzrock R et al (2012) Dabrafenib in patients with melanoma, untreated brain metastases, and other solid tumours: a phase 1 dose-escalation trial. Lancet 379(9829):1893–1901
111. Rudin CM, Hong K, Streit M (2013) Molecular characterization of acquired resistance to the BRAF inhibitor dabrafenib in a patient with BRAF-mutant non-small-cell lung cancer. J Thorac Oncol 8(5):e41–e42
112. McCourt CM, McArt DG, Mills K et al (2013) Validation of next generation sequencing technologies in comparison to current diagnostic gold standards for BRAF, EGFR and KRAS mutational analysis. PLoS One 8(7), e69604
113. Tuononen K, Maki-Nevala S, Sarhadi VK et al (2013) Comparison of targeted next-generation sequencing (NGS) and real-time PCR in the detection of EGFR, KRAS, and BRAF mutations on formalin-fixed, paraffin-embedded tumor material of non-small cell lung carcinoma-superiority of NGS. Genes Chromosomes Cancer 52(5):503–511
114. Ilie M, Long E, Hofman V et al (2013) Diagnostic value of immunohistochemistry for the detection of the BRAFV600E mutation in primary lung adenocarcinoma Caucasian patients. Ann Oncol 24(3):742–748
115. Sasaki H, Shimizu S, Tani Y et al (2013) Usefulness of immunohistochemistry for the detection of the BRAF V600E mutation in Japanese lung adenocarcinoma. Lung Cancer 82(1):51–54

Epithelial Mesenchymal Transition in Aggressive Lung Cancers

Vivek Mittal

Abstract The progression of a cancer cell into a metastatic entity contributes to more than 90 % of cancer related deaths. Therefore, the prevention and treatment of metastasis is an unmet clinical need. Epithelial to mesenchymal transition (EMT) is an evolutionary conserved developmental program, which is induced during cancer progression and contributes to metastatic colonization. EMT endows metastatic properties upon cancer cells by enhancing mobility, invasion, and resistance to apoptotic stimuli. Furthermore, EMT-derived tumor cells acquire stem cell properties and exhibit therapeutic resistance. The disseminated tumor cells recruited to distant organs are suggested to subsequently undergo an EMT reversion through mesenchymal to epithelial transition (MET), necessary for efficient colonization and macrometastasis. A major focus of cancer research is to determine the cellular and molecular mechanisms underlying EMT/MET in tumor invasion, dissemination and metastasis. In this chapter, we will focus on the contribution of the EMT signaling pathways in lung cancer progression, cancer stem cells and acquired resistance to EGFR tyrosine kinase inhibitors and chemotherapy. We will also discuss the potential of targeting EMT pathways as an attractive strategy for the treatment of lung cancer.

Keywords Epithelial mesenchymal transition • Lung cancer • Therapy • Resistance • Cancer stem cells • Metastasis

---

V. Mittal (✉)
Department of Cardiothoracic Surgery, Neuberger Berman Foundation Lung Cancer Center, New York, NY 10065, USA

Department of Cell and Developmental Biology, Weill Medical College of Cornell University, 1300 York Avenue, New York, NY 10065, USA
e-mail: vim2010@med.cornell.edu

A. Ahmad, S.M. Gadgeel (eds.), *Lung Cancer and Personalized Medicine: Novel Therapies and Clinical Management*, Advances in Experimental Medicine and Biology 890, DOI 10.1007/978-3-319-24932-2_3

1 Epithelial Mesenchymal Transition in Cancer: Overview

Epithelial–mesenchymal transition (EMT), an evolutionarily conserved process, is essential for embryonic development, gastrulation, neural crest formation, and organ development [1]. EMT has been established as an important step in tissue repair, organ fibrosis, and cancer progression [2–4]. EMT is a dynamic and reversible process, during which epithelial cells transition from polarized, cobblestone-like cells to migratory, spindle-shaped mesenchymal cells. In addition to morphological changes, cells undergoing EMT also exhibit changes at the molecular level by losing expression of epithelial markers such as E-cadherin, ZO-1 and occludin, and gaining expression of mesenchymal markers including N-cadherin, vimentin, and fibronectin. Several signaling pathways regulate EMT including TGFs, BMPs, FGF, EGF, HGF, Wnt/beta-catenin and Notch, in which both transcriptional and post-transcriptional processes are involved [5, 6].

The similarities between transcriptional and epigenetic regulatory pathways in developmental and pathological EMTs suggest that the developmental EMT program is hijacked during tumor invasion and metastasis [3, 7–10]. To identify key EMT molecular pathways that govern the metastatic process, many studies have focused on cell-based experimental models. These studies have shown that EMT confers tumor cells with invasive and metastatic abilities, resistance to therapies, as well as cancer stem cell (CSC) phenotypes that have a major impact on cancer progression [11]. Consistent with the demonstration that EMT activators such as Twist, can induce EMT and breast CSC phenotypes [12, 13], enrichment of CSC/EMT signatures in residual tumors remaining after neoadjuvant chemotherapy was demonstrated [14]. However, a recent study showed that the homeobox factor "paired-related homeobox transcription factor 1" (Prrx1) is an EMT inducer conferring migratory and invasive properties. However, in contrast to other EMT-activators, Prrx1 suppresses CSC phenotypes [15]. This study suggests that unlike the classical EMT transcription factors, Prrx1 contributes to metastasis by uncoupling stemness from EMT.

While cancer cell intrinsic EMT signaling pathways have been well elucidated, the contribution of the tumor microenvironment (TME) in providing EMT activating signals to the cancer cells have only recently been investigated [16, 17]. Several paracrine and autocrine signals trigger induction of EMT resulting in mesenchymal and CSC states in cancer [18–20]. Following EMT, the disseminated mesenchymal cells undergo mesenchymal to epithelial transition (MET) at the site of metastasis [1, 21, 22].

The clinical relevance of EMT has been an area of long standing controversy, mainly due to the lack of evidence of EMT in clinical carcinomas and metastasis [23–26]. More recent efforts have been directed towards demonstrating EMT directly in vivo in mice and humans, and until now the direct role of EMT in vivo has remained elusive. In this chapter, we will focus on EMT in cancer progression, with emphasis on lung cancer, and discuss opportunities for novel anti-EMT therapeutic approaches.

2 Epithelial Mesenchymal Transition in Physiological Processes and Cancer

Three types of EMT have been proposed [27]. Type 1 EMT describes the transition of cells into the mesenchyme during embryogenesis and organ development, and does not involve pathological events [1]. Type 2 EMT is important for wound healing, tissue repair and organ fibrosis, where inflammatory cells produce EMT-inducing factors including TGFβ, PDGF, FGF and Matrix metalloproteinases (MMPs), which induce EMT in normal epithelial cells leading to extensive organ fibrosis [27, 28]. Type 3 EMT is associated with cancer progression and metastases [3, 8, 9]. In addition, following primary EMT, mesenchymal cells are capable of reversing back to epithelial phenotypes through mesenchymal to epithelial transition (MET), which is critical for organ formation including kidney organogenesis and somitogenesis [3, 29]. In cancer, histological analysis has revealed morphological similarities between primary tumors and their metastatic lesions [29], and it has been reported that E-cadherin levels are elevated in lymph node metastases relative to matched primary tumor samples. These data suggest that EMT in primary tumors may be followed by MET at distant metastatic sites [30, 31]. Consistent with these correlative clinical findings, recent studies have demonstrated that re-differentiation of disseminated tumor cells in the metastatic site through MET is critical for colonization [21, 24, 32]. The involvement of EMT in cancer progression is widely recognized; however, the potential role of MET is unclear, and constitutes an area of intense investigation.

3 Epithelial Mesenchymal Transition in Primary Tumor and Metastatic Dissemination

Since the first description of EMT in cancer progression, EMT has been inherently related to metastasis [27, 33]. Accumulating evidence from in vitro experiments have shown that EMT represents a major mechanism for tumor cells to acquire critical metastatic features including enhanced mobility, invasion, and resistance to apoptotic stimuli. Furthermore, as a result of EMT, tumor cells acquire chemoresistance and exhibit increased potential for initiating secondary tumors [34]. More importantly, EMT has also been implicated in conferring CSC properties [12, 35], a rare subpopulation of cancer cells with capacity of self-renewal, regeneration and differentiation into diverse types of cancer cells.

With the identification of a mesenchymal phenotype in the highly malignant breast CSCs, research focus has recently progressed towards understanding the role of EMT in metastasis in vivo. Using intravital imaging approaches, it was shown that single breast cancer cells gained mobility for hematogenous metastasis by activating EMT-promoting TGFβ-Smad2/3 signaling [36]. Indeed, EMT was also observed during metastasis in spontaneous tumor models in mice, where disseminated tumor cells in the lungs of MMTV-PyMT transgenic mice expressed a mesenchymal marker, FSP1, suggesting involvement of EMT in tumor dissemination [37]. Using a squamous cell carcinoma mouse model, activation of EMT-inducing transcription factor Twist was sufficient to promote carcinoma cells to undergo EMT and disseminate into blood circulation [38]. However, at the distant sites, turning off Twist1 to allow reversion of EMT was essential for disseminated tumor cells to proliferate and form overt metastases. Direct evidence of EMT has also been shown in a K-Ras mediated spontaneous pancreatic tumor model, which develops liver metastases [39]. Remarkably, EMT-positive cells were found in primary lesions, in the circulation, and as single cell deposits in the liver at a very early stage of primary tumor development, even before malignancy could be detected by rigorous histologic analysis. These post-EMT tumor cells gained expression of typical mesenchymal markers including fibronectin, Zeb1 and FSP1 and lost expression of E-cadherin. Importantly, the post-EMT tumor cells represent the majority of metastatic tumor cells that seeded the metastatic liver. However, more rigorous lineage tracing approaches are being developed to actually demonstrate the process of EMT in vivo. For example, using an EMT-lineage tracing strategy of mesenchymal specific (FSP1) Cre mediated β-galactosidase activity, Trimboli et al. compared the incidence of EMT events in three different oncogene-driven breast tumor models [40]. Significantly, post-EMT tumor cells were detected in the Myc-driven tumors, but not in the PyMT- or Neu-driven tumors. Notably, lung metastases were formed in almost all MMTV-PyMT and MMTV-neu mice, but not in MMTV-myc animals, suggesting that the contribution of EMT in metastasis may be tumor type specific. It is also possible that the β-galactosidase activity was not sensitive enough to monitor the relatively rare EMT events, and that better EMT-lineage tracing systems are required to clarify the biological contributions of post-EMT tumor cells in metastasis.

4 Epithelial Mesenchymal Transition in Lung Cancer

Lung cancer is a global public health problem with an estimated 1.3 million new cases each year [41]. In the United States, approximately 226,160 new cases of lung cancer are diagnosed per year with over 160,000 deaths. Despite advances in treatment options, including minimally invasive surgical resection, stereotactic radiation, and novel chemotherapeutic regimens, the 5-year survival rate in NSCLC remains only at approximately 15 %. Available targeted therapies such as EGFR tyrosine kinase inhibitors (TKIs, erlotinib and gefitinib) and EML4-ALK inhibitor (crizotinib) benefit only 15–20 % of NSCLC patients who carry specific drug-sensitive mutations. Even in these patients, acquired resistance is a major impediment to a durable therapeutic response [42–44]. Notably, EMT has been implicated in mediating resistance to therapy in lung cancer. A growing body of evidence supports the role of EMT in the progression of many cancers [2], and transcriptional factors and microRNAs involved in the EMT process have been identified in a number of signaling pathways. However, the role of EMT in lung cancer has not been extensively characterized.

4.1 *Epithelial Mesenchymal Transition and Prognosis in Lung Cancer*

Several studies have suggested an association between EMT factors including E-cadherin, hypoxia inducible factor 1α (HIF-1α), twist, snail and poor prognosis in lung cancer [45]. Notably, expression of Twist, Slug, and Foxc2 was an independent predictor of recurrence-free and overall survival in stage I NSCLC [46]. Analysis of archived tissue from primary human lung tumors, brain metastases and adjacent bronchial epithelial specimens showed high expression of EMT associated markers in progressing primary lung cancer specimens, particularly in squamous cell carcinoma [47]. Compared to primary NSCLC, brain metastases showed decreased EMT phenotype expression, consistent with the notion that disseminated tumor cells undergo MET at the site of metastasis [1, 21]. It was suggested that overexpression of Forkhead box M1 (FOXM1), a member of the Fox family of transcriptional factors, may have prognostic value for patients with NSCLC, and FOXM1 was shown to promote metastasis by inducing EMT through activation of the AKT/p70S6K pathway [48].

In NSCLC, invasive tumor growth is accompanied by desmoplastic stroma reaction and concomitant upregulation of EMT markers at the invasive front [49]. Previously, an analysis of surgically resected 533 NSCLC specimens by immunohistochemistry showed that EMT proteins periostin, versican and elastin confer prognostic value [50, 51]. Clinically relevant EMT biomarkers with significant prognostic value in lung adenocarcinoma were identified recently [52]. In this study, analysis of the secretome from a TGF-β induced model of EMT by mass spectrometry unraveled a 97-gene EMT signature with positive correlations to lymph node metastasis, advanced tumor stage and histological grade. Moreover, a refined 20-gene signature predicted survival of both adenocarcinoma and squamous carcinoma patients. Increased expression of BRF2, a RNA polymerase II transcription factor was significantly associated with the poor prognosis of NSCLC patients by virtue of promoting EMT [53]. In another study, downregulation of BRAF activated non-coding RNA promoted EMT, which was associated with poor prognosis in NSCLC [54]. Importantly, in some studies, survival data related to the EMT profile is lacking.

4.2 *Epithelial Mesenchymal Transition and Lung Cancer Progression*

The association of EMT and cancer progression has been shown in several types of cancer, including breast cancer, prostate cancer, pancreatic cancer and hepatocellular carcinoma. However, the role of EMT in lung cancer has not been extensively studied, and the role of EMT in the pathogenesis of several lung disorders is currently intensely debated. More recently, a number of signaling pathways and biomarkers have been implicated in EMT-induced lung cancer progression (Fig. 1).

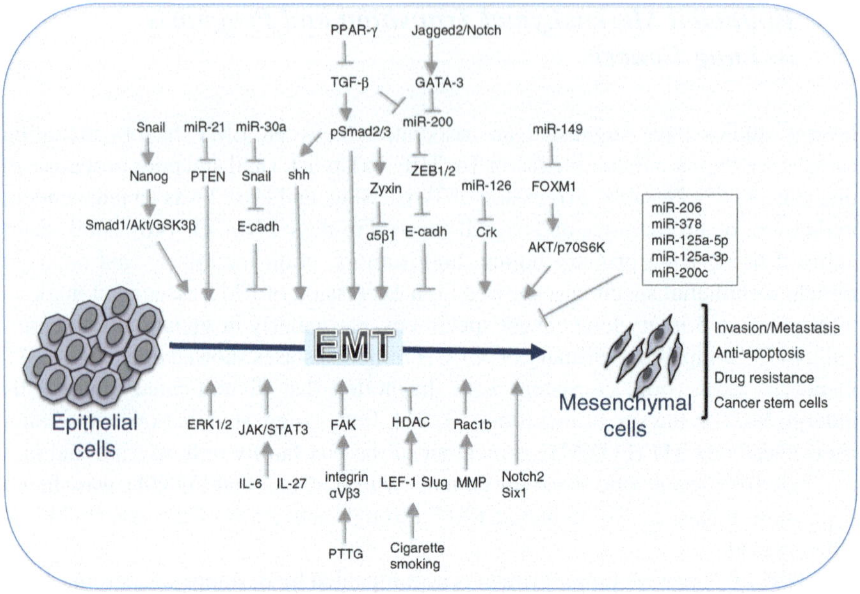

Fig. 1 Schema depicting potential EMT pathways in lung cancer

EMT is orchestrated by several signaling pathways, including TGF-β/Smad and IL-6/JAK/STAT3 (signal transducer and activator of transcription 3) signaling. The JAK/STAT3 pathway was required for TGF-β-induced EMT and cancer cell migration and invasion via upregulation of p-Smad3 and Snail, and the IL-6/JAK/STAT3 and TGF-β/Smad signaling synergistically enhanced EMT in lung carcinomas [55]. In another study, activation of peroxisome proliferator-activated receptor-gamma (PPAR-γ) inhibited TGF-β-induced EMT in lung cancer cells and prevented metastasis by antagonizing Smad3 function [56]. TGF-β1-induced EMT in lung cancer cells resulted in the acquisition of a mesenchymal profile associated with elevated levels of stem cell markers [57–59]. In a related study, TGF-β1-induced EMT in lung cancer cells upregulated Neuropilin (NRP)-2, the high-affinity receptor for SEMA3F [60]. Notably, NRP2 blocked invasive potential of tumor xenografts and reversed TGF-β1-mediated growth inhibition. In NSCLC, Snail was shown to regulate Nanog during EMT via the Smad1/Akt/GSK3β signaling pathway [61].

Notch-1 signaling is critical in lung development and disease [62, 63], and has been shown to promote EMT [64]. It has been demonstrated that blocking Notch-1 signaling by Hey-1 or Jagged1 knockdown or a γ-secretase inhibitor (GSI) attenuates EMT [65]. Radiation-induced Notch-1 overexpression promoted survival and EMT in NSCLC via miR-34a [66]. In this context, induction of miR-34a decreased the expression of Notch-1 and its downstream targets including Hes-1, Cyclin D1, Survivin and Bcl-2 and blocked proliferation and invasion in NSCLC cells [67]. Analysis of the Kras (G12D)-driven NSCLC mouse model showed that conditional Notch1 and Notch2 receptor deletion revealed opposing roles in NSCLC progression [68].

In another study, transcriptional factors Notch2 and Six1 induced EMT and conferred malignant phenotypes to lung adenocarcinomas [69].

MicroRNAs have been shown to contribute to EMT in NSCLC. miR-132 suppressed the migration and invasion of NSCLC cells through targeting ZEB2 [70]. Expression of miR-149, downregulated in lung cancer, was inversely correlated with invasive and EMT phenotypes in NSCLC cells [71]. miR-149 targeted Forkhead box M1 (FOXM1), and FOXM1 was involved in the EMT induced by TGF-β1. miR-200s have recently been shown to inhibit EMT and promote MET by direct targeting of E-cadherin transcriptional repressors ZEB1 and ZEB2 [72–75]. The observation that the miR-200 family enforces the epithelial phenotype and inhibits EMT and invasion in vitro suggests that these miRNAs are likely to suppress metastasis. Recently, it was shown that, while re-differentiation induced by expression of miR-200 is required for metastatic colonization in a lung tumor xenograft model, miR-200 also directly targets SEC23A, which stimulates the secretion of metastasis-suppressive proteins [32]. Interestingly, cancer cells established from a mouse model of lung adenocarcinoma, driven by oncogenic K-Ras and loss of function p53 mutations, display epithelial plasticity [76], and undergo EMT following TGF-β exposure, which is dependent on downregulation of mir-200 with concomitant stabilization of ZEB1 expression. Ceppi and colleagues have shown that miR-200c expression induces an aggressive, invasive, and chemoresistant phenotype, and that lower mir-200c levels were associated with poor grade of differentiation and higher metastatic potential in NSCLC patients [77]. In another study, immortalized human bronchial epithelial cells (HBECs) exposed to tobacco carcinogens exhibited EMT and stem-like features associated with miR-200 and miR-205. Notably, EMT was driven both by chromatin remodeling and promoter DNA methylation [78]. Some studies have reported conflicting roles of miR-200s in metastatic progression [76, 79, 80], possibly invalidating the therapeutic utility of miR-200s. Furthermore, it remains unclear whether metastasis-related functions of the miR-200s are mediated entirely or only partially through the ZEB–E-cadherin axis.

Osteopontin (OPN), a prognostic marker in NSCLC [81, 82], through integrin αVβ3, activated the FAK, PI3K, Akt, ERK and NF-kB pathways, contributing to the migration of lung cancer cells [83]. Similarly, a role of pituitary tumor transforming gene (PTTG), in regulating EMT by inducing expression of integrin αVβ3 and adhesion-complex proteins (FAK) in lung cancer cells was shown [84]. Zyxin was identified as a novel functional target and effector of TGF-β/Smad3 signaling that regulates lung cancer cell motility and EMT via Integrin α5β1 [85].

Inflammation is an important contributor of lung carcinogenesis. The inflammatory component of the TME has been shown to stimulate EMT in lung cancer by contributing to hypoxia, angiogenesis and differential regulation of miRNAs [86, 87]. Paracrine and autocrine contribution of signaling molecules in inducing EMT in lung cancer has been documented. For example, a role for IL-27 in regulating EMT and angiogenesis through modulation of the STAT pathways in human NSCLC was demonstrated [88]. Similarly, COX-2-dependent pathways via modulation of transcriptional repressors of E-cadherin, ZEB1 and Snail regulated EMT in NSCLC [89].

Although association between cigarette smoking and lung cancer is well documented, the molecular mechanisms underlying cigarette smoke-induced EMT processes that are critical for the progression and metastasis of lung cancer are not well understood. Cigarette smoking was shown to induce the repression of E-cadherin via transcription factors LEF-1 and Slug-mediated recruitment of histone deacetylase, HDAC [90]. In another study, cigarette smoke induced EMT through Rac1/Smad2 and Rac1/PI3K/Akt signaling pathways in pulmonary epithelial cells [91].

MMPs that degrade components of the extracellular matrix have been shown to induce EMT. MMP-3, MMP-7, and MMP-28 induce EMT in human A549 lung adenocarcinoma cells [92–94]. Recently MMP-induced upregulation of Rac1b contributed to EMT in a transgenic mice model of lung cancer [95].

4.3 Epithelial Mesenchymal Transition and Drug Resistance in Lung Cancer

Drug resistance constitutes a major challenge for the successful treatment of cancer patients. Cancer therapy is often associated with two major forms of drug resistance—*de novo* or acquired. Patients who are initially refractory to therapy display intrinsic or "*de novo*" drug resistance. Patients that initially respond to therapy typically relapse as a consequence of "acquired" drug resistance. EMT has been associated with resistance to chemotherapy, EGFR inhibitors, and other targeted drugs in cancers of the lung [96–98], bladder [99], head and neck [100], pancreas [101], and breast [102]. Intriguingly, EMT can trigger reversion to a CSC-like phenotype [12, 35], providing an association between EMT, CSCs and drug resistance.

In NSCLC, despite the initial response, patients with EGFR-mutant NSCLC eventually develop acquired resistance to EGFR TKIs. The EGFR-T790M secondary mutation is responsible for approximately half of acquired resistance cases, while MET amplification has been associated with acquired resistance in about 5–15 % of NSCLCs [43, 103]. Accumulating evidence suggests that reversible epigenetic changes that emerge during acquired drug resistance reflect changes in the differentiation state of the tumor, which is likely to reflect EMT and the emergence of chemoresistant cells with stem cell-like features [104, 105]. Notably, gefitinib inhibited invasive phenotype and EMT in drug-resistant NSCLC cells with MET amplification [106].

Overcoming *de novo* and acquired resistance to drug therapy remains a challenge in the clinical management of NSCLC, and approaches to reverse or inhibit EMT as a strategy for drug sensitization are being considered. For example, Buonato and colleagues showed that ERK 1/2 signaling maintained a mesenchymal phenotype in NSCLC cells, and prolonged exposure to MEK or ERK inhibitors restored epithelial phenotypes and overcome resistance to EGFR-targeted therapy [107]. Consistent with these observations, simultaneous EGFR and MEK inhibition are being considered in gastric cancer [108] and pancreatic cancer cells [109], and current clinical trials are evaluating erlotinib combined with MEK inhibitors in NSCLC.

In an attempt to explain resistance to EGFR TKIs, Sordella and colleagues have uncovered the existence of a subpopulation of lung cancer cells that are intrinsically resistant to erlotinib and display EMT phenotypes. These cells by virtue of secreting elevated amounts of TGF-β and IL-6 resisted Tarceva treatment independently of the EGFR pathway [110]. In a previous study, lung adenocarcinomas harboring EGFR mutations were shown to exhibit upregulated IL-6 which activated the gp130/JAK/STAT3 pathway [111]. In this context, Varmus and colleagues showed that inducible expression of EGFR kinase domain–activating mutations targeted to the lung epithelium gave rise to adenocarcinomas containing pSTAT3 and pAKT, demonstrating an association between this oncogene and activated STAT3 [112]. Interestingly, metformin that suppress the IL-6/STAT3 pathway mediated EMT, and sensitized EGFR-TKI-resistant human lung cancer cells to erlotinib or gefitinib [113]. In another study, the expression of Ras-related nuclear protein (Ran) GTPase was elevated in invasive NSCLC. Ran induced EMT and enhanced invasion in NSCLC cells through the activation of PI3K-AKT signaling [114].

In EGFR-TKI resistant lung cancer, activated Notch-1 was found to promote EMT associated with increased Snail and Vimentin expression, suggesting that gefitinib resistance was secondary to Notch-activated EMT [115]. Consistent with this observation, cisplatin was shown to induce the enrichment of multidrug resistant CD133+ CSCs by the activation of Notch signaling [116]. Consistent with this observation, Notch pathway activity identified cells with CSC-like properties and correlated with worse survival in human lung adenocarcinoma [117]. High Notch activity has also been shown to induce radiation resistance in NSCLC [118]. The Hedgehog (Hh) pathway is implicated in lung squamous cell carcinomas (SCC). Notably, activated Hh signaling was shown to regulate metastasis through EMT, and the Shh/Gli pathway was implicated in SCC recurrence, metastasis and resistance to chemotherapy [119]. In NSCLC, TGF-β1-mediated upregulation of shh induced EMT in NSCLC cells [120], and conferred resistance to EGFR-TKIs [121]. Importantly, both genetic and pharmacological inhibition of the Hh pathway reversed the EMT phenotype and improved the therapeutic efficacy of EGFR-TKIs [121].

The miR-134/487b/655 cluster was shown to regulate TGF-β1-induced EMT and induced resistance to gefitinib by targeting MAGI2 (membrane-associated guanylate kinase, WW, and PDZ domain-containing protein 2) in which suppression subsequently caused loss of PTEN stability in lung cancer cells [122].

Platinum-based chemotherapy is the standard first-line approach for the treatment of NSCLC, but recurrence occurs in most patients [123]. Novel combination of chemotherapeutic agents have enhanced the overall median survival of NSCLC patients [124]. However, chemoresistance of tumor cells continues to be a challenge in the management of NSCLCs. Tumor cells often show initial sensitivity to chemotherapeutic drugs, but acquired resistance develops during the treatment, leading to tumor recurrence and further tumor progression. Analysis of cisplatin resistant lung cancer cells showed acquisition of the EMT phenotype, decreased connexin43 (Cx43) expression, and increased capability of invasion and migration [125]. In a related study, resistance of lung cancer cells to docetaxel was associated with EMT, and inhibition of ZEB1 reversed EMT and chemoresistance [126]. Integrinβ1 induced EGFR TKI resistance in NSCLC tumors was associated with an EMT phenotype. [127].

5 Therapeutic Potential of Targeting Epithelial Mesenchymal Transition in Lung Cancer

In lung cancer, EMT has been associated with key tumorigenic properties including increased invasion, angiogenesis and metastasis. Mechanistic insights on how EMT affects signaling pathways contributing to carcinogenesis is necessary to develop effective therapeutics. A number of signaling pathways including notch, wnt, hedgehog and PI3K-AKT, have been implicated in EMT. Furthermore, a growing body of evidence suggests that epithelial cells are more likely to initially respond to therapy, and that EMT confers acquisition of therapeutic resistance. As such, EMT, CSCs, and drug resistance have been described as an emerging axis of evil in cancer [128]. Targeting EMT has been considered a promising strategy against lung cancer, as it would provide novel translational and clinical studies for the benefit of advanced stage cancer patients with metastatic disease [129]. NSCLCs resistant to EGFR TKIs have been shown to downregulate EGFR and increase expression of platelet-derived growth factor receptor (PDGFR), fibroblast growth factor receptor (FGFR), and AXL [130].

EMT is currently being investigated as a therapeutic target for overcoming drug resistance in lung cancer. For example, HGF-mediated activation of Met receptor induced EMT conferred an aggressive phenotype and induced chemoresistance in preclinical models. Notably, treatment with Met inhibitor resensitized cells to chemotherapy [131]. These findings have clinical relevance, as human NSCLC specimens expressing mesenchymal markers were associated with Met activation, predicted worse survival, and were upregulated in chemorefractory disease. These results support the rationale for Met inhibitor and chemotherapy-centered clinical trials, and suggest that the selection of SCLC patients based on mesenchymal biomarkers in combination with Met expression may be a superior alternative for clinical trials of Met inhibitors plus chemotherapy. Similarly, in drug-resistant NSCLC cells with MET amplification, gefitinib was shown to inhibit invasive phenotype and EMT [106].

ERK1/2 signaling was shown to maintain a mesenchymal phenotype in NSCLC cells associated with resistance to EGFR-TKIs. Prolonged exposure to MEK or ERK inhibitors restored epithelial phenotypes and overcame resistance of NSCLC to EGFR-targeted therapy [107]. For example, combination treatment with gefitinib and MEK inhibitors was effective in the treatment of gefitinib-resistant lung adenocarcinoma cells harboring EGFR mutations [132]. Indeed, current clinical trials have begun to evaluate erlotinib in combination with MEK inhibitors in NSCLC (NCT01229150). Similarly, the IL-6/STAT3 pathway-mediated EMT is also being exploited in EGFR-TKI-resistant NSCLC. Suppression of this pathway with metformin sensitized resistant lung cancer cells to erlotinib or gefitinib [113].

Metformin also inhibited IL-6-induced EMT and lung adenocarcinoma growth and metastasis [133].

A 76-gene EMT signature was found to predict resistance to EGFR and PI3K/Akt inhibitors, and AXL (a member of the RTK family), was identified as a potential therapeutic target for overcoming EGFR inhibitor resistance associated with the mesenchymal phenotype [134]. In this context, activated phospho-AXL was detected in 59.8 % of adenocarcinoma cases examined and correlated significantly with larger tumor size and with overall survival of the patients [135]. A recent study has shown that EMT rewires the mechanism of PI3K pathway activation-dependent proliferation in NSCLC cells [136, 137]. In epithelial cells, autocrine ERBB3 activation maintained PI3K signaling; however EMT altered the proliferative potential of cells by modulating ERBB3 expression.

The CXCR4/CXCL12 axis contributes to the pathology of NSCLC, and targeting this axis has been considered as a potential therapeutic approach for the treatment of NSCLC [138]. Importantly, elevated CXCR4 levels were observed in NSCLC cells high in self-renewal capacity and increased chemotherapeutic resistance [139]. Inhibition of CXCR4 suppressed the self renewal capacity of NSCLC cells [140], and a previous study had shown that the transcription factor 5T4 via CXCR4 may induce EMT and increase migration of NSCLC [141]. The therapeutic potential of CXCR4/CXCL12 axis is being considered for cancer treatment [142–144]. EMT-induced CSC phenotypes have been implicated in resistance to cisplatin, as cisplatin-treated patients with lung cancer showed enrichment of $CD133^+$ stem cells due to activated Notch signaling, suggesting that blocking Notch signaling may reduce the recurrence of NSCLCs [116]. Similarly, the AKT/β-catenin/Snail signaling pathway has been associated with CSC-like properties and EMT features in NSCLC cells, implying the therapeutic potential of this pathway for the treatment of NSCLC [145].

6 Future Perspectives

Current EMT research efforts are directed towards understanding the interplay of multiple regulatory networks that contribute to the conversion of an epithelial tumor cell to a mesenchymal state resulting in acquisition of various acquired capabilities such as resistance to anoikis, oncogene-induced senescence, and resistance to apoptosis/chemotherapy and CSC properties. Various transcriptional and post-transcriptional processes have been identified; however, the mechanisms by which these pathways are interconnected during cancer progression are not completely understood. A variety of contextual paracrine and autocrine signaling factors that maintain mesenchymal and CSC phenotypes have begun to emerge [20], and recent studies have implicated the contribution of chromatin modification as a mechanism to attain widespread changes in gene expression that accompany the EMT process [9]. In lung cancer, EMT is associated with metastatic progression, resistance to EGFR inhibitors, chemotherapy, and other targeted drugs [96–98]. Acquired resistance to the EGFR inhibitor erlotinib resulted from the selection and expansion of a mesenchymal subpopulation [110], and restoring E-cadherin expression in mesenchymal-like NSCLC cells potentiated sensitivity to EGFR inhibitors [146] suggesting that a treatment approach eliciting a mesenchymal to epithelial transition (MET) may be useful for expanding the efficacy of EGFR inhibitors. In addition, growing evidence for AXL-mediated EGFR inhibitor resistance has been linked to EMT [147]. EMT regulators are being considered as potential molecular biomarkers and therapeutic targets for developing multi-targeted strategies for improving current cancer therapies and preventing disease relapse. For example, TGF-β has been shown to induce EMT in NSCLC [57], and clinical benefits of TGF-β signaling inhibitors is being considered [148]. Consistent with this notion, IN-1130, a novel inhibitor of TGF-β type I receptor, was shown to impair breast cancer lung metastasis through inhibition of EMT [149]. Similarly, Wnt signaling has emerged as a critical pathway in lung carcinogenesis, and Wnt pathway antagonists are being explored in NSCLC [150, 151]. Given that EMT contributes to resistance of EGFR-TKIs, inhibition of EMT constitutes a critical therapeutic strategy for overcoming to EGFR-TKis resistance in lung cancer.

Despite the significant and rapid progress in the EMT field, several issues have still remained unresolved. For example, circulating tumor cell (CTC) number in metastatic cancer patients is being considered as prognostic markers consistent with enhanced cell migration and invasion via loss of adhesion, a feature of EMT. Evidence of prognostic significance of CTC number emerged from a study of resectable NSCLC, demonstrating an association between increased CTC number and shorter disease free survival [152]. A hybrid EMT phenotype of CTCs was also demonstrated in patients with metastatic NSCLC [153]. In light of these studies, multiplex analysis and further detailed exploration of metastatic potential and EMT in CTCs is now warranted in a larger patient cohort.

Finally, the role of EMT in cancer progression has been a topic of debate in the scientific community mainly due to paucity of robust in vivo data demonstrating the importance of EMT in tumorigenesis. Furthermore, the clinical relevance of EMT is often questionable due to the lack of evidence of EMT in clinical carcinomas and metastasis [23, 25] [24, 26]. More recent efforts are directed towards EMT demonstration directly in vivo using lineage tracing approaches and live intravital microscopy imaging. These analyses may establish a more direct role of EMT in vivo during tumorigenesis.

Acknowledgments We thank Sharrell Lee for reading the manuscript. VM is supported by NIH grants and by Cornell Center on the Microenvironment and Metastasis through Award Number U54CA143876 from the National Cancer Institute, and the Neuberger Berman Lung Cancer Center. The authors apologize for studies that could not be included due to space limitations.

References

1. Lim J, Thiery JP (2012) Epithelial-mesenchymal transitions: insights from development. Development 139:3471–3486
2. Hugo H, Ackland ML, Blick T, Lawrence MG, Clements JA, Williams ED, Thompson EW (2007) Epithelial–mesenchymal and mesenchymal–epithelial transitions in carcinoma progression. J Cell Physiol 213:374–383
3. Thiery JP, Acloque H, Huang RY, Nieto MA (2009) Epithelial-mesenchymal transitions in development and disease. Cell 139:871–890

4. Yang J, Weinberg RA (2008) Epithelial-mesenchymal transition: at the crossroads of development and tumor metastasis. Dev Cell 14:818–829
5. Lamouille S, Xu J, Derynck R (2014) Molecular mechanisms of epithelial-mesenchymal transition. Nat Rev Mol Cell Biol 15:178–196
6. Said NA, Williams ED (2011) Growth factors in induction of epithelial-mesenchymal transition and metastasis. Cells Tissues Organs 193:85–97
7. De Craene B, Berx G (2013) Regulatory networks defining EMT during cancer initiation and progression. Nat Rev Cancer 13:97–110
8. Nieto MA (2011) The ins and outs of the epithelial to mesenchymal transition in health and disease. Annu Rev Cell Dev Biol 27:347–376
9. Tam WL, Weinberg RA (2013) The epigenetics of epithelial-mesenchymal plasticity in cancer. Nat Med 19:1438–1449
10. Thomson S, Petti F, Sujka-Kwok I, Mercado P, Bean J, Monaghan M, Seymour SL, Argast GM, Epstein DM, Haley JD (2011) A systems view of epithelial-mesenchymal transition signaling states. Clin Exp Metastasis 28:137–155
11. Dave B, Mittal V, Tan NM, Chang JC (2012) Epithelial-mesenchymal transition, cancer stem cells and treatment resistance. Breast Cancer Res 14:202
12. Mani SA, Guo W, Liao MJ, Eaton EN, Ayyanan A, Zhou AY, Brooks M, Reinhard F, Zhang CC, Shipitsin M et al (2008) The epithelial-mesenchymal transition generates cells with properties of stem cells. Cell 133:704–715
13. Morel AP, Lièvre M, Thomas C, Hinkal G, Ansieau S, Puisieux A (2008) Generation of breast cancer stem cells through epithelial-mesenchymal transition. PLoS One 3, e2888
14. Creighton CJ, Li X, Landis M, Dixon JM, Neumeister VM, Sjolund A, Rimm DL, Wong H, Rodriguez A, Herschkowitz JI et al (2009) Residual breast cancers after conventional therapy display mesenchymal as well as tumor-initiating features. Proc Natl Acad Sci U S A 106:13820–13825
15. Ocaña OH, Córcoles R, Fabra A, Moreno-Bueno G, Acloque H, Vega S, Barrallo-Gimeno A, Cano A, Nieto MA (2012) Metastatic colonization requires the repression of the epithelial-mesenchymal transition inducer Prrx1. Cancer Cell 22:709–724
16. Gao D, Mittal V (2012) Tumor microenvironment regulates epithelial-mesenchymal transitions in metastasis. Expert Rev Anticancer Ther 12:857–859
17. Gao D, Vahdat LT, Wong S, Chang JC, Mittal V (2012) Microenvironmental regulation of epithelial-mesenchymal transitions in cancer. Cancer Res 72:4883–4889
18. Katoh Y, Katoh M (2008) Hedgehog signaling, epithelial-to-mesenchymal transition and miRNA (review). Int J Mol Med 22:271–275
19. Moustakas A, Heldin CH (2007) Signaling networks guiding epithelial-mesenchymal transitions during embryogenesis and cancer progression. Cancer Sci 98:1512–1520
20. Scheel C, Eaton EN, Li SH, Chaffer CL, Reinhardt F, Kah KJ, Bell G, Guo W, Rubin J, Richardson AL et al (2011) Paracrine and autocrine signals induce and maintain mesenchymal and stem cell states in the breast. Cell 145:926–940
21. Gao D, Joshi N, Choi H, Ryu S, Hahn M, Catena R, Sadik H, Argani P, Wagner P, Vahdat LT et al (2012) Myeloid progenitor cells in the premetastatic lung promote metastases by inducing mesenchymal to epithelial transition. Cancer Res 72:1384–1394
22. Sheng W, Wang G, La Pierre DP, Wen J, Deng Z, Wong CK, Lee DY, Yang BB (2006) Versican mediates mesenchymal-epithelial transition. Mol Biol Cell 17:2009–2020
23. Bastid J (2012) EMT in carcinoma progression and dissemination: facts, unanswered questions, and clinical considerations. Cancer Metastasis Rev 31:277–283
24. Brabletz T (2012) To differentiate or not–routes towards metastasis. Nat Rev Cancer 12:425–436
25. Ledford H (2011) Cancer theory faces doubts. Nature 472:273
26. Tarin D, Thompson EW, Newgreen DF (2005) The fallacy of epithelial mesenchymal transition in neoplasia. Cancer Res 65:5996–6000, discussion 6000–5991
27. Kalluri R, Weinberg RA (2009) The basics of epithelial-mesenchymal transition. J Clin Invest 119:1420–1428

28. Zeisberg M, Kalluri R (2013) Cellular mechanisms of tissue fibrosis. 1. Common and organ-specific mechanisms associated with tissue fibrosis. Am J Physiol Cell Physiol 304:C216–C225
29. Chaffer CL, Thompson EW, Williams ED (2007) Mesenchymal to epithelial transition in development and disease. Cells Tissues Organs 185:7–19
30. Jeschke U, Mylonas I, Kuhn C, Shabani N, Kunert-Keil C, Schindlbeck C, Gerber B, Friese K (2007) Expression of E-cadherin in human ductal breast cancer carcinoma in situ, invasive carcinomas, their lymph node metastases, their distant metastases, carcinomas with recurrence and in recurrence. Anticancer Res 27:1969–1974
31. Park D, Kåresen R, Axcrona U, Noren T, Sauer T (2007) Expression pattern of adhesion molecules (E-cadherin, alpha-, beta-, gamma-catenin and claudin-7), their influence on survival in primary breast carcinoma, and their corresponding axillary lymph node metastasis. APMIS 115:52–65
32. Korpal M, Ell BJ, Buffa FM, Ibrahim T, Blanco MA, Celià-Terrassa T, Mercatali L, Khan Z, Goodarzi H, Hua Y et al (2011) Direct targeting of Sec23a by miR-200s influences cancer cell secretome and promotes metastatic colonization. Nat Med 17:1101–1108
33. Scheel C, Weinberg RA (2011) Phenotypic plasticity and epithelial-mesenchymal transitions in cancer and normal stem cells? Int J Cancer 129:2310–2314
34. Hennessy BT, Gonzalez-Angulo AM, Stemke-Hale K, Gilcrease MZ, Krishnamurthy S, Lee JS, Fridlyand J, Sahin A, Agarwal R, Joy C et al (2009) Characterization of a naturally occurring breast cancer subset enriched in epithelial-to-mesenchymal transition and stem cell characteristics. Cancer Res 69:4116–4124
35. Polyak K, Weinberg RA (2009) Transitions between epithelial and mesenchymal states: acquisition of malignant and stem cell traits. Nat Rev Cancer 9:265–273
36. Giampieri S, Manning C, Hooper S, Jones L, Hill CS, Sahai E (2009) Localized and reversible TGFbeta signalling switches breast cancer cells from cohesive to single cell motility. Nat Cell Biol 11:1287–1296
37. Xue C, Plieth D, Venkov C, Xu C, Neilson EG (2003) The gatekeeper effect of epithelial-mesenchymal transition regulates the frequency of breast cancer metastasis. Cancer Res 63:3386–3394
38. Tsai JH, Donaher JL, Murphy DA, Chau S, Yang J (2012) Spatiotemporal regulation of epithelial-mesenchymal transition is essential for squamous cell carcinoma metastasis. Cancer Cell 22:725–736
39. Rhim AD, Mirek ET, Aiello NM, Maitra A, Bailey JM, McAllister F, Reichert M, Beatty GL, Rustgi AK, Vonderheide RH et al (2012) EMT and dissemination precede pancreatic tumor formation. Cell 148:349–361
40. Trimboli AJ, Fukino K, de Bruin A, Wei G, Shen L, Tanner SM, Creasap N, Rosol TJ, Robinson ML, Eng C et al (2008) Direct evidence for epithelial-mesenchymal transitions in breast cancer. Cancer Res 68:937–945
41. Siegel R, Naishadham D, Jemal A (2012) Cancer statistics, 2012. CA Cancer J Clin 62:10–29
42. Choi YL, Soda M, Yamashita Y, Ueno T, Takashima J, Nakajima T, Yatabe Y, Takeuchi K, Hamada T, Haruta H et al (2010) EML4-ALK mutations in lung cancer that confer resistance to ALK inhibitors. N Engl J Med 363:1734–1739
43. Engelman JA, Zejnullahu K, Mitsudomi T, Song Y, Hyland C, Park JO, Lindeman N, Gale CM, Zhao X, Christensen J et al (2007) MET amplification leads to gefitinib resistance in lung cancer by activating ERBB3 signaling. Science 316:1039–1043
44. Pao W, Miller VA, Politi KA, Riely GJ, Somwar R, Zakowski MF, Kris MG, Varmus H (2005) Acquired resistance of lung adenocarcinomas to gefitinib or erlotinib is associated with a second mutation in the EGFR kinase domain. PLoS Med 2, e73
45. Xiao D, He J (2010) Epithelial mesenchymal transition and lung cancer. J Thorac Dis 2:154–159
46. Jiang W, Pang XG, Wang Q, Shen YX, Chen XK, Xi JJ (2012) Prognostic role of Twist, Slug, and Foxc2 expression in stage I non-small-cell lung cancer after curative resection. Clin Lung Cancer 13:280–287

47. Prudkin L, Liu DD, Ozburn NC, Sun M, Behrens C, Tang X, Brown KC, Bekele BN, Moran C, Wistuba II (2009) Epithelial-to-mesenchymal transition in the development and progression of adenocarcinoma and squamous cell carcinoma of the lung. Mod Pathol 22:668–678
48. Kong FF, Qu ZQ, Yuan HH, Wang JY, Zhao M, Guo YH, Shi J, Gong XD, Zhu YL, Liu F et al (2014) Overexpression of FOXM1 is associated with EMT and is a predictor of poor prognosis in non-small cell lung cancer. Oncol Rep 31:2660–2668
49. Soltermann A (2012) Epithelial-mesenchymal transition in non-small cell lung cancer. Pathologe 33(suppl 2):311–317
50. Morra L, Moch H (2011) Periostin expression and epithelial-mesenchymal transition in cancer: a review and an update. Virchows Arch 459:465–475
51. Soltermann A, Tischler V, Arbogast S, Braun J, Probst-Hensch N, Weder W, Moch H, Kristiansen G (2008) Prognostic significance of epithelial-mesenchymal and mesenchymal-epithelial transition protein expression in non-small cell lung cancer. Clin Cancer Res 14:7430–7437
52. Reka AK, Chen G, Jones RC, Amunugama R, Kim S, Karnovsky A, Standiford TJ, Beer DG, Omenn GS, Keshamouni VG (2014) Epithelial-mesenchymal transition-associated secretory phenotype predicts survival in lung cancer patients. Carcinogenesis 35:1292–1300
53. Tian Y, Lu M, Yue W, Li L, Li S, Gao C, Si L, Qi L, Hu W, Tian H (2014) TFIIB-related factor 2 is associated with poor prognosis of nonsmall cell lung cancer patients through promoting tumor epithelial-mesenchymal transition. Biomed Res Int 2014:530786
54. Sun M, Liu XH, Wang KM, Nie FQ, Kong R, Yang JS, Xia R, Xu TP, Jin FY, Liu ZJ et al (2014) Downregulation of BRAF activated non-coding RNA is associated with poor prognosis for non-small cell lung cancer and promotes metastasis by affecting epithelial-mesenchymal transition. Mol Cancer 13:68
55. Liu RY, Zeng Y, Lei Z, Wang L, Yang H, Liu Z, Zhao J, Zhang HT (2014) JAK/STAT3 signaling is required for TGF-β-induced epithelial-mesenchymal transition in lung cancer cells. Int J Oncol 44:1643–1651
56. Reka AK, Kurapati H, Narala VR, Bommer G, Chen J, Standiford TJ, Keshamouni VG (2010) Peroxisome proliferator-activated receptor-gamma activation inhibits tumor metastasis by antagonizing Smad3-mediated epithelial-mesenchymal transition. Mol Cancer Ther 9:3221–3232
57. Pirozzi G, Tirino V, Camerlingo R, Franco R, La Rocca A, Liguori E, Martucci N, Paino F, Normanno N, Rocco G (2011) Epithelial to mesenchymal transition by TGFβ-1 induction increases stemness characteristics in primary non small cell lung cancer cell line. PLoS One 6, e21548
58. Pirozzi G, Tirino V, Camerlingo R, La Rocca A, Martucci N, Scognamiglio G, Franco R, Cantile M, Normanno N, Rocco G (2013) Prognostic value of cancer stem cells, epithelial-mesenchymal transition and circulating tumor cells in lung cancer. Oncol Rep 29:1763–1768
59. Tirino V, Camerlingo R, Bifulco K, Irollo E, Montella R, Paino F, Sessa G, Carriero MV, Normanno N, Rocco G et al (2013) TGF-β1 exposure induces epithelial to mesenchymal transition both in CSCs and non-CSCs of the A549 cell line, leading to an increase of migration ability in the CD133+ A549 cell fraction. Cell Death Dis 4, e620
60. Nasarre P, Gemmill RM, Potiron VA, Roche J, Lu X, Barón AE, Korch C, Garrett-Mayer E, Lagana A, Howe PH et al (2013) Neuropilin-2 Is upregulated in lung cancer cells during TGF-β1-induced epithelial-mesenchymal transition. Cancer Res 73:7111–7121
61. Liu CW, Li CH, Peng YJ, Cheng YW, Chen HW, Liao PL, Kang JJ, Yeng MH (2014) Snail regulates Nanog status during the epithelial-mesenchymal transition via the Smad1/Akt/GSK3β signaling pathway in non-small-cell lung cancer. Oncotarget 5:3880–3894
62. Westhoff B, Colaluca IN, D'Ario G, Donzelli M, Tosoni D, Volorio S, Pelosi G, Spaggiari L, Mazzarol G, Viale G et al (2009) Alterations of the Notch pathway in lung cancer. Proc Natl Acad Sci U S A 106:22293–22298
63. Xu K, Moghal N, Egan SE (2012) Notch signaling in lung development and disease. Adv Exp Med Biol 727:89–98
64. Sahlgren C, Gustafsson MV, Jin S, Poellinger L, Lendahl U (2008) Notch signaling mediates hypoxia-induced tumor cell migration and invasion. Proc Natl Acad Sci U S A 105: 6392–6397

65. Zavadil J, Cermak L, Soto-Nieves N, Böttinger EP (2004) Integration of TGF-beta/Smad and Jagged1/Notch signalling in epithelial-to-mesenchymal transition. EMBO J 23:1155–1165
66. Kang J, Kim E, Kim W, Seong KM, Youn H, Kim JW, Kim J, Youn B (2013) Rhamnetin and cirsiliol induce radiosensitization and inhibition of epithelial-mesenchymal transition (EMT) by miR-34a-mediated suppression of Notch-1 expression in non-small cell lung cancer cell lines. J Biol Chem 288:27343–27357
67. Ji X, Wang Z, Geamanu A, Goja A, Sarkar FH, Gupta SV (2012) Delta-tocotrienol suppresses Notch-1 pathway by upregulating miR-34a in nonsmall cell lung cancer cells. Int J Cancer 131:2668–2677
68. Baumgart A, Mazur PK, Anton M, Rudelius M, Schwamborn K, Feuchtinger A, Behnke K, Walch A, Braren R, Peschel C et al (2015) Opposing role of Notch1 and Notch2 in a Kras(G12D)-driven murine non-small cell lung cancer model. Oncogene 34:578–588
69. Mimae T, Okada M, Hagiyama M, Miyata Y, Tsutani Y, Inoue T, Murakami Y, Ito A (2012) Upregulation of notch2 and six1 is associated with progression of early-stage lung adenocarcinoma and a more aggressive phenotype at advanced stages. Clin Cancer Res 18:945–955
70. You J, Li Y, Fang N, Liu B, Zu L, Chang R, Li X, Zhou Q (2014) MiR-132 suppresses the migration and invasion of lung cancer cells via targeting the EMT regulator ZEB2. PLoS One 9, e91827
71. Ke Y, Zhao W, Xiong J, Cao R (2013) miR-149 inhibits non-small-cell lung cancer cells EMT by targeting FOXM1. Biochem Res Int 2013:506731
72. Burk U, Schubert J, Wellner U, Schmalhofer O, Vincan E, Spaderna S, Brabletz T (2008) A reciprocal repression between ZEB1 and members of the miR-200 family promotes EMT and invasion in cancer cells. EMBO Rep 9:582–589
73. Gregory PA, Bert AG, Paterson EL, Barry SC, Tsykin A, Farshid G, Vadas MA, Khew-Goodall Y, Goodall GJ (2008) The miR-200 family and miR-205 regulate epithelial to mesenchymal transition by targeting ZEB1 and SIP1. Nat Cell Biol 10:593–601
74. Korpal M, Lee ES, Hu G, Kang Y (2008) The miR-200 family inhibits epithelial-mesenchymal transition and cancer cell migration by direct targeting of E-cadherin transcriptional repressors ZEB1 and ZEB2. J Biol Chem 283:14910–14914
75. Park SM, Gaur AB, Lengyel E, Peter ME (2008) The miR-200 family determines the epithelial phenotype of cancer cells by targeting the E-cadherin repressors ZEB1 and ZEB2. Genes Dev 22:894–907
76. Gibbons DL, Lin W, Creighton CJ, Rizvi ZH, Gregory PA, Goodall GJ, Thilaganathan N, Du L, Zhang Y, Pertsemlidis A et al (2009) Contextual extracellular cues promote tumor cell EMT and metastasis by regulating miR-200 family expression. Genes Dev 23:2140–2151
77. Ceppi P, Mudduluru G, Kumarswamy R, Rapa I, Scagliotti GV, Papotti M, Allgayer H (2010) Loss of miR-200c expression induces an aggressive, invasive, and chemoresistant phenotype in non-small cell lung cancer. Mol Cancer Res 8:1207–1216
78. Tellez CS, Juri DE, Do K, Bernauer AM, Thomas CL, Damiani LA, Tessema M, Leng S, Belinsky SA (2011) EMT and stem cell-like properties associated with miR-205 and miR-200 epigenetic silencing are early manifestations during carcinogen-induced transformation of human lung epithelial cells. Cancer Res 71:3087–3097
79. Dykxhoorn DM, Wu Y, Xie H, Yu F, Lal A, Petrocca F, Martinvalet D, Song E, Lim B, Lieberman J (2009) miR-200 enhances mouse breast cancer cell colonization to form distant metastases. PLoS One 4:e7181
80. Olson P, Lu J, Zhang H, Shai A, Chun MG, Wang Y, Libutti SK, Nakakura EK, Golub TR, Hanahan D (2009) MicroRNA dynamics in the stages of tumorigenesis correlate with hallmark capabilities of cancer. Genes Dev 23:2152–2165
81. Boldrini L, Donati V, Dell'Omodarme M, Prati MC, Faviana P, Camacci T, Lucchi M, Mussi A, Santoro M, Basolo F et al (2005) Prognostic significance of osteopontin expression in early-stage non-small-cell lung cancer. Br J Cancer 93:453–457
82. Donati V, Boldrini L, Dell'Omodarme M, Prati MC, Faviana P, Camacci T, Lucchi M, Mussi A, Santoro M, Basolo F et al (2005) Osteopontin expression and prognostic significance in non-small cell lung cancer. Clin Cancer Res 11:6459–6465

83. Fong YC, Liu SC, Huang CY, Li TM, Hsu SF, Kao ST, Tsai FJ, Chen WC, Chen CY, Tang CH (2009) Osteopontin increases lung cancer cells migration via activation of the alphavbeta3 integrin/FAK/Akt and NF-kappaB-dependent pathway. Lung Cancer 64:263–270
84. Shah PP, Fong MY, Kakar SS (2012) PTTG induces EMT through integrin αVβ3-focal adhesion kinase signaling in lung cancer cells. Oncogene 31:3124–3135
85. Mise N, Savai R, Yu H, Schwarz J, Kaminski N, Eickelberg O (2012) Zyxin is a transforming growth factor-β (TGF-β)/Smad3 target gene that regulates lung cancer cell motility via integrin α5β1. J Biol Chem 287:31393–31405
86. Heinrich EL, Walser TC, Krysan K, Liclican EL, Grant JL, Rodriguez NL, Dubinett SM (2012) The inflammatory tumor microenvironment, epithelial mesenchymal transition and lung carcinogenesis. Cancer Microenviron 5:5–18
87. Krysan K, Lee JM, Dohadwala M, Gardner BK, Reckamp KL, Garon E, St John M, Sharma S, Dubinett SM (2008) Inflammation, epithelial to mesenchymal transition, and epidermal growth factor receptor tyrosine kinase inhibitor resistance. J Thorac Oncol 3:107–110
88. Kachroo P, Lee MH, Zhang L, Baratelli F, Lee G, Srivastava MK, Wang G, Walser TC, Krysan K, Sharma S et al (2013) IL-27 inhibits epithelial-mesenchymal transition and angiogenic factor production in a STAT1-dominant pathway in human non-small cell lung cancer. J Exp Clin Cancer Res 32:97
89. Dohadwala M, Yang SC, Luo J, Sharma S, Batra RK, Huang M, Lin Y, Goodglick L, Krysan K, Fishbein MC et al (2006) Cyclooxygenase-2-dependent regulation of E-cadherin: prostaglandin E(2) induces transcriptional repressors ZEB1 and snail in non-small cell lung cancer. Cancer Res 66:5338–5345
90. Nagathihalli NS, Massion PP, Gonzalez AL, Lu P, Datta PK (2012) Smoking induces epithelial-to-mesenchymal transition in non-small cell lung cancer through HDAC-mediated downregulation of E-cadherin. Mol Cancer Ther 11:2362–2372
91. Shen HJ, Sun YH, Zhang SJ, Jiang JX, Dong XW, Jia YL, Shen J, Guan Y, Zhang LH, Li FF et al (2014) Cigarette smoke-induced alveolar epithelial-mesenchymal transition is mediated by Rac1 activation. Biochim Biophys Acta 1840:1838–1849
92. Illman SA, Lehti K, Keski-Oja J, Lohi J (2006) Epilysin (MMP-28) induces TGF-beta mediated epithelial to mesenchymal transition in lung carcinoma cells. J Cell Sci 119:3856–3865
93. McGuire JK, Li Q, Parks WC (2003) Matrilysin (matrix metalloproteinase-7) mediates E-cadherin ectodomain shedding in injured lung epithelium. Am J Pathol 162:1831–1843
94. Radisky DC, Przybylo JA (2008) Matrix metalloproteinase-induced fibrosis and malignancy in breast and lung. Proc Am Thorac Soc 5:316–322
95. Stallings-Mann ML, Waldmann J, Zhang Y, Miller E, Gauthier ML, Visscher DW, Downey GP, Radisky ES, Fields AP, Radisky DC (2012) Matrix metalloproteinase induction of Rac1b, a key effector of lung cancer progression. Sci Transl Med 4:142ra195
96. Garofalo M, Romano G, Di Leva G, Nuovo G, Jeon YJ, Ngankeu A, Sun J, Lovat F, Alder H, Condorelli G et al (2012) EGFR and MET receptor tyrosine kinase-altered microRNA expression induces tumorigenesis and gefitinib resistance in lung cancers. Nat Med 18:74–82
97. Thomson S, Petti F, Sujka-Kwok I, Epstein D, Haley JD (2008) Kinase switching in mesenchymal-like non-small cell lung cancer lines contributes to EGFR inhibitor resistance through pathway redundancy. Clin Exp Metastasis 25:843–854
98. Yauch RL, Januario T, Eberhard DA, Cavet G, Zhu W, Fu L, Pham TQ, Soriano R, Stinson J, Seshagiri S et al (2005) Epithelial versus mesenchymal phenotype determines in vitro sensitivity and predicts clinical activity of erlotinib in lung cancer patients. Clin Cancer Res 11:8686–8698
99. Shrader M, Pino MS, Brown G, Black P, Adam L, Bar-Eli M, Dinney CP, McConkey DJ (2007) Molecular correlates of gefitinib responsiveness in human bladder cancer cells. Mol Cancer Ther 6:277–285
100. Frederick BA, Helfrich BA, Coldren CD, Zheng D, Chan D, Bunn PA, Raben D (2007) Epithelial to mesenchymal transition predicts gefitinib resistance in cell lines of head and neck squamous cell carcinoma and non-small cell lung carcinoma. Mol Cancer Ther 6: 1683–1691

101. Yin T, Wang C, Liu T, Zhao G, Zha Y, Yang M (2007) Expression of snail in pancreatic cancer promotes metastasis and chemoresistance. J Surg Res 141:196–203
102. Li X, Lewis MT, Huang J, Gutierrez C, Osborne CK, Wu MF, Hilsenbeck SG, Pavlick A, Zhang X, Chamness GC et al (2008) Intrinsic resistance of tumorigenic breast cancer cells to chemotherapy. J Natl Cancer Inst 100:672–679
103. Bean J, Brennan C, Shih JY, Riely G, Viale A, Wang L, Chitale D, Motoi N, Szoke J, Broderick S et al (2007) MET amplification occurs with or without T790M mutations in EGFR mutant lung tumors with acquired resistance to gefitinib or erlotinib. Proc Natl Acad Sci U S A 104:20932–20937
104. Sharma SV, Lee DY, Li B, Quinlan MP, Takahashi F, Maheswaran S, McDermott U, Azizian N, Zou L, Fischbach MA et al (2010) A chromatin-mediated reversible drug-tolerant state in cancer cell subpopulations. Cell 141:69–80
105. Voulgari A, Pintzas A (2009) Epithelial-mesenchymal transition in cancer metastasis: mechanisms, markers and strategies to overcome drug resistance in the clinic. Biochim Biophys Acta 1796:75–90
106. La Monica S, Caffarra C, Saccani F, Galvani E, Galetti M, Fumarola C, Bonelli M, Cavazzoni A, Cretella D, Sirangelo R et al (2013) Gefitinib inhibits invasive phenotype and epithelial-mesenchymal transition in drug-resistant NSCLC cells with MET amplification. PLoS One 8, e78656
107. Buonato JM, Lazzara MJ (2014) ERK1/2 blockade prevents epithelial-mesenchymal transition in lung cancer cells and promotes their sensitivity to EGFR inhibition. Cancer Res 74:309–319
108. Yoon YK, Kim HP, Han SW, Hur HS, Oh DY, Im SA, Bang YJ, Kim TY (2009) Combination of EGFR and MEK1/2 inhibitor shows synergistic effects by suppressing EGFR/HER3-dependent AKT activation in human gastric cancer cells. Mol Cancer Ther 8:2526–2536
109. Diep CH, Munoz RM, Choudhary A, Von Hoff DD, Han H (2011) Synergistic effect between erlotinib and MEK inhibitors in KRAS wild-type human pancreatic cancer cells. Clin Cancer Res 17:2744–2756
110. Yao Z, Fenoglio S, Gao DC, Camiolo M, Stiles B, Lindsted T, Schlederer M, Johns C, Altorki N, Mittal V et al (2010) TGF-beta IL-6 axis mediates selective and adaptive mechanisms of resistance to molecular targeted therapy in lung cancer. Proc Natl Acad Sci U S A 107:15535–15540
111. Gao SP, Mark KG, Leslie K, Pao W, Motoi N, Gerald WL, Travis WD, Bornmann W, Veach D, Clarkson B et al (2007) Mutations in the EGFR kinase domain mediate STAT3 activation via IL-6 production in human lung adenocarcinomas. J Clin Invest 117:3846–3856
112. Politi K, Zakowski MF, Fan PD, Schonfeld EA, Pao W, Varmus HE (2006) Lung adenocarcinomas induced in mice by mutant EGF receptors found in human lung cancers respond to a tyrosine kinase inhibitor or to down-regulation of the receptors. Genes Dev 20:1496–1510
113. Li L, Han R, Xiao H, Lin C, Wang Y, Liu H, Li K, Chen H, Sun F, Yang Z et al (2014) Metformin sensitizes EGFR-TKI-resistant human lung cancer cells in vitro and in vivo through inhibition of IL-6 signaling and EMT reversal. Clin Cancer Res 20:2714–2726
114. Ning J, Liu W, Zhang J, Lang Y, Xu S (2014) Ran GTPase induces EMT and enhances invasion in non-small cell lung cancer cells through activation of PI3K-AKT pathway. Oncol Res 21:67–72
115. Xie M, Zhang L, He CS, Xu F, Liu JL, Hu ZH, Zhao LP, Tian Y (2012) Activation of Notch-1 enhances epithelial-mesenchymal transition in gefitinib-acquired resistant lung cancer cells. J Cell Biochem 113:1501–1513
116. Liu YP, Yang CJ, Huang MS, Yeh CT, Wu AT, Lee YC, Lai TC, Lee CH, Hsiao YW, Lu J et al (2013) Cisplatin selects for multidrug-resistant CD133+ cells in lung adenocarcinoma by activating Notch signaling. Cancer Res 73:406–416
117. Hassan KA, Wang L, Korkaya H, Chen G, Maillard I, Beer DG, Kalemkerian GP, Wicha MS (2013) Notch pathway activity identifies cells with cancer stem cell-like properties and correlates with worse survival in lung adenocarcinoma. Clin Cancer Res 19:1972–1980

118. Theys J, Yahyanejad S, Habets R, Span P, Dubois L, Paesmans K, Kattenbeld B, Cleutjens J, Groot AJ, Schuurbiers OC et al (2013) High NOTCH activity induces radiation resistance in non small cell lung cancer. Radiother Oncol 108:440–445
119. Yue D, Li H, Che J, Zhang Y, Tseng HH, Jin JQ, Luh TM, Giroux-Leprieur E, Mo M, Zheng Q et al (2014) Hedgehog/Gli promotes epithelial-mesenchymal transition in lung squamous cell carcinomas. J Exp Clin Cancer Res 33:34
120. Maitah MY, Ali S, Ahmad A, Gadgeel S, Sarkar FH (2011) Up-regulation of sonic hedgehog contributes to TGF-β1-induced epithelial to mesenchymal transition in NSCLC cells. PLoS One 6, e16068
121. Ahmad A, Maitah MY, Ginnebaugh KR, Li Y, Bao B, Gadgeel SM, Sarkar FH (2013) Inhibition of Hedgehog signaling sensitizes NSCLC cells to standard therapies through modulation of EMT-regulating miRNAs. J Hematol Oncol 6:77
122. Kitamura K, Seike M, Okano T, Matsuda K, Miyanaga A, Mizutani H, Noro R, Minegishi Y, Kubota K, Gemma A (2014) MiR-134/487b/655 cluster regulates TGF-β-induced epithelial-mesenchymal transition and drug resistance to gefitinib by targeting MAGI2 in lung adenocarcinoma cells. Mol Cancer Ther 13:444–453
123. Thatcher N, Faivre-Finn C, Blackhall F, Anderson H, Lorigan P (2005) Sequential platinum-based chemotherapy-thoracic radiotherapy in early stage non-small cell lung cancer. Clin Cancer Res 11:5051s–5056s
124. Socinski MA (2004) Clinical issues in the management of non-small-cell lung cancer and the role of platinum-based therapy. Clin Lung Cancer 5:274–289
125. Yu M, Zhang C, Li L, Dong S, Zhang N, Tong X (2014) Cx43 reverses the resistance of A549 lung adenocarcinoma cells to cisplatin by inhibiting EMT. Oncol Rep 31:2751–2758
126. Ren J, Chen Y, Song H, Chen L, Wang R (2013) Inhibition of ZEB1 reverses EMT and chemoresistance in docetaxel-resistant human lung adenocarcinoma cell line. J Cell Biochem 114:1395–1403
127. Ju L, Zhou C (2013) Integrin beta 1 enhances the epithelial-mesenchymal transition in association with gefitinib resistance of non-small cell lung cancer. Cancer Biomark 13:329–336
128. Singh A, Settleman J (2010) EMT, cancer stem cells and drug resistance: an emerging axis of evil in the war on cancer. Oncogene 29:4741–4751
129. Ginnebaugh KR, Ahmad A, Sarkar FH (2014) The therapeutic potential of targeting the epithelial-mesenchymal transition in cancer. Expert Opin Ther Targets 18:731–745
130. Niederst MJ, Engelman JA (2013) Bypass mechanisms of resistance to receptor tyrosine kinase inhibition in lung cancer. Sci Signal 6:re6
131. Cañadas I, Rojo F, Taus Á, Arpí O, Arumí-Uría M, Pijuan L, Menéndez S, Zazo S, Dómine M, Salido M et al (2014) Targeting epithelial-to-mesenchymal transition with Met inhibitors reverts chemoresistance in small cell lung cancer. Clin Cancer Res 20:938–950
132. Huang MH, Lee JH, Chang YJ, Tsai HH, Lin YL, Lin AM, Yang JC (2013) MEK inhibitors reverse resistance in epidermal growth factor receptor mutation lung cancer cells with acquired resistance to gefitinib. Mol Oncol 7:112–120
133. Zhao Z, Cheng X, Wang Y, Han R, Li L, Xiang T, He L, Long H, Zhu B, He Y (2014) Metformin inhibits the IL-6-induced epithelial-mesenchymal transition and lung adenocarcinoma growth and metastasis. PLoS One 9, e95884
134. Byers LA, Diao L, Wang J, Saintigny P, Girard L, Peyton M, Shen L, Fan Y, Giri U, Tumula PK et al (2013) An epithelial-mesenchymal transition gene signature predicts resistance to EGFR and PI3K inhibitors and identifies Axl as a therapeutic target for overcoming EGFR inhibitor resistance. Clin Cancer Res 19:279–290
135. Iida S, Miki Y, Suzuki T, Mori K, Saito M, Niikawa H, Kondo T, Yamada-Okabe H, Sasano H (2014) Activation of AXL and antitumor effects of a monoclonal antibody to AXL in lung adenocarcinoma. Anticancer Res 34:1821–1827
136. Niederst MJ, Benes CH (2014) EMT twists the road to PI3K. Cancer Discov 4:149–151
137. Salt MB, Bandyopadhyay S, McCormick F (2014) Epithelial-to-mesenchymal transition rewires the molecular path to PI3K-dependent proliferation. Cancer Discov 4:186–199

138. Wald O, Shapira OM, Izhar U (2013) CXCR4/CXCL12 axis in non small cell lung cancer (NSCLC) pathologic roles and therapeutic potential. Theranostics 3:26–33
139. Bertolini G, Roz L, Perego P, Tortoreto M, Fontanella E, Gatti L, Pratesi G, Fabbri A, Andriani F, Tinelli S et al (2009) Highly tumorigenic lung cancer CD133+ cells display stem-like features and are spared by cisplatin treatment. Proc Natl Acad Sci U S A 106:16281–16286
140. Jung MJ, Rho JK, Kim YM, Jung JE, Jin YB, Ko YG, Lee JS, Lee SJ, Lee JC, Park MJ (2013) Upregulation of CXCR4 is functionally crucial for maintenance of stemness in drug-resistant non-small cell lung cancer cells. Oncogene 32:209–221
141. Damelin M, Geles KG, Follettie MT, Yuan P, Baxter M, Golas J, DiJoseph JF, Karnoub M, Huang S, Diesl V et al (2011) Delineation of a cellular hierarchy in lung cancer reveals an oncofetal antigen expressed on tumor-initiating cells. Cancer Res 71:4236–4246
142. Fahham D, Weiss ID, Abraham M, Beider K, Hanna W, Shlomai Z, Eizenberg O, Zamir G, Izhar U, Shapira OM et al (2012) In vitro and in vivo therapeutic efficacy of CXCR4 antagonist BKT140 against human non-small cell lung cancer. J Thorac Cardiovasc Surg 144:1167–1175.e1161
143. Otani Y, Kijima T, Kohmo S, Oishi S, Minami T, Nagatomo I, Takahashi R, Hirata H, Suzuki M, Inoue K et al (2012) Suppression of metastases of small cell lung cancer cells in mice by a peptidic CXCR4 inhibitor TF14016. FEBS Lett 586:3639–3644
144. Peled A, Wald O, Burger J (2012) Development of novel CXCR4-based therapeutics. Expert Opin Investig Drugs 21:341–353
145. Wang H, Zhang G, Zhang H, Zhang F, Zhou B, Ning F, Wang HS, Cai SH, Du J (2014) Acquisition of epithelial-mesenchymal transition phenotype and cancer stem cell-like properties in cisplatin-resistant lung cancer cells through AKT/β-catenin/Snail signaling pathway. Eur J Pharmacol 723:156–166
146. Witta SE, Gemmill RM, Hirsch FR, Coldren CD, Hedman K, Ravdel L, Helfrich B, Dziadziuszko R, Chan DC, Sugita M et al (2006) Restoring E-cadherin expression increases sensitivity to epidermal growth factor receptor inhibitors in lung cancer cell lines. Cancer Res 66:944–950
147. Zhang Z, Lee JC, Lin L, Olivas V, Au V, LaFramboise T, Abdel-Rahman M, Wang X, Levine AD, Rho JK et al (2012) Activation of the AXL kinase causes resistance to EGFR-targeted therapy in lung cancer. Nat Genet 44:852–860
148. Nagaraj NS, Datta PK (2010) Targeting the transforming growth factor-beta signaling pathway in human cancer. Expert Opin Investig Drugs 19:77–91
149. Park CY, Min KN, Son JY, Park SY, Nam JS, Kim DK, Sheen YY (2014) An novel inhibitor of TGF-β type I receptor, IN-1130, blocks breast cancer lung metastasis through inhibition of epithelial-mesenchymal transition. Cancer Lett 351:72–80
150. Stewart DJ (2014) Wnt signaling pathway in non-small cell lung cancer. J Natl Cancer Inst 106:djt356
151. Stewart DJ, Chang DW, Ye Y, Spitz M, Lu C, Shu X, Wampfler JA, Marks RS, Garces YI, Yang P et al (2014) Wnt signaling pathway pharmacogenetics in non-small cell lung cancer. Pharmacogenomics J 14:509–522
152. Hofman V, Ilie MI, Long E, Selva E, Bonnetaud C, Molina T, Vénissac N, Mouroux J, Vielh P, Hofman P (2011) Detection of circulating tumor cells as a prognostic factor in patients undergoing radical surgery for non-small-cell lung carcinoma: comparison of the efficacy of the Cell Search Assay™ and the isolation by size of epithelial tumor cell method. Int J Cancer 129:1651–1660
153. Lecharpentier A, Vielh P, Perez-Moreno P, Planchard D, Soria JC, Farace F (2011) Detection of circulating tumour cells with a hybrid (epithelial/mesenchymal) phenotype in patients with metastatic non-small cell lung cancer. Br J Cancer 105:1338–1341

The Role of Cancer Stem Cells in Recurrent and Drug-Resistant Lung Cancer

Raagini Suresh, Shadan Ali, Aamir Ahmad, Philip A. Philip, and Fazlul H. Sarkar

Abstract Lung cancer is the leading cause of cancer-related deaths worldwide with a 5-year overall survival rate of less than 20 %. Considering the treatments currently available, this statistics is shocking. A possible explanation for the disconnect between sophisticated treatments and the survival rate can be related to the post-treatment enrichment of Cancer Stem Cells (CSCs), which is one of a sub-set of drug resistant tumor cells with abilities of self-renewal, cancer initiation, and further maintenance of tumors. Lung CSCs have been associated with resistance to radiation and chemotherapeutic treatments. CSCs have also been implicated in tumor recurrence because CSCs are not typically killed after conventional therapy. Investigation of CSCs in determining their role in tumor recurrence and drug-resistance relied heavily on the use of specific markers present in CSCs, including CD133, ALDH, ABCG2, and Nanog. Yet another cell type that is also associated with increased resistance to treatment is epithelial-to-mesenchymal transition (EMT) phenotypic cells. Through the processes of EMT, epithelial cells lose their epithelial phenotype and gain mesenchymal properties, rendering EMT phenotypic cells acquire drug-resistance. In this chapter, we will further discuss the role of microRNAs (miRNAs) especially because miRNA-based therapies are becoming attractive target with respect to therapeutic resistance and CSCs. Finally, the potential role of the natural agents and synthetic derivatives of natural compounds with

R. Suresh
Department of Pathology, Karmanos Cancer Institute, Wayne State University School of Medicine, Detroit, MI 48201, USA

S. Ali • P.A. Philip
Department of Oncology, Karmanos Cancer Institute, Wayne State University School of Medicine, Detroit, MI 48201, USA

A. Ahmad
Karmanos Cancer Institute, Wayne State University, Detroit, MI 48201, USA

F.H. Sarkar (✉)
Department of Pathology, Karmanos Cancer Institute, Wayne State University School of Medicine, Detroit, MI 48201, USA

Department of Oncology, Karmanos Cancer Institute, Wayne State University School of Medicine, Detroit, MI 48201, USA
e-mail: fsarkar@med.wayne.edu

A. Ahmad, S.M. Gadgeel (eds.), *Lung Cancer and Personalized Medicine: Novel Therapies and Clinical Management*, Advances in Experimental Medicine and Biology 890, DOI 10.1007/978-3-319-24932-2_4

anti-cancer activity, e.g. curcumin, CDF, and BR-DIM is highlighted in overcoming therapeutic resistance, suggesting that the above mentioned agents could be important for better treatment of lung cancer in combination therapy.

Keywords Lung cancer • Cancer stem cells • Drug-resistant • microRNAs • BR-DIM • Curcumin • CDF

1 Introduction

Lung cancer has two main pathological entities. These are small cell lung cancer (SCLC) and non-small cell lung cancer (NSCLC). Cases of NSCLC make up 75–80 % of all lung cancer cases [1]. NSCLC can be further subdivided into squamous cell carcinoma, adenocarcinoma, and large cell carcinoma. Most originating sites of the various types of lung cancer are located at or near identified airway stem cell niches, which suggests their stem cell origin [2]. The discovery of a group of cells with self-renewing abilities in tumors was groundbreaking, which prompted further studies. These cells, called cancer stem cells (CSCs), may be the primary cause of chemotherapy resistance, and thus the role of CSCs in tumor recurrence in patients with multiple types of cancer including lung cancer [3] became the area of cutting-edge research. In order to gain better understanding of lung CSCs, and develop new treatments, a fundamental understanding of CSC markers, their therapeutic targets, the biology of drug-resistant properties of CSCs, and the role of novel molecular markers such as microRNAs (miRNAs) must be considered. Based on current understanding, combined with further research novel insight, one would be able to develop better treatment option that could be designed for targeted eradication of CSCs which will aid in the prevention of tumor recurrence in part mediated through overcoming drug-resistance of lung cancer.

2 Cancer Stem Cells of the Lungs

2.1 Markers Defining Lung CSCs and Their Potential Biological Implications

In order to research CSCs, they must first be identified. Among the common markers used to isolate and study CSCs are CD133, ALDH, ABCG2 and Nanog, as presented in Fig. 1. These markers provide ways to assess how effective different treatments are at eradicating CSCs. The markers also have prognostic applications. Furthermore, the markers have been specifically targeted to reduce functionality—or even induce apoptosis—in CSCs, increasing the specificity and thus improving treatment outcome.

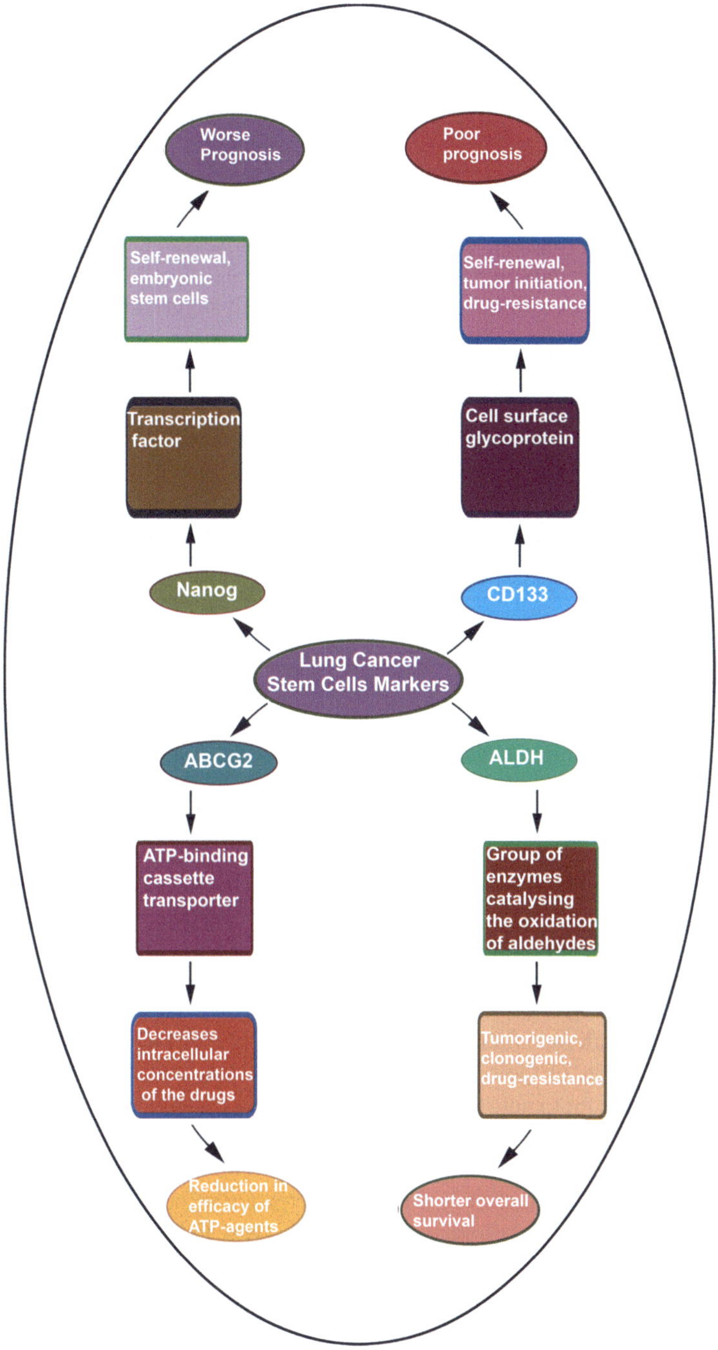

Fig. 1 A schematic presentation of stem cell markers studied and their signaling pathways involved in the development and progression of lung cancer

2.1.1 CD133

CD133 is a commonly demonstrated lung CSC marker [2]. It is a cell surface glycoprotein that consists of five transmembrane domains and two large glycosylated extracellular loops [4]. Researchers tested ten NSCLC cell lines in an attempt to verify that cells positive for CD133 possessed properties of CSCs. Findings suggested that CD133 positive (CD133$^+$) cells showed significantly higher abilities of self-renewal, tumor initiation, and drug resistance characteristics when compared to CD133$^-$ cells [5, 6]. In addition to these findings in NSCLC cell lines, CD133$^+$ cells with similar CSC properties have been found in SCLC, suggesting that CD133 may be a pan-lung cancer stem cell marker [2].

In terms of the potential implications of this marker, high CD133 expression has been linked to poor prognosis in patients with NSCLC [7, 8]. This may result from the fact that CD133 expression has also been associated with higher tumor stage in adenocarcinoma [7]. However, these results are not completely conclusive yet and cannot be generalized for all patients with NSCLC, as indicated by one study that did not find any link between CD133 expression and NSCLC prognosis [9].

2.1.2 ALDH

Another marker useful for identifying and isolating CSCs has to do with the high aldehyde dehydrogenase activity of stem cells. Aldehyde dehydrogenase (ALDH)'s enzymes control the differentiation of normal stem cells, suggesting a link between ALDH and CSC differentiation [10]. Furthermore, the ALDH family of intracellular enzymes was found to participate in cellular detoxification and drug resistance in CSCs [2]. ALDH1, a cytosolic isoenzyme, is a member of the ALDH family. Lung cancer cells that expressed ALDH1 demonstrated highly tumorigenic and clonogenic properties [11]. Moreover, ALDH1A1$^+$ CSCs displayed resistance to chemotherapy drugs and EGFR-TKI (epidermal growth factor receptor tyrosine kinase inhibitors), both treatments are typically used to fight lung cancer [12]. Specifically, the drugs to which ALDH1A1$^+$ CSCs displayed resistance are the common chemotherapeutic drugs such as cisplatin, etoposide, and fluorouracil, as well as the EGFR-TKI gefitinib [12].

Combined effects of the overexpression of CD133 in conjunction with that of ALDH, it is important to note that this combination has been related to an increased risk of recurrence in early-stage NSCLC [13]. Furthermore, the concomitant expression of CD133 and ALDH1A1 was correlated with shortest overall survival among 205 stage-1 NSCLC patients [13]. Thus, the detection of both CD133 and ALDH could potentially serve as a prognosis indicator for NSCLC patients.

2.1.3 ABCG2

Another marker of lung CSCs is ABCG2, an ATP-binding cassette transporter. ABCG2 has the ability to pump chemotherapeutic drugs out of the cell, ultimately resulting in decreased intracellular concentrations of the drugs [4]. The transporter works by using energy from ATP to drive the active transport of drug metabolites and other compounds across the cell membrane. The ATP-binding cassette (ABC) superfamily, of which ABCG2 is a part, is a powerful resistance mechanism that greatly contributes to chemoresistance of CSCs [14, 15]. Looking at the implications of the presence of the ABCG2 marker, the source of the energy driving its active transport becomes important. Since ABC transporters are ATP-dependent, ATP-competitive agents could target them and could potentially reduce their efficacy.

2.1.4 Nanog

The Nanog transcription factor plays a key role in maintaining the self-renewal capacity of embryonic stem cells in embryonic development [16, 17]. It plays a similar role in CSCs. Since its role is directly related to such a key phenotypic characteristic of CSCs, it has been used as a marker in lung CSCs [17, 18]. The overexpression of the Nanog protein predicted worse prognosis for lung cancer patients, suggesting its possible use as a prognostic indicator [19]. The relationship between Nanog and lung CSCs needs to be further examined in order to continue whether Nanog could be useful for the development of novel therapeutics.

2.2 Therapeutic Targeting of Lung CSC Markers

Therapeutic treatments have been developed for specifically targeting the CSCs. Such treatments have made use of CSC markers by either using them to find CSCs or by actually targeting the markers themselves. The therapeutic targeting of lung CSC markers has not been studied to the depth it merits in lung cancer. However, markers of lung CSCs have indeed been established and studied in great detail. Thus, this section will entail the discussion of therapeutic targeting of lung CSC markers in any type of cancer. Some lung CSC markers that have been targeted include the aforementioned CD133, ALDH, ABCG2, and Nanog.

CD133 targeting in human metastatic melanoma has been effective. Short hairpin RNAs were used to down-regulate CD133. This led to decreased movement ability, spheroid-forming ability, and capacity of metastasis [20]. The down-regulation also led to slower overall cell growth. An efficient method in the elimination of $CD133^+$ tumors has been reported by the use of antibody-drug conjugates [21]. This method has been used with success in hepatocellular and gastric cancers, and its efficiency when applied to lung cancer should be further studied.

Another marker targeted in lung cancer is the ALDH family. The ALDH family has been targeted in colorectal cancer and breast cancer, among others as well. In both colorectal and breast cancer, ALDH1 activity inhibition with DEAB was successful. In breast cancer cells, the ALDH1 inhibition resulted in the suppression of tumor-initiating ability and a reduction of metastasis to the lungs [22]. In colorectal cancer cells, ALDH1 inhibition led to increased sensitivity to the cytotoxic effects of a chemotherapeutic drug, CPA [16]. Another method used in colorectal cancer cells was the down-regulation of ALDH through the use of shRNA, which reduced the number of detected CSCs [16].

As previously discussed, the ABC multidrug efflux pumps are important for the chemoresistance of CSCs. In order to increase the potency of treatment, the ABCG2 transporter has been targeted. Inhibitors of the transporter are still waiting comprehensive clinical assessment, but they include phosphodiesterase-5 inhibitors and Ko143 [23]. Dietary flavonoids may also work to inhibit ABCG2-mediated cellular drug efflux [24]. Such inhibitors will hopefully eventually work synergistically with conventional chemotherapeutics to eliminate tumors and reduce possibilities of cancer recurrence.

Finally, Nanog mRNA knock-down has resulted in decreased mobility and invasion abilities of choriocarcinoma cells [25]. Since the therapeutic targeting of Nanog has proven successful in one type of cancer, it has the potential to be successful in the treatment of lung cancer, suggesting that further studies are warranted.

3 Drug-Resistance

Therapeutic resistance (intrinsic and extrinsic) is one of the primary causes of failure in cancer treatment [26]. Drug-resistant properties of cancer can result in either an immediate re-initiation of the disease or re-initiation after a significant lapse of time [27]. Some common treatments of lung cancer that have faced the problem of treatment resistance include Epidermal Growth Factor Tyrosine Kinase Inhibitors (EGFR-TKI), chemotherapy, anti-proliferative treatments, and radiation treatment [27–29]. The drug resistance has been linked with a cellular process named epithelial-to-mesenchymal transition (EMT) whose characteristics closely mimic the cellular and molecular characteristics of CSCs.

3.1 Role of EMT in Drug-Resistance

Epithelial cells can become invasive, migratory mesenchymal cells. This process, known as epithelial-to-mesenchymal transition, EMT, gives cancer cells the ability to migrate, invade, and spread through the vascular system. Furthermore, EMT may result in the production of CSCs, as evidenced by differences in cell surface marker expression and increased tumor formation [30–32]. Typical progression of EMT involves losing epithelial markers and gaining mesenchymal markers [33]. A distinctive feature of EMT is the loss of E-cadherin, a glycoprotein that is involved in epithelial cell-cell adhesion and cytoskeletal organization [26]. Considering its primary functions, it is clear that E-cadherin would not be useful for a migratory mesenchymal cell.

The loss of function of E-cadherin is thought to enable cancer cells undergo the processes of metastasis by giving rise to significant transcriptional and functional changes. One particular study focused on the role of E-cadherin in EMT was sought to determine whether E-cadherin loss could result solely in the loss of cell-cell contacts or if E-cadherin loss could activate multiple transcriptional pathways. Results showed that E-cadherin loss contributed to the action of multiple transcriptional pathways [26, 34]. In fact, after E-cadherin loss, 19 transcription factors were highly induced. Moreover, E-cadherin loss alone was enough to confer metastatic abilities to non-metastatic breast cancer cells [35].

Emerging evidence has shown that EMT plays a key role in making cancer cells drug-resistant to commonly used therapeutics, such as EGFR-TKI. EGFR is an oncogenic pathway that could be inhibited through the use of tyrosine kinase inhibitors (TKIs) [29]. EGFR-TKI has been used to treat the adenocarcinoma subset of NSCLC [29]. Though patients respond to the treatment initially, most patients face the potential of relapse [36]. Adenocarcinoma cells resistant to EGFR inhibitors such as gefitinib and erlotinib showed a decrease in their expression of E-cadherin, an epithelial cell marker, and an increase in their expression of vimentin, a mesenchymal cell marker. Since the drug-resistant lung cancer cells display the mesenchymal phenotype, EMT might be an indicator of insensitivity to EGFR inhibition in lung cancer [26]. Furthermore, restoration of E-cadherin increased the sensitivity of the drug-resistant cancer cells to EGFR-TKIs such as gefitinib, further suggesting a relationship between EMT and resistance to EGFR-inhibitors [29]. Though support for the relationship between EMT and resistance to these inhibitors in adenocarcinoma is present, the evidence is still inconclusive. For example, one particular study found that only 50 % of samples had undergone EMT after exposure to gefitinib [37]. Further research is required to fully understand the relationship between EGFR-TKI resistance and EMT. Such research may help increase the efficacy of EGFR-TKI in patients who have shown resistance to this treatment method.

3.2 Role of CSCs in Drug-Resistance

Some therapies that are currently in place are effective in that they are able to remove bulky disease; however, therapies that fail to employ a strategic elimination of CSCs are often ineffective, and results in cancer recurrence [27]. A specific example of such an instance can be seen in platinum-based combination chemotherapy, a first-line treatment for NSCLC in advanced stages [28]. This type of treatment works by inhibiting DNA repair and/or DNA synthesis in cancer cells. Notably, a significant number of patients face the problem of tumor recurrence after platinum-based combination chemotherapy [38]. When first-line agents fail, second-line agents (such as Docetaxel and Pemetrexed) are used. Unfortunately, the second-line agents tend to be ineffective in patients who have received typical first-line chemotherapy. A recent study discovered that cisplatin treatment, a platinum-based first-line treatment, elevated the ratio of cells expressing the CSC markers CD133 and Nanog [14, 28], suggesting enrichment of these drug resistant cells after conventional therapy. The cisplatin treatment appears to select for CSCs, resulting in the high rate of paclitaxel resistance as well in patients who had been treated with cisplatin.

CSCs have special properties that contribute to their drug-resistance phenotype. Some of the more significant contributing properties include CSCs' relative dormancy, their high capacity for DNA repair, and their high expression of multiple drug resistance membrane transporters [27]. The relative dormancy of CSCs is important when considering anti-proliferative treatments, such as Imatinib and Nilotinib [27]. CSCs are often in a state of dormancy, or quiescence, where they are non-proliferative [39]. While CSCs are not in the cell cycle, they are protected from chemo-radiotherapy. The use of specific agents (like As_2O_3) to force the CSCs to re-enter the cell cycle can restore chemo- and radio-sensitivity and should be employed in conjunction with anti-proliferative treatments [40], suggesting that further proof-of-concept studies are warranted.

CSCs express a significant number of multiple drug resistance membrane transporters, including those of the ABC family [27, 41]. As previously discussed, these transporters use active transport to efflux drugs, hence reducing the drugs' impact on CSCs [14]. However, CSCs rely on still other mechanisms for drug resistance, limiting the efficacy of ABC transporter inhibitors.

Furthermore, CSCs have a high capacity for DNA repair, yet another factor contributing to their drug-resistance [27]. In a study of human glioblastomas, $CD133^+$ cells were found to survive radiation treatment better than cells without this CSC marker [42]. This survival difference can be attributed to the efficient DNA repair mechanisms present in CSCs, such as the role of Chk1 and Chk2 checkpoint kinases [42]. These kinases pauses the cell cycle to allow DNA repair to happen, and thus these strategies could be useful for overcoming therapeutic resistance. In addition to the role cellular processes and the genes that are involved in therapeutic resistance, there are many regulatory networks that may be equally responsible for therapeutic resistance including microRNA (miRNAs) that regulate the expression of many functional genes as discussed below.

4 The Role of miRNAs

MicroRNAs (miRNAs), are non-coding RNAs made up of 19–22 nucleotides that help regulate gene expression during translational control [43]. The miRNAs play very important roles in numerous biological processes of cancer cells, including development, proliferation, and apoptosis [44]. The miRNAs are endogenous post-transcriptional regulators that negatively regulate the expression of their target genes [45]. The miRNAs can be either oncogenic or tumor suppressing, depending on the subsequent pathways they influence. The role of miRNAs will be discussed in terms of their impact on chemoresistance and the maintenance of CSCs in general in the following section. New therapies take advantage of knowledge gained from miRNA research, making the understanding of how miRNAs are critically involved in cancer development, treatment and therapeutic resistance.

4.1 MicroRNAs Associated with Chemoresistance

Since miRNAs are useful in so many different arenas, it is only natural that they be discussed in relation to chemoresistance. Much research has been focused on miRNAs, and continues to focus on the up-regulation or down-regulation of miRNAs in relation to treatment resistance. This research can result in attempts to up-regulate the miRNAs to reverse treatment resistance or developments of new treatments altogether. Since miRNAs are associated with chemoresistance, they can also prove to be useful as prognostic indicators. The miR-212, the let-7 family, and various other miRNAs are associated with EGFR signaling should be further researched in order to identify new treatments or improving the effectiveness of currently used common treatments for lung cancer.

4.1.1 miR-212

miR-212 is considered a tumor suppressor, and its down-regulation has been correlated with chemoresistance [46]. When the expression of miR-212 levels is normal, it increases tumor necrosis factor-related apoptosis-inducing ligand (TRAIL)-induced cell death in NSCLC cells [47]. The down-regulation of miR-212 leads to the up-regulation of the anti-apoptotic PED, and PED has been implicated in inducing resistance to chemotherapeutic treatment, meaning that miR-212 down-regulation is in part responsible for chemoresistance. Another way miR-212 may be involved in chemoresistance is through its relationship with ABC multidrug efflux transporters. In CML, or chronic myeloid leukemia, miR-212 down-regulation has been found to be associated with decreased ABCG2 protein expression [48]. The use of reporter gene assays established that miR-212 targeted the 3′-UTR region of ABCG2 [48]. Finally, miR-212 down-regulation has also been suggested to be responsible for docetaxel resistance in NSCLC adenocarcinoma cells [49].

4.1.2 The let-7 Family

Let-7 (lethal-7) refers to a family that consists of 12 miRNAs. The let-7 family is a known inhibitor of EMT [50]. Accordingly, let-7 has been found to be down-regulated in A549 NSCLC cells treated with TGF-β1. These cells were also found to be resistant to the drug erlotinib. The re-expression of let-7b and let-7c led to the reversal of EMT and was accompanied by increased erlotinib sensitivity [51]. Since let-7 down-regulation results in drug resistance, it follows as logical that reduced levels of let-7 have been associated with poor patient outcome for patients with lung cancer [52].

4.1.3 miRNAs Associated with EGFR

Acquired resistance of NSCLC to EGFR has been found to be in part due to the acquisition of secondary mutations in EGFR itself. An example of such a mutation is the EGFR T790M "gatekeeper" mutation, which has been responsible for 50 %

of resistant cases [53]. Another mechanism of acquired resistance, the amplification of the MET oncogene, has been associated with tumor growth and metastasis. This mechanism has been observed in 20 % of resistant cases [54]. The study of miRNAs through a microRNA microarray identified that miR-30b, miR-30c, miR-221, and miR-222 target both epidermal growth factor (EGF) and MET receptors [55]. The microarray also found that miR-103 and miR-203 target solely the MET oncogene. These microRNAs collectively had a large impact on the response to gefitinib-induced apoptosis of NSCLC cells. The miRNAs inhibited the expression of genes encoding BCL2-like 11 (BIM), apoptotic peptidase activating factor 1 (APAF-1), protein kinase C-ε, and sarcoma viral oncogene homolog (SRC) [56]. Modulating these miRNAs, in conjunction with chemotherapy, could provide a better outlook for NSCLC patients treated with EGFR-TKIs.

4.2 *MicroRNAs Associated with CSCs*

MiRNAs, important regulators of CSCs, are inappropriately regulated in many cancers. Such incorrect regulation could include the deregulation of miRNAs, as seen in miR-34a, miR-21, and the miR-200 family (Table 1). This process raises a question on whether re-introduction or inhibition of these miRNAs would restore normal tumor suppressing/oncogenic ability as discussed in the following sections.

4.2.1 miR-34a

MiR-34a is a known tumor suppressor, and its up-regulation led to increased apoptosis [46]. The tumor suppressor p53 transcriptionally induces miR-34a [57]. When miR-34a expression is reduced, lung CSCs take on a more aggressive phenotype [58]. When miR-34a expression is increased again, this increased aggressive phenotype is lost [58]. Since miR-34a is frequently down-regulated in lung cancer, it is being evaluated as a replacement therapy candidate [55]. The delivery of a miR-34a mimic has been shown to reduce tumor growth [59]. This suggests that miRNA replacement therapy may prove extremely useful, and encourages further research into the field of miRNAs related to CSCs—and cancer in general.

Table 1 miRNAs as regulators of cancer stem cells

MiRNA	Up or down-regulated in cancer	Target genes	Reference numbers
MiR-212	Down-regulated	PED	[46–49]
Let-7 family	Down-regulated	RAS, HMGA2	[50–52]
MiR-34a	Down-regulated	c-Met, CDK4, Bcl-2	[46, 55, 57–59]
MiR-21	Up-regulated	PTEN	[45, 60, 61]
MiR-200 family	Down-regulated	E2F3	[55, 60, 62]
MiR-30b/30c	Up-regulated	BIM/APAF-1, EGFR	[46, 55, 56]
MiR-221/222	Up-regulated	BIM/APAF-1, EGFR	[55, 56, 63]
MiR-103/203	Down-regulated	PKC-ε, SRC, MET	[55, 56]

4.2.2 miR-21

MiR-21 expression was greatly increased in colon cancer CSCs [45]. The down-regulation of miR-21 caused the differentiation of CSCs, as evidenced by a decrease in CSC markers. Since differentiated CSCs are more susceptible to treatments, and thus down-regulation of miR-21 in conjunction with other treatment was investigated. When the down-regulation of miR-21 preceded other treatments such as 5-fluorouracil + oxaliplatin (FUOX) and CDF (a novel synthetic agent), the treatments were more effective [45]. Taking a more detailed look at miR-21, it is important to consider its targets. Phosphatase and tension homolog (PTEN) is a tumor suppressor gene that is a target of miR-21 [60]. When miR-21 is suppressed, PTEN is up-regulated, resulting in tumor suppression [60]. In relation to lung cancer, miR-21-3p relative expressions were found to be higher in NSCLC tissues as compared to non-cancerous tissues [61]. However, miR-21 has a lower prognostic value when compared to other miRNAs, so while down-regulation of miR-21 should be attempted in lung cancer, the expectations for its impact on lung CSCs should require further in-depth mechanistic studies.

4.2.3 The miR-200 Family

The miR-200 family is a known inhibitor of EMT, a process that is responsible for some of the production of CSCs [30–32, 51]. The loss of expression of the miR-200 family is associated with an increase in EMT phenotypic cells, and consequently drug resistance and enrichment of CSCs [60]. MiR-200b, a member of the miR-200 family, targets Suz12 a subunit of a polycomb repressor complex (PRC2) among others. The expression of Suz12 is enough to generate CSCs [62]. The re-expression of miR-200 would inhibit Suz12, helping to suppress tumor growth and stop the generation of CSCs [62]. This re-expression of miR-200 through the use of drugs such as CDF could also potentially reverse EMT, leading to the differentiation of CSCs, and thus improve prognosis of lung cancer [63] although further studies are warranted.

5 Natural Agents and Their Synthetic Derivative as Anti-cancer Compounds

The discovery of anti-cancer compounds, both natural and synthetic, is very interesting in that though we may be searching for compounds with astounding effects on cancer; we are also interested in learning how these compounds may function. The increased understanding of both natural and synthetic anti-cancer compounds can result in the discovery or synthesis of novel compounds that may have a profound impact on cancer treatment worldwide especially for overcoming therapeutic resistance. In this section, a natural compound, BR-DIM, will be discussed, as will another natural compound, curcumin, and its synthetic analog, CDF to highlight the area of research that certainly require further cutting-edge research.

5.1 BR-DIM

One treatment that has been shown to be effective in the growth inhibition of cancer cells is the BR-DIM treatment [64]. This natural agent works in part by inducing apoptosis in lung cancer cells by down-regulating Survivin and Bcl-2, decreasing Bax, and enhancing procaspase cleavage [65, 66]. This agent also induces apoptosis through activation of the p38 MAPK pathway [67]. In NSCLC, BR-DIM has been shown to inhibit the growth of drug-resistant cell lines that exhibited mutant EGFR [66]. Even cancer cells resistant to targeted therapies, chemotherapy or radiation exhibited growth inhibition in the presence of BR-DIM [66]. Met, which has been linked to poor patient prognosis in lung cancer, showed reduced expression in lung cancer cells when they were treated with BR-DIM [66].

Most significantly, BR-DIM may be able to reduce cancer metastasis or recurrence. Such an outcome is possible due to BR-DIM's ability to decrease invasive abilities of EGFR signaling. A possible mechanism for this is the suppression of the pro-metastatic chemokine receptor CXCR4 [68, 69]. Therefore this compound should be studied in combination with other forms of therapy to find best treatment regimen that will improve patient prognosis.

5.2 Curcumin

One example of another natural anti-cancer compound is curcumin. Curcumin is a non-toxic substance extracted from turmeric [43]. Curcumin has proven effective in inducing apoptosis as well as inhibition of proliferation of drug-resistant CSCs. Some ways by which curcumin has been shown to be effective including EGFR-mediated processes of cell survival and apoptosis, increasing CSC treatment sensitivity that maybe interacting with miRNAs to induce apoptosis [43].

As previously discussed, the EGFR-TKI method of NSCLC treatment is prone to resistance. However, when curcumin is present, the EGFR protein undergoes ubiquitination and degradation [70]. Decreasing the EGFR protein on the cell membrane results in eventual cancer cell apoptosis and death [70]. Part of what makes this method successful is the fact that it is not susceptible to EGFR mutation.

Furthermore, curcumin may increase the therapeutic effectiveness of existing treatment modalities. Curcumin was able to induce the sensitivity of $CD133^+$ CSCs in laryngeal carcinoma to cisplatin. This resulted in the reduction of the percentage of $CD133^+$ CSCs, which were previously resistant to treatment [71]. Curcumin was able to reduce drug-resistant properties by down-regulating the expression and/or activity of ABC multidrug transporters in leukemic cells [43]. ABCG2, a member of this family of transporters, is also a marker for lung CSCs, suggesting curcumin's potential efficacy in reducing drug-resistant properties of lung CSCs. Curcumin has also reduced amounts of $CD133^+$ medulloblastoma, glioblastoma, pancreatic and colon CSC proliferation through Hedgehog, insulin growth factor (IGF-), STAT3-, and histone methyltransferase EZH2-dependent mechanisms [70]. CD133 is also a marker used for the identification of lung CSCs in both NSCLC and SCLC, again suggesting curcumin's potential effectiveness in lung cancer. Curcumin could be useful to reduce drug-resistant properties of cancer by targeting CSCs and their markers. This may indirectly result in the reduction of tumor recurrence, since CSCs have been linked as being responsible for this phenomenon [27, 72].

Curcumin has also been able to induce apoptosis in a multi-drug resistant lung adenocarcinoma cell line, A549 [73]. By down-regulating miR-186 in A549 (lung adenocarcinoma) cells, curcumin was able to promote lung cancer cell apoptosis [74]. Discoveries of the efficiency of curcumin in lung cancer treatment and cancer treatment in general in pre-clinical model suggested activity; however, based on the lack of optimal bioavailability of curcumin the clinical trial results has been disappointing, which prompted research into the field of curcumin analogs, some of which have been useful in pre-clinical studies, and thus warrant further investigation.

5.3 CDF

The low bioavailability of curcumin prompted the synthesis of CDF, a difluorinated synthetic analog of curcumin with greater bioavailability [3, 60]. CDF works in a manner similar to curcumin. It down-regulates the expression and/or activity of EGFR, IGF-1R, NF-κB, c-Myc, β-catenin, COX-2, and the ABCG2 multidrug transporter [3]. In order to ensure that the efficiency of CDF in killing CSCs is consistent with that of curcumin, tests were conducted comparing the two in terms of their ability to reduce the presence of CSC markers in chemo-resistant colon cancer cells that were highly enriched in CSCs [3]. These tests discovered that CDF was more effective than curcumin in killing CSCs.

CDF has also been found to cause a greater induction of overall apoptosis [43]. CDF mediated induction of apoptosis was in part mediated by activating the pro-apoptotic factor Bax [3]. Furthermore, CDF was able to inhibit and disintegrate colonospheres containing over 80 % of CSCs, as determined by the presence of the colon CSC marker CD44 [3]. Curcumin failed to show similar biological activity. In a study comparing CDF and curcumin in the pancreatic cancer cell lines AsPc-1 and MIAPaCa-2, similar results were observed [60]. The determination of which agent is superior in terms of killing lung CSCs has not been done yet, and thus further research needs to be conducted. Furthermore, the specificities of the mechanisms of CDF in the elimination of CSCs have not been fully elucidated.

6 Conclusions: The Future of CSCs and CSC-Targeted Treatment

Research on CSCs has shed enormous light on why so many cancers are drug-resistant and leads to tumor recurrence. With this powerful information, treatments can be modified to include agents that could kill CSCs as well as bulk of cancer cells in a tumor mass. Understanding the processes of how CSCs acquire drug-resistance can lead to the development of novel treatment strategies with the objective of elimination or reversal of drug-resistant characteristics of cancer cells prior to the administration of conventional therapeutics.

CSCs have already changed the face of cancer treatment. Already, the use of antibody-drug conjugates that target markers of CSCs in addition to normal drug function have been successfully employed [21]. Such ideas are delightfully simple, but they could not have ever come into existence without countless hours in the laboratory determining the very existence of CSCs, pinpointing their markers, finding an antibody, and creating the antibody-drug conjugate. The antibody-drug conjugate is just one example of a success story but the future looks brighter especially for miRNA-targeting therapeutics in the context of CSCs.

To that end, novel natural agents or their synthetic analogs that are designed to target CSCs and miRNAs are beginning to be appreciated. These natural compounds can help us as human beings make lifestyle choices and changes, where possible, to reduce risk of cancer and more importantly assist in overcoming therapeutic resistance so that conventional treatment modalities become much more effective in eradicating tumors. Prevention is always more efficient than treatment. For example, BR-DIM and curcumin can be added to the standard diet fairly easily [7] although further research into these compounds may result in the eventual synthesis of a compound that maybe superior to all existing compounds. The possibilities are endless and the future looks brighter.

CSCs driven research should be at the forefront of cancer research. The practical applications surrounding their research are absolutely astounding. Future research should focus on new ways to target CSC markers, methods to induce CSC differentiation to reduce drug-resistance, and the potential use of miRNAs as a target for therapy which underscore the importance of natural compounds as anti-cancer agents. By continuing to amalgamate more knowledge, there is hope for improvement in the treatment outcome of patients afflicted with cancers and especially lung cancer.

References

1. Pathak AK, Bhutani M, Mohan A, Guleria R, Bal S, Kochupillai V (2004) Non small cell lung cancer (NSCLC): current status and future prospects. Indian J Chest Dis Allied Sci 46:191–203
2. Singh S, Chellappan S (2014) Lung cancer stem cells: molecular features and therapeutic targets. Mol Aspects Med 39:50–60
3. Kanwar SS, Yu Y, Nautiyal J, Patel BB, Padhye S, Sarkar FH et al (2011) Difluorinated-curcumin (CDF): a novel curcumin analog is a potent inhibitor of colon cancer stem-like cells. Pharm Res 28:827–838
4. Hu Y, Fu L (2012) Targeting cancer stem cells: a new therapy to cure cancer patients. Am J Cancer Res 2:340–356
5. Chen YC, Hsu HS, Chen YW, Tsai TH, How CK, Wang CY et al (2008) Oct-4 expression maintained cancer stem-like properties in lung cancer-derived CD133-positive cells. PLoS One 3, e2637

6. Wu Y, Wu PY (2009) CD133 as a marker for cancer stem cells: progresses and concerns. Stem Cells Dev 18:1127–1134
7. Mizugaki H, Sakakibara-Konishi J, Kikuchi J, Moriya J, Hatanaka KC, Kikuchi E et al (2014) CD133 expression: a potential prognostic marker for non-small cell lung cancers. Int J Clin Oncol 19:254–259
8. Shien K, Toyooka S, Ichimura K, Soh J, Furukawa M, Maki Y et al (2012) Prognostic impact of cancer stem cell-related markers in non-small cell lung cancer patients treated with induction chemoradiotherapy. Lung Cancer 77:162–167
9. Herpel E, Jensen K, Muley T, Warth A, Schnabel PA, Meister M et al (2011) The cancer stem cell antigens CD133, BCRP1/ABCG2 and CD117/c-KIT are not associated with prognosis in resected early-stage non-small cell lung cancer. Anticancer Res 31:4491–4500
10. Russo JE, Hilton J (1988) Characterization of cytosolic aldehyde dehydrogenase from cyclophosphamide resistant L1210 cells. Cancer Res 48:2963–2968
11. Sullivan JP, Spinola M, Dodge M, Raso MG, Behrens C, Gao B et al (2010) Aldehyde dehydrogenase activity selects for lung adenocarcinoma stem cells dependent on notch signaling. Cancer Res 70:9937–9948
12. Huang CP, Tsai MF, Chang TH, Tang WC, Chen SY, Lai HH et al (2013) ALDH-positive lung cancer stem cells confer resistance to epidermal growth factor receptor tyrosine kinase inhibitors. Cancer Lett 328:144–151
13. Alamgeer M, Ganju V, Szczepny A, Russell PA, Prodanovic Z, Kumar B et al (2013) The prognostic significance of aldehyde dehydrogenase 1A1 (ALDH1A1) and CD133 expression in early stage non-small cell lung cancer. Thorax 68:1095–1104
14. Bertolini G, Roz L, Perego P, Tortoreto M, Fontanella E, Gatti L et al (2009) Highly tumorigenic lung cancer CD133+ cells display stem-like features and are spared by cisplatin treatment. Proc Natl Acad Sci U S A 106:16281–16286
15. Sung JM, Cho HJ, Yi H, Lee CH, Kim HS, Kim DK et al (2008) Characterization of a stem cell population in lung cancer A549 cells. Biochem Biophys Res Commun 371:163–167
16. Dylla SJ, Beviglia L, Park IK, Chartier C, Raval J, Ngan L et al (2008) Colorectal cancer stem cells are enriched in xenogeneic tumors following chemotherapy. PLoS One 3, e2428
17. Li L, Yu H, Wang X, Zeng J, Li D, Lu J et al (2013) Expression of seven stem-cell-associated markers in human airway biopsy specimens obtained via fiberoptic bronchoscopy. J Exp Clin Cancer Res 32:28
18. Yi H, Cho HJ, Cho SM, Jo K, Park JA, Kim NH et al (2012) Blockade of interleukin-6 receptor suppresses the proliferation of H460 lung cancer stem cells. Int J Oncol 41:310–316
19. Du Y, Ma C, Wang Z, Liu Z, Liu H, Wang T (2013) Nanog, a novel prognostic marker for lung cancer. Surg Oncol 22:224–229
20. Rappa G, Fodstad O, Lorico A (2008) The stem cell-associated antigen CD133 (Prominin-1) is a molecular therapeutic target for metastatic melanoma. Stem Cells 26:3008–3017
21. Smith LM, Nesterova A, Ryan MC, Duniho S, Jonas M, Anderson M et al (2008) CD133/prominin-1 is a potential therapeutic target for antibody-drug conjugates in hepatocellular and gastric cancers. Br J Cancer 99:100–109
22. Kim RJ, Park JR, Roh KJ, Choi AR, Kim SR, Kim PH et al (2013) High aldehyde dehydrogenase activity enhances stem cell features in breast cancer cells by activating hypoxia-inducible factor-2alpha. Cancer Lett 333:18–31
23. Stacy AE, Jansson PJ, Richardson DR (2013) Molecular pharmacology of ABCG2 and its role in chemoresistance. Mol Pharmacol 84:655–669
24. Mimeault M, Hauke R, Batra SK (2008) Recent advances on the molecular mechanisms involved in the drug resistance of cancer cells and novel targeting therapies. Clin Pharmacol Ther 83:673–691
25. Siu MK, Wong ES, Chan HY, Ngan HY, Chan KY, Cheung AN (2008) Overexpression of NANOG in gestational trophoblastic diseases: effect on apoptosis, cell invasion, and clinical outcome. Am J Pathol 173:1165–1172
26. Xiao D, He J (2010) Epithelial mesenchymal transition and lung cancer. J Thorac Dis 2:154–159

27. Trumpp A, Wiestler OD (2008) Mechanisms of disease: cancer stem cells–targeting the evil twin. Nat Clin Pract Oncol 5:337–347
28. Liu YP, Yang CJ, Huang MS, Yeh CT, Wu AT, Lee YC et al (2013) Cisplatin selects for multidrug-resistant CD133+ cells in lung adenocarcinoma by activating Notch signaling. Cancer Res 73:406–416
29. Witta SE, Gemmill RM, Hirsch FR, Coldren CD, Hedman K, Ravdel L et al (2006) Restoring E-cadherin expression increases sensitivity to epidermal growth factor receptor inhibitors in lung cancer cell lines. Cancer Res 66:944–950
30. Mani SA, Guo W, Liao MJ, Eaton EN, Ayyanan A, Zhou AY et al (2008) The epithelial-mesenchymal transition generates cells with properties of stem cells. Cell 133:704–715
31. Rhim AD, Mirek ET, Aiello NM, Maitra A, Bailey JM, McAllister F et al (2012) EMT and dissemination precede pancreatic tumor formation. Cell 148:349–361
32. Zhang Y, Wei J, Wang H, Xue X, An Y, Tang D et al (2012) Epithelial mesenchymal transition correlates with CD24+ CD44+ and CD133+ cells in pancreatic cancer. Oncol Rep 27:1599–1605
33. Giarnieri E, De VC, Noto A, Roscilli G, Salerno G, Mariotta S et al (2013) EMT markers in lung adenocarcinoma pleural effusion spheroid cells. J Cell Physiol 228:1720–1726
34. Singh A, Settleman J (2010) EMT, cancer stem cells and drug resistance: an emerging axis of evil in the war on cancer. Oncogene 29:4741–4751
35. Onder TT, Gupta PB, Mani SA, Yang J, Lander ES, Weinberg RA (2008) Loss of E-cadherin promotes metastasis via multiple downstream transcriptional pathways. Cancer Res 68:3645–3654
36. Zhang WC, Shyh-Chang N, Yang H, Rai A, Umashankar S, Ma S et al (2012) Glycine decarboxylase activity drives non-small cell lung cancer tumor-initiating cells and tumorigenesis. Cell 148:259–272
37. Uramoto H, Iwata T, Onitsuka T, Shimokawa H, Hanagiri T, Oyama T (2010) Epithelial-mesenchymal transition in EGFR-TKI acquired resistant lung adenocarcinoma. Anticancer Res 30:2513–2517
38. Azzoli CG, Baker S Jr, Temin S, Pao W, Aliff T, Brahmer J et al (2010) American Society of Clinical Oncology Clinical Practice Guideline update on chemotherapy for stage IV non-small-cell lung cancer. Zhongguo Fei Ai Za Zhi 13:171–189
39. Kusumbe AP, Bapat SA (2009) Cancer stem cells and aneuploid populations within developing tumors are the major determinants of tumor dormancy. Cancer Res 69:9245–9253
40. Kim EY, Lee SS, Shin JH, Kim SH, Shin DH, Baek SY (2014) Anticancer effect of arsenic trioxide on cholangiocarcinoma: in vitro experiments and in vivo xenograft mouse model. Clin Exp Med 14:215–224
41. Patel P, Chen EI (2012) Cancer stem cells, tumor dormancy, and metastasis. Front Endocrinol (Lausanne) 3:125
42. Bao S, Wu Q, McLendon RE, Hao Y, Shi Q, Hjelmeland AB et al (2006) Glioma stem cells promote radioresistance by preferential activation of the DNA damage response. Nature 444:756–760
43. Mimeault M, Batra SK (2011) Potential applications of curcumin and its novel synthetic analogs and nanotechnology-based formulations in cancer prevention and therapy. Chin Med 6:31
44. Liu C, Tang DG (2011) MicroRNA regulation of cancer stem cells. Cancer Res 71:5950–5954
45. Yu Y, Sarkar FH, Majumdar AP (2013) Down-regulation of miR-21 induces differentiation of chemoresistant colon cancer cells and enhances susceptibility to therapeutic regimens. Transl Oncol 6:180–186
46. Sarkar FH, Li Y, Wang Z, Kong D, Ali S (2010) Implication of microRNAs in drug resistance for designing novel cancer therapy. Drug Resist Updat 13:57–66
47. Incoronato M, Garofalo M, Urso L, Romano G, Quintavalle C, Zanca C et al (2010) miR-212 increases tumor necrosis factor-related apoptosis-inducing ligand sensitivity in non-small cell lung cancer by targeting the antiapoptotic protein PED. Cancer Res 70:3638–3646
48. Turrini E, Haenisch S, Laechelt S, Diewock T, Bruhn O, Cascorbi I (2012) MicroRNA profiling in K-562 cells under imatinib treatment: influence of miR-212 and miR-328 on ABCG2 expression. Pharmacogenet Genomics 22:198–205

49. Rui W, Bing F, Hai-Zhu S, Wei D, Long-Bang C (2010) Identification of microRNA profiles in docetaxel-resistant human non-small cell lung carcinoma cells (SPC-A1). J Cell Mol Med 14:206–214
50. Ahmad A, Aboukameel A, Kong D, Wang Z, Sethi S, Chen W et al (2011) Phosphoglucose isomerase/autocrine motility factor mediates epithelial-mesenchymal transition regulated by miR-200 in breast cancer cells. Cancer Res 71:3400–3409
51. Ahmad A, Maitah MY, Ginnebaugh KR, Li Y, Bao B, Gadgeel SM et al (2013) Inhibition of Hedgehog signaling sensitizes NSCLC cells to standard therapies through modulation of EMT-regulating miRNAs. J Hematol Oncol 6:77
52. Takamizawa J, Konishi H, Yanagisawa K, Tomida S, Osada H, Endoh H et al (2004) Reduced expression of the let-7 microRNAs in human lung cancers in association with shortened postoperative survival. Cancer Res 64:3753–3756
53. Takezawa K, Okamoto I, Tanizaki J, Kuwata K, Yamaguchi H, Fukuoka M et al (2010) Enhanced anticancer effect of the combination of BIBW2992 and thymidylate synthase-targeted agents in non-small cell lung cancer with the T790M mutation of epidermal growth factor receptor. Mol Cancer Ther 9:1647–1656
54. Engelman JA, Zejnullahu K, Mitsudomi T, Song Y, Hyland C, Park JO et al (2007) MET amplification leads to gefitinib resistance in lung cancer by activating ERBB3 signaling. Science 316:1039–1043
55. Garofalo M, Croce CM (2013) MicroRNAs as therapeutic targets in chemoresistance. Drug Resist Updat 16:47–59
56. Garofalo M, Romano G, Di LG, Nuovo G, Jeon YJ, Ngankeu A et al (2012) EGFR and MET receptor tyrosine kinase-altered microRNA expression induces tumorigenesis and gefitinib resistance in lung cancers. Nat Med 18:74–82
57. Bommer GT, Gerin I, Feng Y, Kaczorowski AJ, Kuick R, Love RE et al (2007) p53-mediated activation of miRNA34 candidate tumor-suppressor genes. Curr Biol 17:1298–1307
58. Basak SK, Veena MS, Oh S, Lai C, Vangala S, Elashoff D et al (2013) The CD44(high) tumorigenic subsets in lung cancer biospecimens are enriched for low miR-34a expression. PLoS One 8, e73195
59. Wiggins JF, Ruffino L, Kelnar K, Omotola M, Patrawala L, Brown D et al (2010) Development of a lung cancer therapeutic based on the tumor suppressor microRNA-34. Cancer Res 70:5923–5930
60. Bao B, Ali S, Kong D, Sarkar SH, Wang Z, Banerjee S et al (2011) Anti-tumor activity of a novel compound-CDF is mediated by regulating miR-21, miR-200, and PTEN in pancreatic cancer. PLoS One 6, e17850
61. Jiang M, Zhang P, Hu G, Xiao Z, Xu F, Zhong T et al (2013) Relative expressions of miR-205-5p, miR-205-3p, and miR-21 in tissues and serum of non-small cell lung cancer patients. Mol Cell Biochem 383:67–75
62. Iliopoulos D, Lindahl-Allen M, Polytarchou C, Hirsch HA, Tsichlis PN, Struhl K (2010) Loss of miR-200 inhibition of Suz12 leads to polycomb-mediated repression required for the formation and maintenance of cancer stem cells. Mol Cell 39:761–772
63. Dandawate P, Padhye S, Ahmad A, Sarkar FH (2013) Novel strategies targeting cancer stem cells through phytochemicals and their analogs. Drug Deliv Transl Res 3:165–182
64. Soubani O, Ali AS, Logna F, Ali S, Philip PA, Sarkar FH (2012) Re-expression of miR-200 by novel approaches regulates the expression of PTEN and MT1-MMP in pancreatic cancer. Carcinogenesis 33:1563–1571
65. Ichite N, Chougule MB, Jackson T, Fulzele SV, Safe S, Singh M (2009) Enhancement of docetaxel anticancer activity by a novel diindolylmethane compound in human non-small cell lung cancer. Clin Cancer Res 15:543–552
66. Rahimi M, Huang KL, Tang CK (2010) 3,3′-Diindolylmethane (DIM) inhibits the growth and invasion of drug-resistant human cancer cells expressing EGFR mutants. Cancer Lett 295:59–68
67. Xue L, Firestone GL, Bjeldanes LF (2005) DIM stimulates IFNgamma gene expression in human breast cancer cells via the specific activation of JNK and p38 pathways. Oncogene 24:2343–2353

68. Hsu EL, Chen N, Westbrook A, Wang F, Zhang R, Taylor RT et al (2008) CXCR4 and CXCL12 down-regulation: a novel mechanism for the chemoprotection of 3,3′-diindolylmethane for breast and ovarian cancers. Cancer Lett 265:113–123
69. Jung MJ, Rho JK, Kim YM, Jung JE, Jin YB, Ko YG et al (2013) Upregulation of CXCR4 is functionally crucial for maintenance of stemness in drug-resistant non-small cell lung cancer cells. Oncogene 32:209–221
70. Ye MX, Li Y, Yin H, Zhang J (2012) Curcumin: updated molecular mechanisms and intervention targets in human lung cancer. Int J Mol Sci 13:3959–3978
71. Zhang H, Yu T, Wen L, Wang H, Fei D, Jin C (2013) Curcumin enhances the effectiveness of cisplatin by suppressing CD133 cancer stem cells in laryngeal carcinoma treatment. Exp Ther Med 6:1317–1321
72. Mimeault M, Batra SK (2014) Altered gene products involved in the malignant reprogramming of cancer stem/progenitor cells and multitargeted therapies. Mol Aspects Med 39:3–32
73. Zhang J, Zhang T, Ti X, Shi J, Wu C, Ren X et al (2010) Curcumin promotes apoptosis in A549/DDP multidrug-resistant human lung adenocarcinoma cells through an miRNA signaling pathway. Biochem Biophys Res Commun 399:1–6
74. Zhang J, Du Y, Wu C, Ren X, Ti X, Shi J et al (2010) Curcumin promotes apoptosis in human lung adenocarcinoma cells through miR-186* signaling pathway. Oncol Rep 24:1217–1223

The Microenvironment of Lung Cancer and Therapeutic Implications

Vivek Mittal, Tina El Rayes, Navneet Narula, Timothy E. McGraw, Nasser K. Altorki, and Mary Helen Barcellos-Hoff

Abstract The tumor microenvironment (TME) represents a milieu that enables tumor cells to acquire the hallmarks of cancer. The TME is heterogeneous in composition and consists of cellular components, growth factors, proteases, and extracellular matrix. Concerted interactions between genetically altered tumor cells and genetically stable intratumoral stromal cells result in an "activated/reprogramed" stroma that promotes carcinogenesis by contributing to inflammation, immune suppression, therapeutic resistance, and generating premetastatic niches that support the initiation and establishment of distant metastasis. The lungs present a unique milieu in which tumors progress in collusion with the TME, as evidenced by regions of aberrant angiogenesis, acidosis and hypoxia. Inflammation plays an important role in the pathogenesis of lung cancer, and pulmonary disorders in lung cancer patients such as chronic obstructive pulmonary disease (COPD) and emphysema, constitute comorbid conditions and are independent risk factors for lung cancer. The TME also contributes to immune suppression, induces epithelial-to-mesenchymal

V. Mittal (✉)
Department of Cell and Developmental Biology, Weill Medical College of Cornell University, 1300 York Avenue, New York, NY 10065, USA

Department of Cardiothoracic Surgery, Weill Medical College of Cornell University, 1300 York Avenue, New York, NY 10065, USA

Neuberger Berman Lung Cancer Research Center, Weill Medical College of Cornell University, 1300 York Avenue, New York, NY 10065, USA
e-mail: vim2010@med.cornell.edu

T. El Rayes
Department of Cardiothoracic Surgery, Weill Medical College of Cornell University, 1300 York Avenue, New York, NY 10065, USA

Neuberger Berman Lung Cancer Research Center, Weill Medical College of Cornell University, 1300 York Avenue, New York, NY 10065, USA

Department of Cell and Developmental Biology, Weill Medical College of Cornell University, 1300 York Avenue, New York, NY 10065, USA

Weill Cornell Graduate School of Medical Sciences, Weill Medical College of Cornell University, 1300 York Avenue, New York, NY 10065, USA

A. Ahmad, S.M. Gadgeel (eds.), *Lung Cancer and Personalized Medicine: Novel Therapies and Clinical Management*, Advances in Experimental Medicine and Biology 890, DOI 10.1007/978-3-319-24932-2_5

transition (EMT) and diminishes efficacy of chemotherapies. Thus, the TME has begun to emerge as the "Achilles heel" of the disease, and constitutes an attractive target for anti-cancer therapy. Drugs targeting the components of the TME are making their way into clinical trials. Here, we will focus on recent advances and emerging concepts regarding the intriguing role of the TME in lung cancer progression, and discuss future directions in the context of novel diagnostic and therapeutic opportunities.

Keywords Microenvironment • Lung cancer • Inflammation • Immune cells • Angiogenesis • Endothelial cells • Bone marrow • Hypoxia • Therapy • Immunotherapy • Radiation • Resistance

1 The Tumor Microenvironment: An Overview

The TME has been recognized as a major contributor to tumor progression and metastasis [1–4]. The TME is heterogeneous in composition, and concerted heterotypic reciprocal interactions between genetically altered tumor epithelial cells and intratumoral stromal cells regulate major hallmarks of cancer including angiogenesis, inflammation, immune suppression, epithelial-to-mesenchymal transition (EMT), and metastasis [1, 3]. Importantly, strategies that target the TME are being considered in cancer prevention [5–7].

N. Narula
Department of Pathology, Weill Medical College of Cornell University, 1300 York Avenue, New York, NY 10065, USA

T.E. McGraw
Department of Cardiothoracic Surgery, Weill Medical College of Cornell University, 1300 York Avenue, New York, NY 10065, USA

Neuberger Berman Lung Cancer Research Center, Weill Medical College of Cornell University, 1300 York Avenue, New York, NY 10065, USA

Department of Biochemistry, Weill Medical College of Cornell University, 1300 York Avenue, New York, NY 10065, USA

N.K. Altorki
Department of Cardiothoracic Surgery, Weill Medical College of Cornell University, 1300 York Avenue, New York, NY 10065, USA

Neuberger Berman Lung Cancer Research Center, Weill Medical College of Cornell University, 1300 York Avenue, New York, NY 10065, USA

M. Helen Barcellos-Hoff (✉)
Department of Radiation Oncology, New York University School of Medicine, 566 First Avenue, New York, NY 10016, USA
e-mail: MHBarcellos-Hoff@nyumc.org

The stromal cells recruited to the tumor beds are "educated" and "reprogramed" by the paracrine activity of tumor epithelial cells to acquire an "activated" protumorigenic phenotype [8–10]. Examples of tumor-activated stromal cells include macrophages (classically activated M1 to alternatively-activated M2 phenotype) [11, 12], neutrophils (N1 to N2 conversion) [11], fibroblasts (conversion to activated cancer-associated fibroblasts (CAFs)) [13], endothelial cells [14] and immune cells [15]. These activated stromal cells promote tumor growth and have begun to emerge as attractive targets for anti-cancer therapy [1, 5, 16, 17].

The "angiogenic switch" is a critical step in tumor growth and in the progression of micrometastasis to lethal macrometastasis [1, 18, 19]. The molecular players and mechanisms underlying the angiogenic switch have been intensely investigated, and a variety of pro-angiogenic factors and angiogenic inhibitors that play critical roles during the angiogenic switch have been identified and characterized. Insights from these investigations have led to the development of various pro- and anti-angiogenic therapies that are currently tested in clinical trials or are already in clinical use. Inhibition of angiogenesis by neutralizing antibodies against vascular endothelial growth factor (VEGF) is effective at reducing progression of certain tumors despite having little effect on most tumor cells [7]. In addition to endothelial cells, the inflammatory cells, particularly cells of the myeloid lineages (monocytes, macrophages, and neutrophils) and CAFs progressively accumulate in tumors, where they establish an inflammatory protumorigenic TME [12, 20]. Inflammation is now accepted as an underlying or enabling characteristic that contributes to key hallmarks of cancer, and non-steroidal anti-inflammatory drugs have shown a reduction in cancer risk [21, 22] and may prevent distant metastasis [23]. Myeloid cells also secrete VEGF, basic fibroblast growth factor (bFGF), platelet-derived growth factor (PDGF), placental growth factor (PIGF), and Bv8, that contribute to vascular remodeling during tumor progression [24, 25]. Myeloid cells also secrete proteases such as urokinase-type plasminogen activator (uPA) and matrix metalloproteinases (MMPs), which degrade extracellular matrix (ECM) components to release VEGF and other sequestered mitogenic factors that facilitate endothelial migration and tumor invasion [26].

Tumor-associated macrophages (TAMs) accumulate in regions of hypoxia [27] and support multiple aspects of tumor progression [28]. Studies from breast cancer and glioblastoma have shown that TAMs promote invasive cellular phenotypes [29], through a paracrine signaling loop that involves tumor-derived colony-stimulating factor 1 (CSF-1) and macrophage-derived epidermal growth factor (EGF) [30–32]. TAMs also secrete proteases, such as cysteine cathepsins, which support tumor progression and confer therapeutic resistance [33, 34]. The therapeutic potential of targeting TAMs has been demonstrated in breast cancer and in glioblastoma [6, 34, 35].

The stromal cells also generate inflammatory conditions that contribute to tumorigenesis [20, 36, 37]. The inflammation-responsive Ikappa B kinase (IKK)-beta and its target nuclear factor kappa B (NF-κB) have important tumor-promoting functions within malignant cells and inflammatory cells (macrophages, lymphocytes) [38]. From a clinical perspective, a strong tumor-associated inflammatory response can be initiated by cancer therapy. For example, radiation and chemotherapy cause massive necrotic death of cancer cells and surrounding tissues, which in turn trigger an inflammatory reaction. Therapy-induced inflammation may have tumor-promoting functions [39, 40], or may enhance the cross-presentation of tumor antigens and subsequent induction of an anti-tumor immune response [41].

Cells and molecules of the immune system are a fundamental component of the TME. The tumor-infiltrating immune cells constitute two distinct compartments mediating the innate and adaptive immune responses. The innate immune system consists of phagocytes including neutrophils, mast cells/macrophages ($CD68^+$), dendritic cells (DC), natural killer NK cells ($CD56^+$ $CD3^-$), and NK T cells ($CD56^+$ $CD3^+$), and mainly serves as the first-line defense against both foreign pathogens and transformed cells. However, the tumor "reprogramed" innate immune system stimulates tumor growth by promoting tumor angiogenesis, invasion, and metastasis; whereas the adaptive immune system tends to repress tumor growth. The adaptive immune system is mediated by two major T lymphocyte subsets; cytotoxic T cells (CTL) ($CD8^+$) and helper T cells (Th) ($CD4^+$), and B cells ($CD20^+$). The adaptive immune system is the second-line defense, acting via antigen-specific molecules and requiring clonal expansion following the recognition of foreign antigens. However, in the TME, cancer cells often induce an immunosuppressive microenvironment, which favors the development of immunosuppressive populations of immune cells, such as myeloid-derived suppressor cells (MDSCs) and regulatory T cells (Treg). Understanding the complexity of immunomodulation by tumors is important for the development of immunotherapy, and among the most promising approaches to activating therapeutic antitumor immunity is the blockade of immune checkpoint pathways [42].

MDSCs are a heterogeneous population of immature myeloid progenitors, and precursors of macrophages, granulocytes and dendritic cells [43, 44]. In general, MDSCs from cancer patients express the common myeloid markers CD33 and CD11b, display heterogeneous expression of CD14 (monocytic) and CD15 (granulocytic) markers, but lack mature myeloid or lymphoid markers such as HLA-DR [45, 46]. Clinical correlation studies in breast, colorectal, pancreatic, esophageal, and gastric cancer patients demonstrated that MDSC levels confer an independent prognostic factor for survival [47, 48]. Since MDSCs the major regulators of the immune response due to their ability to suppress both the cytotoxic activities of natural killer (NK) and NKT cells, and the adaptive immune response mediated by $CD4^+$ and $CD8^+$ T cells [44, 49, 50], this cell type has generated much attention. While the mechanism of NK cell inhibition is currently not well understood, multiple pathways are responsible for MDSC-mediated T cell suppression including: (1) production of Arginase 1 (ARG1), which depletes L-Arginine from the microenvironment, and (2) production of nitric oxide synthase 2 (NOS2). Both pathways block translation of the T cell CD3 zeta chain, inhibit T cell proliferation, and promote T cell apoptosis [51]. Not much is known regarding upstream regulators of these suppressive mediators. However recent studies have demonstrated the importance of key signaling pathways such as PI3K, Ras, JAK-STAT, and TGFβ—STAT3 signaling [52, 53]. In mice, MDSCs have been defined as $CD11b^+$ $Gr1^+$ cells and can be subdivided into granulocytic ($CD11b^+$ $Ly6G^+$ $Ly6C^{low}$) or monocytic ($CD11b^+$ $Ly6G^-$ $Ly6C^{hi}$) [54]. The mechanisms by which MDSCs are generated and contribute to immune suppression is being exploited for developing anti-MDSC agents [55]. Approaches to inhibit MDSCs include use of phosphodiesterase (PDE) inhibitors, nitroaspirins, synthetic triterpenoids, COX2 inhibitors, ARG1 inhibitors, anti-glycan antibodies, CSF-1R antagonists, IL-17 inhibitors, and histamine-based approaches. In another approach, MDSCs differentiate by using all-trans retinoic acid (ATRA), vitamins A or D3, or IL-12 [56]. Some compounds, such as ATRA, PDE5 inhibitors, nitroaspirins (e.g. NCX-4016), or tyrosine kinase inhibitors, are being tested in clinical trials to mediate suppression of MDSCs, and improve the efficacy of immune modulating therapies (immune checkpoint inhibitors or cancer vaccines). Notably, pre-clinical evidence suggests that cancer vaccines are more effective in tumor-bearing mice that have been depleted of MDSCs.

2 TME in Lung Cancer Prognosis

Lung cancer is the leading cause of cancer-related deaths worldwide [57]. Lung cancer is generally classified into two histopathological subtypes, small-cell lung carcinoma (SCLC) and non–small cell lung carcinoma (NSCLC). NSCLC accounts for 80% of all lung malignancies, and the overall 5-year survival of patients with this disease remains approximately 15% [58]. A major research focus in lung cancer has been directed to cancer cell intrinsic properties [59–61], which has led to the discovery of important driver mutations and the development of targeted therapies, such as the receptor tyrosine kinase (RTK) inhibitors gefitinib/erlotinib (EGFR inhibitors) and crizotinib (EML4-ALK inhibitor) [62–64]. However, these treatments benefit only a small proportion (15–20%) of patients harboring these driver mutations, and acquired resistance to these therapies presents a major impediment to the effective treatment of NSCLC patients with these mutations [65–67]. More recent studies have begun to elucidate the prognostic and pathophysiological role of the TME in lung cancer.

Many studies have examined the contribution of tumor epithelial molecular markers for prognosis and guidance of cancer therapy, yet only a few have focused on the analysis of the tumor-associated stroma for the identification of prognostic and predictive markers in cancer therapy. More recent studies have begun to demonstrate the prognostic role of TME in cancer with the promise to advance discovery of prognostic and predictive molecular markers for patient management and cancer therapy. For example, stromal gene signatures have been shown to predict clinical outcome and resistance to therapy in breast cancer [68, 69], and fibroblast-derived transcriptional signatures were associated with cancer progression and poor outcome in human breast and lung cancer [70, 71]. In patients with stage I NSCLC, the presence of CAFs is a poor prognostic indicator typically associated with nodal metastases and a higher risk of recurrence [72]. Interestingly, a specific 11-gene expression signature in CAFs stratified NSCLC patients into low and high-risk groups, and was associated with survival [71]. Similarly, prognostic gene signatures from bulk NSCLC tissue analysis included prominent stromal genes such as glypican 3, ICAM-1, laminin B1, L-selectin, P-selectin, and SPARC [73, 74]. High numbers of circulating endothelial cells (CECs) and high levels of soluble CD146 (sCD146) in the plasma have been shown to correlate with poor prognosis and may be useful for the prediction of clinical outcome in patients undergoing surgery for NSCLC [75].

Recently, several groups have demonstrated that the immune fraction of the TME has prognostic value in lung cancer. Elevated numbers of MDSCs have been associated with poor clinical outcomes [76, 77]. Similarly, leukocyte infiltrates, particularly increased numbers of neutrophils, were significantly associated with a worse outcome in patients with bronchioalveolar carcinoma [78–80]. Tumor-infiltrating mature dendritic cells have been suggested to identify patients with early-stage NSCLC who have a high risk of relapse [81, 82]. High density of stromal $CD56^+$ NK cells was shown to be an independent factor associated with improved prognosis in resected NSCLC [81]. TAMs are abundant components of NSCLC, and clinical data correlating the apoptotic index and/or macrophage densities and polarization status (M1/M2) with outcome in NSCLC patients has been recently reviewed [83]. The number of macrophages in NSCLC stroma is an independent predictor of survival time in NSCLC patients [84]. Similarly, mast cells [85], cytotoxic T cells [86], and helper T cells [87] have been reported as potential prognostic factors following resection in patients with NSCLC. Recently, tumor-infiltrating $FOXP3^+$ Treg cells were positively correlated with intratumoral COX-2 expression and were associated with a worse recurrence-free survival (RFS), especially among patients with node-negative NSCLC [88]. Stromal CD99 expression has been described as a novel prognostic marker in human NSCLC [89], and humoral immune response immunoglobulin kappa C (IGKC) expression in tumor-infiltrating plasma cells was shown to have prognostic value in NSCLC [90].

3 TME in Lung Cancer Progression and Metastasis

The stroma in NSCLC is heterogeneous, comprised of many different populations of cells, including bone marrow-derived immune and inflammatory cells, fibroblasts, and endothelial cells (Fig. 1). The contribution of these cell types to tumor growth is illustrated below.

3.1 Cancer-Associated Fibroblasts (CAFs)

As is the case for many solid tumors, the TME of human NSCLC often demonstrates significant desmoplasia, which is characterized by stromal changes depicted by the presence of activated stromal fibroblasts [91–93]. In addition, several mouse explant studies have suggested a pro-tumorigenic role for tumor-derived lung fibroblasts in NSCLCs [94–96]. CAFs, which differ morphologically and functionally from normal fibroblasts (NFs), exhibit similar activities with wound-activated fibroblasts, suggesting that the supportive and reparative roles of activated fibroblasts in wound healing contribute to the pro-tumorigenic activities of CAFs. The origin of CAFs is not clear, yet it is likely that they arise from a reprogramming of tissue resident fibroblasts [97] as well as differentiate from BM cells recruited to the tumor [98].

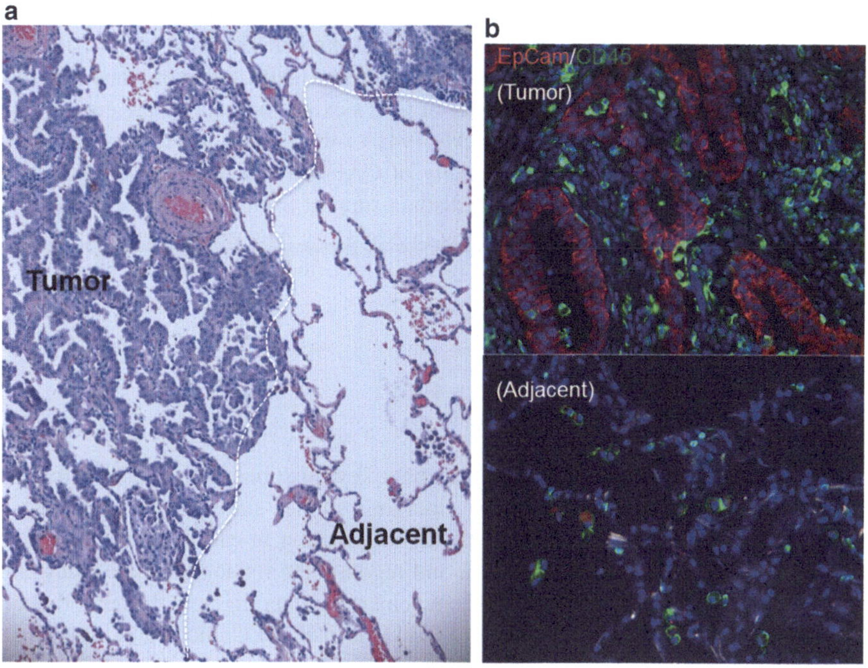

Fig. 1 Infiltration of BM hematopoietic cells in the adenocarcinoma and matched adjacent lung. (**a**) H&E staining of lung tissue from an adenocarcinoma patient (×20 magnification). (**b**) Representative immunofluorescence image of tumor and matched adjacent non-neoplastic lung of adenocarcinoma patient stained for epithelial cells (EpCAM$^+$, *red*) and BM-derived hematopoietic cells (CD45$^+$, *green*). DAPI (*blue*) was used to label cell nuclei

CAFs have been reported to support tumor progression, metastasis, and chemotherapy resistance by a wide variety of mechanisms, including direct paracrine support of cancer cells via the secretion of growth factors, cytokines, and chemokines, through pro-angiogenic effects, as well as by remodeling the extracellular matrix [99–102].

A number of different mechanisms have been specifically reported for the pro-tumorigenic activity of CAFs in NSCLC. A paracrine crosstalk between fibroblasts and NSCLC cells involves IL-6 and TGFβ-enhanced EMT and tumor progression [97, 103]. Cross-species functional characterization of mouse and human lung CAFs identified a secreted gene signature, and functional studies identified important roles for cardiotrophin-like cytokine factor 1 (CLCF1)-Ciliary Neurotrophic Factor Receptor (CNTFR) and interleukin (IL)-6–IL-6R signaling in promoting growth of NSCLCs [104]. A paracrine network was described, involving Insulin-like growth factor-II (IGFII)/IGF1 receptor (IGF1R)-Nanog signaling pathway by which CAFs contributed to cancer stem cell enrichment in NSCLC [105]. Importantly, this paracrine signaling predicted overall and relapse-free survival in stage I NSCLC patients. Similarly, pulmonary fibroblasts induced EMT and stem cell potential in NSCLC [106]. Fibroblast-derived hepatocyte growth factor (HGF) was shown to induce EGFR-tyrosine kinase inhibitor (TKI) resistance in NSCLC with EGFR-activating mutations [107, 108].

The lack of a single pro-tumorigenic activity likely reflects the heterogeneity of CAFs within a tumor. Although there are several markers of CAFs (e.g. α-smooth muscle actin (αSMA), fibroblast-activating protein (FAP), and fibroblast-specific protein (FSP)), no distinct single marker of CAFs exist, and none of the commonly used markers for CAFs are unique to CAFs [94]. Compounding this heterogeneity of CAFs within a tumor is the heterogeneity of CAFs among different tumors. It is likely that specific cancer cells require distinct support from CAFs. For example, in a recent study, metabolic reprogramming in NSCLC-CAFs was shown to correlate with increased glycolytic metabolism of the tumor, indicating tumor-specific specialization of CAFs [109].

3.2 *Endothelial Cells*

Endothelial cells that form the vasculature have key functions in providing nutrients and oxygen to the tumor. However, emerging studies have begun to describe "angiocrine" regulation as a major endothelial function in cancer [110]. Vascular endothelial cells actively participate in and regulate the inflammatory response in both normal and diseased tissues [111], and emerging data suggests that endothelial cells directly influence tumor behavior [18, 112]. In NSCLC, the degree of tumor-associated angiogenesis correlates with disease progression and predicts unfavorable survival outcome [113]. In particular, high vascularity at the tumor periphery has been correlated with tumor progression [114]. However, high steady state vessel density in the lung has imposed challenges in accurate identification and quantification of neoangiogenic microvessels in the tumor tissue. Notably, some NSCLCs do not display an angiogenic phenotype and these tumors are invasive, exploiting the pre-existing alveolar vessels for growth [115, 116].

In a recent study, endothelial-derived angiocrine signals were shown to induce regenerative lung alveolarization. Particularly, activation of VEGFR2 and FGFR1 in pulmonary capillary endothelial cells induced MMP14 expression that unmasked EGF receptor ligands to enhance alveologenesis [117]. Lung endothelial cells also control lung stem cell differentiation, as bone morphogenetic protein 4 (BMP4)-BMPR1A signaling triggers calcineurin/NFATc1-dependent expression of thrombospondin-1 (Tsp-1) in lung endothelial cells to promote alveolar lineage-specific bronchioalveolar stem cell differentiation [118]. Using a mouse model of lung adenocarcinoma, it was shown that perlecan, a component of the ECM, secreted by endothelial cells in a paracrine fashion blocked proliferation and invasiveness of lung cancer by impacting pro-inflammatory pathways [112].

3.3 *Hypoxia in Lung Cancer*

Hypoxia is typically present in solid tumors, like lung cancer, and is known to enhance tumor progression and therapy resistance [119]. The effects of hypoxia are largely mediated by the hypoxia-inducible factors (HIFs) HIF-1α and HIF-2α, as they activate the transcription of genes implicated in tumor angiogenesis, cell survival, and resistance to chemotherapeutic drugs [120]. The overexpression of HIF-1α confers cellular resistance to the EGFR-blocking mAb cetuximab in epidermoid carcinoma cells. In addition, knocking down HIF-1α substantially restores cellular sensitivity to cetuximab-mediated antitumor activities [121]. These findings suggest that HIF-1α expression is associated with the therapeutic responses of cancer cells to EGFR-targeted therapies. More recently, the involvement of hypoxia in the resistance to EGFR-TKIs, such as gefitinib and erlotinib, in NSCLC with an EGFR-sensitive mutation was shown to be mediated by TGFβ [122]. The hypoxic microenvironment is an important stem cell niche that promotes the persistence of cancer stem cells (CSCs) in tumors. Importantly, hypoxia was shown to increase the population of lung CSCs resistant to gefitinib in EGFR mutation-positive NSCLC by activating IGF1R [123].

3.4 Inflammation

Chronic lung inflammation has been associated with an increased risk of lung cancer. Carcinogens including asbestos, cigarette smoke, and other pollutants are known to cause a chronic inflammatory state, which in turn promotes tumorigenesis [20]. Moreover, pulmonary disorders such as COPD/emphysema and pulmonary fibrosis, which are associated with greater risk for developing lung cancer, are characterized by copious inflammation [124–126]. It remains unclear whether inflammation affects the incidence of driver oncogenic mutations. However, inflammation has been shown to enhance tumor progression. Lipopolysaccharide (LPS), a potent endotoxin eliciting chronic lung inflammation, significantly increased the risk of carcinogen-mediated lung tumorigenesis in mice through K-ras gene activation by point mutations [127]. Recently, it was demonstrated that mucin 1 (MUC1) contributes to smoking-induced lung cancers that are driven by inflammatory signals from macrophages, and a signaling pathway involving PPAR-γ, ERK, and MUC1 resulted in TNFα secretion in macrophages [128].

Inflammation has also been described in the generation of lung metastasis from extrapulmonary neoplasms. Clinical studies suggested a correlation between smoking and an increased risk of lung metastasis in patients with breast cancer [129, 130] and esophageal cancer [131]. In addition, inflammation caused by smoke inhalation in mice was also correlated with increased incidence of lung metastasis [132]. Data on autoimmune arthritis showed that lung inflammation in arthritic mice, characterized by neutrophil and mast cell infiltration, as well as increase in circulating levels of pro-inflammatory cytokines, was associated with enhanced lung metastasis [133, 134]. Recently, several mechanisms explaining the metastasis-promoting effects of inflammation have been elucidated. LPS-induced acute lung inflammation dramatically increased breast cancer cell metastasis to lung via a ubiquitin/CXCR4-dependent mechanism [135]. Systemic LPS-induced inflammation led to elevated levels of E-selectin expression in lung tissue and enhanced lung metastasis of breast cancer cells [136]. Induction of lung inflammation by specific NF-κB activation in airway epithelial cells increased lung metastasis via a macrophage-dependent mechanism [137]. Bladder cancer cells expressing the proteoglycan versican metastasize to the lungs via a mechanism involving increased lung CCL2 chemokine expression and macrophage infiltration [138]. The recruitment of CCR2 (the receptor for chemokine CCL2)-expressing monocytes/macrophages to the metastatic site in response to CCL2 enhances breast tumor metastasis to lungs [139]. Lewis lung carcinoma (LLC) cells express versican and subsequently activate TLR2: TLR6 complexes on myeloid cells, inducing TNFα secretion and thus enhancing LLC metastatic growth [140]. Another study showed that $CD11^+$ $Gr1^+$ $Ly6C^{high}$ myeloid progenitor cells express versican in the premetastatic lung, leading to stimulation of mesenchymal-to-epithelial transition of metastatic tumor cells, increasing cell proliferation and accelerating metastasis [8]. Furthermore, these pre-metastatic niches are characterized by the induction of chemoattractants such as, S100A8, growth factors, ECM proteins including fibronectin, and ECM-modifying proteins like lysyl oxidase [141–144], creating a permissive microenvironment for metastasis [145]. Importantly, S100A8/A9 expression in the pre-metastatic niche in turn induces expression of serum amyloid A (SAA) 3, which through the Toll-like receptor 4 (TLR4) leads to the activation of NF-κB signaling and further amplification of inflammatory responses, accelerating lung metastasis [146].

3.5 *Immune Cells*

Tumors utilize various mechanisms to evade destruction by the immune system. One of the key immunomodulatory mechanisms is via immune checkpoint pathways, which play a key role in regulating T-cell responses. Under normal circumstances, the immune checkpoints are important to maintain self-tolerance by preventing autoimmunity and protecting the tissue from damage when the immune system is activated. The expression of immune checkpoint proteins are usually exploited by the tumor cells to develop resistance mechanisms.

3.5.1 T-Cells

Tumor-infiltrating lymphocytes (TILs) are often found in the TME, suggesting an immune response against the tumor. Among the TILs, $CD8^+$ cytotoxic T lymphocytes (CTLs) are directly capable of killing tumor cells, whereas $CD4^+$ T helper lymphocytes (Th) are a heterogeneous cytokine-secreting class of T lymphocytes. Th1 subtypes activate CTLs, whereas Th2 lymphocytes stimulate humoral immunity. Besides the Th1 and Th2 subsets, the $CD4^+$ regulatory T lymphocyte (Treg) subset suppresses effector T lymphocytes. In cancer, Tregs preferentially traffic to tumors, as a result of chemokines produced by tumor cells and microenvironmental macrophages. While active immunotherapy such as adoptive T cell-transfer represents one promising therapeutic approach in lung cancer, more recently, immune checkpoint blockade has received tremendous attention as a potential therapy in solid tumors including lung cancer. The two major immune checkpoint inhibitory pathways involve the programmed cell death-1, PD-1/ PD-L1 pathway and the cytotoxic T-lymphocyte antigen-4, CTLA-4 pathway [147]. PD-1 is a surface receptor member of the B7-CD28 superfamily. It is expressed on many cell types, including activated T cells, B cells, NK cells, and host tissues. PD-1 binds with its ligand PD-L1 (B7-H1, CD274) on antigen presenting cells (APCs), and this interaction inhibits downstream NF-κB transcription and downregulates interferon (IFN)-γ secretion, resulting in T-cell tolerance. Similarly, PD1 can also interact with PD-L2 on dendritic cells, and PD-L2 also has effective inhibitory activity upon T cells. CTLA-4 is expressed on the surface of activated cytotoxic T cells, and it competes with the costimulatory molecule CD28 for mutually shared ligands, B7-1 (CD80) or B7-2 (CD86), and these interactions inhibit the antitumor activity of T-cells.

Recent understanding of the functioning of the immune system and its relation to tumor evasion have led to the development of novel agents that have promising results in the treatment of NSCLC. These agents include immune checkpoint inhibitors such as anti-PD-1 antibodies (nivolumab and MK-3475), anti-PD-L1 antibody (MPDL3280A, MEDI4736), and CTLA-4 inhibitors (tremelimumab and ipilimumab), as well as vaccines.

3.5.2 γδ T Cells

γδ T cells contribute to lymphoid antitumor surveillance and bridge the gap between innate and adaptive immunity [148]. γδ T cells constitute 1%–5% of peripheral blood T lymphocytes and recognize phosphoantigens via polymorphic γδ T-cell antigen receptors (TCR), and develop strong cytolytic and Th1-like effector functions [149]. Therefore, γδ T cells are attractive candidate effector cells for cancer immunotherapy, as they can secrete cytokines abundantly and exert potent cytotoxicity against a wide range of cancer cells. Clinical trials have been conducted to evaluate the safety and efficacy of γδ T-cell-based immunotherapies for non-Hodgkin's lymphoma, multiple myeloma, and solid tumors. In lung cancer, the therapeutic impact of adoptive immunotherapy with expanded γδ T-cells is being assessed [150, 151], and in one study, remission of lung metastasis following adoptive immunotherapy using activated autologous γδ T-cells in a patient with renal cell carcinoma was observed [152].

3.5.3 Myeloid-Derived Suppressor Cells

Increase in the number of MDSCs induces a strong immunosuppressive activity in cancer patients [153–155]. In a mouse model of lung cancer, MDSC depletion increased APC activity and augmented the frequency and activity of NK and T cell effectors that led to impaired tumor growth, enhanced therapeutic vaccination responses, and conferred immunological memory [156, 157]. Immune suppressive MDSCs, defined as $Lin^{-}HLA\text{-}DR^{-}CD33^{+}$ and $CD14^{-}CD11b^{+}$ $CD33^{+}$ [158] were increased in patients with lung cancer. Analysis of 89 patients with NSCLC showed an increase in both frequency and absolute number of MDSCs in the peripheral blood and indicated an association with metastasis, response to chemotherapy, and progression-free survival [159].

4 TME of Premetastatic Niche in the Lung

The lung is one of the most frequent sites of metastasis from extrapulmonary neoplasms including breast and colon cancer. As early as 1889, Steven Paget proposed his "seed" and "soil" hypothesis establishing the concept that primary tumors metastasize to specific organs which harbor a receptive microenvironment [160]. More recently, experimental support for this hypothesis has been provided by studies showing that primary tumors release specific cytokines such as VEGF, SDF-1, TGFβ, and TNFα, which systemically initiate premetastatic niches. These premetastatic niches are characterized by the accumulation of BM-derived cells, and selective induction of organ-specific chemoattractants, growth factors, and ECM-related proteins, which provide permissive local microenvironments for recruiting the incoming tumor cells, leading to the initiation and establishment of micrometastases [145]. Pioneering studies by Lyden and colleagues have shown that the premetastatic niche is comprised of BM-derived $VEGFR1^{+}$ hematopoietic progenitor cells, which express VLA-4 (also known as integrin α4β1), and that tumor-specific growth factors upregulate fibronectin, a VLA-4 ligand in resident fibroblasts, suggesting a possible mechanism by which the permissive niche recruits incoming tumor cells [143, 161]. Similarly, Hiratuska et al. have demonstrated that tumor-secreted factors including VEGF-A, TGFβ, and TNFα induce expression of chemoattractants, such as S100A8 and S100A9 by lung endothelial cells and $Mac1^{+}$ myeloid cells [143, 161], that facilitate the homing of tumor cells to the premetastatic sites, via induction of serum amyloid A3 (SAA3). Notably, SAA3 stimulated NF-κB signaling in the macrophages via TLR4 and facilitated metastasis [146], suggesting the therapeutic potential of blocking SAA3-TLR4 for the prevention of pulmonary metastasis. Giaccia and colleagues have shown that lysyl oxidase (LOX) secreted by hypoxic tumors accumulates in the lungs and supports premetastatic niche formation. LOX remodels ECM by crosslinking collagen IV, which recruits $CD11b^{+}$ myeloid cells that cleave collagen by secreting MMP2, enhancing the invasion and recruitment of BM cells and metastasizing tumor cells. LOX inhibition prevents $CD11b^{+}$ cell recruitment and metastatic growth. $CD11b^{+}$ cells and LOX were also shown to colocalize in biopsies of human metastases [142, 162, 163].

In another mechanism, within the premetastatic niche, fibroblasts expressed periostin which contributed to cancer stem cell maintenance and expansion through Wnt signaling leading to metastasis [164]. In a similar study, metastatic tumor cells, by secreting tenascin C, enhanced stem cell signaling via Notch in the metastatic niche [165]. In the premetastatic lung, BM-derived myeloid progenitor cells were shown to secrete the proteoglycan versican, which induced mesenchymal -to-epithelial transition (MET) of disseminated metastatic tumor cells, accelerating tumor outgrowth in the lungs [8, 166]. Notably, this tumor outgrowth was facilitated by BM-derived endothelial progenitor cells (EPCs), which by initiating the angiogenic switch resulted in the progression of micro- to macrometastases [167]. The premetastatic niche has become an exciting area of research in the quest for novel therapeutic and prophylactic strategies against metastasis [168]. In contrast, a novel mechanism was recently described, whereby metastasis-incompetent tumors generate metastasis-suppressive microenvironments in the lungs by inducing the expression of a potent antiangiogenic factor, thrombospondin 1 (Tsp-1), in the recruited BM-derived myeloid cells [169]. Tsp-1 induction is mediated by the activity of prosaposin (PSAP), a protein secreted by poorly metastatic cells, which acts systemically to reprogram myeloid cells into metastasis-inhibitory cells [169].

5 The Contribution of TME to Therapeutic Resistance

A major research focus to determine the mechanisms of therapeutic resistance has largely been the analysis of tumor cells, and resistance mechanisms involving secondary pathway mutations or bypass mechanisms within the tumor cells, such as EGFR (T790M) mutations or MET receptor amplification have been identified. Importantly, more recent studies have begun to unravel that heterologous cell types within tumors can actively influence therapeutic response and elicit resistance [170, 171].

5.1 Contribution of TME to Resistance to Radiation Therapy

Given that lung cancer is one of the leading causes of death from cancer worldwide, new and effective treatments are urgently needed [172, 173]. Approximately 70% of NSCLC patients receive radiotherapy (RT), either alone or in combination with other treatment modalities such as surgery or chemotherapy [174]. In patients who are unable to tolerate surgical resection because of medical co-morbidities, conventional RT is an alternative, but with poor long-term survival of 15–30% and local failure of up to 50% [175–177]. Retrospective and nonrandomized prospective data suggest that further dose escalation in NSCLC may be associated with better outcomes [178–181]. Additional improvement of the therapeutic ratio for NSCLC will likely come from different radiation dosing schedules. However, for patients with locally advanced disease, the benefit of dose escalation beyond 60 Gy has not been supported by level I evidence. A recent randomized study by the Radiation Therapy Oncology Group (RTOG) in patients with locally advanced NSCLC showed worse survival rates for patients receiving 74 Gy versus 60Gy with concurrent chemotherapy [182].

Accurate delivery of the ionizing radiation (IR) that allows more precise deposition of dose in the tumor while progressively reducing any unwanted dose to surrounding normal tissues has motivated hypofractionated radiation schedules [174]. Stereotactic body RT (SBRT) takes advantage of this favorable dose distribution and gained credence recently as a result of phase II studies with promising outcomes for early-stage medically inoperable NSCLC [183]. However, lack of pathological confirmation of primary tumor control, different definitions of NSCLC control after SBRT, and serious toxicity, particularly for centrally placed tumor, raises concerns about the utility of dose escalation [184, 185]. Clinical factors can explain some of the failures, such as a large tumor and/or advanced tumor stage, but many failures still go unexplained, for tumors with apparently similar sizes, stages, grades, and delivered doses.

It is clear from such clinical considerations and from a wealth of experimental research, that biological factors also have a crucial role in determining treatment success. The main biological factors affecting outcome after RT [186] include intrinsic radioresistance of the tumor cells [187], the ability of the surviving cells, including cancer stem cells, to repopulate [188], and the extent of hypoxia. Sensitizing strategies commonly focus on either targeting intrinsic properties of tumor cells or the vasculature. Recently, targeting the TME has become an even more compelling option to impede tumor progression and augment RT responses [189, 190]. For example, the recognition that tumor infiltration by inflammatory cells and other BM-derived cells contributes to RT responses, particularly tumor regrowth, provides a new route to augment RT efficacy [191, 192].

There is considerable evidence that the microenvironment regulates many tumor responses to radiation, thus providing novel routes for manipulating the response to radiotherapy [193–195]. Of particular interest is the activity of TGFβ, which is a critical signal in cancer and plays a detrimental role to tumor responses to RT. In NSCLC, increased TGFβ activity correlates with tumor progression, increased tumor growth and angiogenesis [196]. TGFβ signaling activation in TME has been identified as a key factor for chemotherapy resistance in NSCLC [197]. Although little is known about how TGFβ modulates the irradiated TME, given its pleiotropic roles in NSCLC, TGFβ inhibition may increase tumor cell radiosensitivity and shift the microenvironment to augment NSCLC response to radiotherapy. TGFβ ligands are enriched in the TME, where their production by stromal or tumor cells varies according to tumor phenotype [198]. The use of clinically viable TGFβ inhibitors in oncology is motivated by rationales to reduce metastasis, augment existing cancer therapies, and to improve tumor vaccines [199]. TGFβ signaling blockade enhances glioblastoma (GBM) response to chemoradiation in preclinical models [200, 201], and specifically inhibits GBM cancer stem cell renewal in vitro and in vivo [202].

In addition to a well recognized phenomenon of the impact of TGFβ on tumor-promoting effects and metastasis [203], TGFβ mediates an effective DNA damage response in epithelial cells via control of ATM kinase activity [204]. TGFβ activity is controlled by production as a latent complex that requires extracellular modification to initiate ligand binding to ubiquitous receptors; this activation is efficiently induced by ionizing radiation, in part due to the presence of a redox sensitive motif in the latency associated peptide (reviewed in [189]). As a consequence, we have shown that inhibiting TGFβ promotes clonogenic cell death of mouse and human breast cancer and GBM cells in vitro and that systemically neutralizing TGFβ enhances RT action in GBM and breast cancer preclinical models [205, 206]. Given that radiation-induced TGFβ is also a significant factor in lung fibrosis, a late tissue toxicity that limits effective tumor control [207], the application of TGFβ antagonists in radiation treatment of NSCLC is clinically viable.

Recent preclinical studies support the potential for improving radiotherapy by use of TGFβ inhibitors (Du and Barcellos-Hoff, unpublished data). As observed for brain and breast tumors [205, 208], most murine and human lung cancer cells were sensitized by TGFβ inhibition prior to radiation, as measured by in vitro clonogenic assays. Using the Lewis lung cancer syngeneic subcutaneous tumors, tumor growth control was significantly improved by use of TGFβ neutralizing antibodies concurrent with single or fractionated radiation treatment. Notably, even though irradiated tumors treated with TGFβ inhibition were significantly smaller at experiment termination, hypoxia was higher and vessel density was also significantly more decreased than that of non-irradiated, bigger tumors. Martin Brown has shown that hypoxia promoted mobilization of $CD11b^+$ monocytes, which secrete the pro-angiogenic factor MMP9 into the TME in preclinical GBM, and blockade of this crucial event prevents tumor recurrence [207]. The combined treatment of radiation and TGFβ inhibition decreased $CD11b^+$/MMP9 monocytes, suggesting that TGFβ is necessary for the recruitment of the $CD11b^+$/MMP9 cells and tumor regrowth.

Given that radiation-induced immunity is critical for long term benefit [209], we also studied the effect of combined treatment of fractionated radiation and TGFβ inhibition on the peripheral anti-tumor immune response. Analysis of monocyte maturation and activation markers CD11b and F4/80 in tumors suggests that distinct BM cells are recruited as a function of treatment: the $F4/80^+$ macrophage population is more differentiated, while $CD11b^+$ cells are more immature. TGFβ inhibition concurrent with radiation treatment also affects systemic maturation as evidenced by analysis of cells from spleens of treated mice. These preliminary data suggest that TGFβ inhibition concurrent with fractionated radiation treatment may cooperate in directing both the microenvironment and the immune system towards an anti-tumor response, which could lead not only to better control of primary tumor growth but also to abrogation of relapse.

5.2 Contribution of TME to Resistance to Antiangiogenic Therapies and EGFR-TKIs

BM-derived cells have also been shown to provide resistance to cancer therapeutics. For example, BM-derived $Gr1^+$ myeloid cells [210] have been shown to make tumors refractory to anti-VEGF treatment [211], by obviating the necessity for VEGF signaling and reinitiating angiogenesis. In another study, administration of vascular disruptive agents (VDA) or chemotherapeutics caused acute hypoxia and necrosis in tumors and triggered an accumulation of endothelial progenitor cells at the tumor leading edge to reinitiate angiogenesis [212]. This appears to be an adaptive response of the tumor to develop evasive resistance to potent anti-angiogenesis therapy. In lung cancer, the tumor-stroma cross talk was implicated in mediating resistance to EGFR-TKIs. For example, fibroblast-derived hepatocyte growth factor (HGF) was shown to induce EGFR-TKI (gefitinib) resistance in NSCLC with EGFR-activating mutations [107, 108].

6 The TME as a Therapeutic Target in Lung Cancer

Lung cancer is a global public health problem with an estimated 1.3 million new cases each year [213]. In the United States, approximately 226,160 new cases of lung cancer are diagnosed per year with over 160,000 deaths. Despite advances in treatment options, including minimally invasive surgical resection, stereotactic radiation, and novel chemotherapeutic regimens, the 5-year survival rate in NSCLC remains at approximately 15%. Available targeted therapies such as EGFR TKIs (erlotinib and gefitinib) and EML4-ALK inhibitor (crizotinib) benefit only 15–20% of NSCLC patients who carry specific drug-sensitive mutations. Even in these patients, acquired resistance is a major impediment to a durable therapeutic response [65–67]. Moreover, a majority of the patients with lung cancer patients do not exhibit an actionable molecular aberration. Therefore, traditional standard cytotoxic chemotherapies remain the only treatment option for the majority of advanced NSCLC patients, and these treatments also usually fail, resulting in an aggressive metastatic relapse. As such, there is an unmet medical need for the development of additional targeted therapies for lung cancer patients. In this context, more recent studies have begun to focus on the TME as an unexplored target for drug discovery, with an increased interest in evaluating anti-angiogenic, immunomodulatory, and anti-inflammatory agents in the treatment of various malignancies, including NSCLC [214] (Table 1).

6.1 Antiangiogenic Therapies in Lung Cancer

Drugs that either block tumor vascularization or interfere with the activity of growth factor receptors and molecular pathways that are triggered by activation of these receptors have already been used in clinical practice [215]. Bevacizumab, a humanized monoclonal antibody against VEGF, has been approved in many countries for use in combination with first-line platinum-based chemotherapy (carboplatin and paclitaxel) for the treatment of NSCLC patients with advanced stage disease [216, 217]. Approvals were based upon an improvement in response rate (RR) and progression-free survival (PFS) observed with the addition of bevacizumab to

Table 1 Stromal therapy in lung cancer

Drug	Type	Mode of action	Clinical trials	Results
CTLA-4 antibodies (Ipilimumab)	Immune checkpoint inhibitor	Blocks PD-L1 interaction with PD-1 and allows T cells to perform antitumor activities	Phase III, NSCLC (NCT01285609)	PFS 5.7 months for ipilimumab + chemo vs 4.6 months for placebo + chemo
			Phase III, SCLC (NCT01450761)	
Tremelimumab			Phase II, Mesothelioma	
PD-1 antibodies	Immune checkpoint inhibitor	Blocks PD-L1 interaction with PD-1 and allows T cells to perform antitumor activities	Phase III, NSCLC (NCT01673867)	
Nivolumab			Squamous cell (NCT01642004)	
MK-3475			Phase III, in PD-L1-positive NSCLC (NCT01905657)	
PD-L1 antibodies	Immune checkpoint inhibitor	Targets the ligand PD-L1 and allows T cells to perform antitumor activities		
MPDL3280A			Phase II in PD-L1-positive NSCLC (NCT01846416)	
MEDI4736			Phase I NSCLC (NCT01693562)	
VEGF antibody Bevacizumab	Anti-angiogenic therapy	Targets VEGF ligand	Phase III	PFS and OS positive with Carbo/PXL
VEGF trap	Anti-angiogenic therapy (Soluble decoy receptor)	Targets VEGFA, VEGFB and PIGF	Phase III	PFS positive with DXI
Aflibercept				OS negative
Endostatin	Anti-angiogenic therapy-natural inhibitor of angiogenesis	Targets bFGF, VEGF	Phase III, in combination with chemotherapy (NCT00657423)	
			Phase II, in combination with chemoradiation in NSCLC (NCT01218594)	

(continued)

Table 1 (continued)

Drug	Type	Mode of action	Clinical trials	Results
Pazopanib	TKI, Antiangiogenic	Targets c-KIT, FGFR, PDGFR and VEGFR	Phase II/III in NSCLC patients who have received first line therapy (NCT01208064)	
			Phase II in Refractory small cell lung cancer (NCT01253369)	
Motesanib	TKI, Antiangiogenic	Targets VEGFR-1, 2, 3, PDGFR, RET, kit	Phase III	PFS positive with Carbo or PXL
				OS negative
Sorafenib	TKI, Antiangiogenic	Targets, VEGFR-2, 3 and PDGFR-b	Phase III, Advanced NSCLC in combination with chemo	PFS and OS negative with chemo
				Monotherapy pending
Cediranib	TKI, Antiangiogenic	Targets VEGFR-1,2, 3, c-kit, Flt-3	Phase III, Advanced NSCLC in combination with chemo	PFS pending with DXI
				OS pending with DXI
Vandetanib	TKI, Antiangiogenic	Targets VEGFR-2, VEGFR-3, RET, EGFR	Phase III, in advanced NSCLC in combination with chemo (NCT00312377)	PFS positive with DXI
				OS negative with DXI
Nintedanib	Antiangiogenic	Targets VEGFR, FGFR, PDGFR	Phase III (LUME-Lung-1)	PFS positive with DXI
				OS not significant

References: (1) Hilbe W, Manegold C, Pircher A. Targeting angiogenesis in lung cancer—Pitfalls in drug development. Transl Lung Cancer Res 2012;1(2):122-128. (2) http://www.cancer.gov/clinicaltrials/results/type/lung

DXI docetaxel, *PXL* paclitaxel, *Carbo* carboplatin, *TKI* tyrosine kinase inhibitor

chemotherapy in two large phase III studies, the North American Eastern Cooperative Oncology Group (ECOG) 4599 [218] and the European AVAiL [219]. The encouraging results with bevacizumab has led to approval of Aflibercept (VEGF Trap), which is a recombinant VEGF receptor-antibody protein fusion with affinity for VEGF-A, VEGF-B and placental growth factor (PlGF), which acts as a decoy receptor preventing angiogenesis [220]. Aflibercept, has been approved for metastatic colorectal cancer, and it has been evaluated in second-line therapy of NSCLC. A randomized phase III trial of second-line docetaxel with or without aflibercept in platinum-pretreated patients with advanced non-squamous NSCLC failed its primary endpoint of overall survival, despite higher response rates and progression free survival in the experimental arm [221].

Other promising anti-angiogenic agents include small molecule TKIs targeting the VEGF receptor (VEGFR). Motesanib, a selective oral inhibitor of VEGF receptors-1, 2, and 3, platelet-derived growth factor receptor (PDGFR), and c-Kit was tested in a randomized phase II trial in combination with carboplatin/paclitaxel as frontline therapy for patients with advanced NSCLC, and results showed that RR, PFS, and OS were comparable in those patients receiving either motesanib or bevacizumab [222]. However, an international randomized phase III trial with carboplatin/paclitaxel either alone or in combination with motesanib in patients with advanced NSCLC showed no improvement in overall survival compared with placebo; despite an improvement in PFS and overall response [223, 224]. Another phase III trial evaluated the addition of the multi-kinase inhibitor (including VEGFR2) sorafenib to chemotherapy in patients with advanced non-squamous NSCLC. Again, despite a slight but statistically significant improvement in PFS, there was no improvement in OS, the trial's primary end-point [225]. A recently reported phase III trial assigned patients with advanced NSCLC who failed first-line therapy to docetaxel with and without nintedanib, a multi-angiogenic kinase inhibitor (VEGFR1-3/FGFR1-3/PDGFR/FLT3). Nintedanib in combination with docetaxel was associated with significant improvement in PFS and OS especially in patients with adenocarcinomas [226]. This is the first and only trial to demonstrate an improvement in OS using a targeted agent in the second-line setting. Finally, a phase III placebo-controlled trial of carboplatin and paclitaxel with and without the vascular disrupting agent vadimezan (ASA404) as first-line therapy for patients with advanced lung cancer did not meet the specified primary and secondary endpoints of OS and PFS [227–229]. Results from recently completed and ongoing phase III trials will determine if these newer antiangiogenic agents will be incorporated into clinical practice [230].

6.2 Anti-inflammatory Therapies in Lung Cancer

Compared to advances with antiangiogenic therapies, success with anti-inflammatory treatments have been less impactful. Previous clinical trials have indicated that long-term use of aspirin or other NSAIDs decreases the incidence of colorectal, esophageal, breast, lung, and bladder cancers [231]. While initial studies had focused on various broad-spectrum NSAIDs (which non-specifically inhibit both COX-1 and COX-2), more recent studies have examined COX-2 specific agents, such as celecoxib [125]. Significant pre-clinical and clinical data support the importance of COX-2 in the development and progression of NSCLC. Despite this, a protective effect of NSAIDs was not observed on lung cancer development in either the general or high-risk COPD populations [232]. Moreover, clinical trials of COX-2 inhibition in NSCLC have been disappointing [233]. The lack of clinical benefit in the Cancer and Leukemia Group B (CALGB) 30203 trial may be that COX-2 inhibition would be of value in COX-2-overexpressing tumors, emphasizing the need for a prospective, randomized trial that selects patients for therapy on the basis of COX-2 expression [234]. CALGB 30801 is a randomized phase III double-blind trial evaluating selective COX-2 inhibition in COX-2-expressing advanced NSCLC. However, given the gastrointestinal (GI) toxicity and non-specific activity of NSAIDs, and the cardiotoxicity of specific COX-2 inhibitors, the use of such agents continues to remain controversial [235].

Two recent studies have shed light on the future therapeutic potential of the NF-κB-mediated inflammatory pathway in lung cancer. Logsdon and colleagues found that in the presence of oncogenic Ras, inflammatory stimuli initiate a positive feedback loop involving NF-κB that further amplifies Ras activity to pathological levels [236]. Because a large proportion of lung cancer patients possess Ras mutations, disruption of this positive feedback loop may be an important strategy for cancer prevention. In another study, using mouse models of lung cancer, Verma and colleagues found that therapies targeting the enzyme IKK2 (involved in inflammation) and Timp1, which help activate the body's inflammatory response, may effectively treat certain lung cancers [237].

6.3 Immune Checkpoint Inhibitors in Lung Cancer

Utilizing the immune system to eliminate cancer holds great potential, and therefore understanding the complexity of immunomodulation by tumors is important for the development of immunotherapy. A large numbers of different factors have been implicated in the inhibition of tumor-specific immune responses. These include regulatory T cells (Treg), MDSCs, various soluble factors and cytokines, and inhibitory molecules expressed by immune and tumor cells. As such, various strategies are being developed to enhance anti-tumor immune responses, including DC-based vaccines and antagonists of inhibitory signaling pathways to overcome 'immune checkpoints'. The immune checkpoint pathway is a series of cell-cell interactions that inhibit effector T cells from being overactive under normal conditions [147, 238]. A major arm of the immune checkpoint pathway consists of the T cell surface receptor CTLA-4. CTLA-4 is an inhibitory receptor expressed upon activation of a cytotoxic T cell, competing with the co-stimulatory receptor CD28 for their shared ligands CD80 and CD86 on antigen-presenting cells (APCs) [239]. Lung cancer can co-opt this mechanism to evade immune surveillance by stimulating abnormal expression of CTLA-4 on T-cells, leading to T cell anergy. The monoclonal antibodies, tremelimumab and ipilimumab, which inhibit CTLA-4, are being tested for the treatment of lung cancer. Although tremelimumab treatment did not enhance PFS in a phase II trial, objective radiological responses in 5% of participants was observed using tremelimumab. Ipilimumab treatment, on the other hand, showed slight improvement in immune-related progression-free survival (irPFS) in NSCLC patients when administered in a phased manner with platinum-based chemotherapy [240]. Interestingly, ipilimumab treatment showed high activity in squamous carcinomas

[241]. These results prompted the phase III trial, testing ipilimumab in squamous NSCLC using the phased ipilimumab schedule [147].

PD-1 pathway is a major immune checkpoint by which tumors suppress lymphocyte function within the TME. PD-1 is a surface receptor on activated T cells, B cells, and NK cells. It binds to its ligands PD-L1 and PD-L2 on the surface of APCs or dendritic cells, leading to T cell anergy. Cancers can co-opt this pathway and aberrantly express PD-L1 on their cell surface, leading to T cell inactivation. It has been reported that sarcomatoid and adenocarcinoma subtypes of lung cancer express PD-L1, and its expression correlated with poor prognosis [242, 243].

Antibody blockade of PD-1 with its ligands (B7-H1/PD-L1 and B7-DC/PD-L2) showed promising activity in several malignancies [42]. In particular, blocking antibodies against PD-1 and PD-L1 have shown clinical activity in NSCLC [244, 245]. Nivolumab, a monoclonal antibody targeting PD-1, as been shown to restore cytokine secretion and proliferation of $CD8^+$ T cells within lung tumors [246]. A phase I trial of Nivolumab showed a response rate of 17% in previously treated patients with advanced NSCLC, with responses persisting for a median duration of 17 months [244, 247]. As with any type of therapy, a main consideration for the implementation of an immunotherapy regimen is toxicity. For instance, Ipilimumab in combination with chemotherapy exhibited 14% to 17% higher incidence of all-cause grade 3/4 adverse events (AE) compared to chemotherapy alone [248]. Furthermore, a fatal side effect that occurs in a small proportion of patients following anti-CTLA-4 antibody treatment is hypophysitis, inflammation of the pituitary gland [249]. Nivolumab treatment exhibited 9% rate of treatment-related grade 3/4 AE [250], with three drug-related deaths due to pneumonitis [147]. Nivolumab treatment in combination with platinum-based chemotherapy yielded an objective response rate of 33% and a grade 3/4 AE rate of 49% [147]. A current phase I trial is testing the combination of nivolumab with ipilimumab for SCLC [147]. Another antibody targeting PD-1 is MK-3475. A phase I trial in 38 NSCLC patients showed an objective response rate of 24%, with a median PFS of 9.7 weeks and median OS of 51 weeks. 53% of patients had drug-related AEs, most of which were mild. Another approach to targeting the PD-1/PD-L1 pathway is using antibodies that target PD-L1 on cancer cells. One such antibody, MPDL3280A, yielded a 23% overall response rate, with only 11% drug-related grade 3–4 AEs in a phase I trial that included 85 patients with NSCLC [147].

Another avenue being explored to block tumor-driven immunosuppression is based on NK cell activity. NK cells express killer cell immunoglobulin-like receptors (KIRs) that downregulate NK cytotoxic activity, in response to HLA class I molecules on target cells. A higher incidence of the suppressive KIR2DL3 and its ligand HLA-C2 is observed in NSCLC [251] leading to reduced NK activity and protection of cancer cells from NK-mediated killing. A monoclonal antibody to KIR, Lirilumab (IPH2102), has demonstrated efficacy in combination with nivolumab in preclinical models. A trial combining nivolumab with lirilumab in human solid tumors, including 32 NSCLC patients is being conducted, as well as a trial combining lirilumab with ipilimumab [147].

6.4 MDSC as a Therapeutic Target in Lung Cancer

MDSCs have prognostic importance in multiple solid tumors. Emerging data has begun to support the utility of circulating MDSCs as a predictive marker for cancer immunotherapy and for predicting clinical response to systemic chemotherapy in patients with advanced solid tumors [252]. An increase in the number of MDSCs evokes strong immune suppressive activity in cancer patients [153–155], and greatly limits the efficacy of immune therapy. In a randomized phase II clinical trial of advanced stage SCLC, depletion of MDSCs with ATRA substantially improved the immune response to vaccination, suggesting that this approach can be used to enhance the effect of immune interventions in cancer [253]. These studies are consistent with the demonstration that targeting MDSCs augments antitumor activity against lung cancer in mice [157].

7 Future Directions

Analysis of TME in lung cancer is a relatively new area of investigation. Therefore, major efforts are required to identify individual stromal components and unravel heterotypic reciprocal crosstalk signaling pathways between the stroma and tumor cells in NSCLC. This is a major challenge given the high heterogeneity of genetic and epigenetic alterations present in the tumor, differences in host genetic background, as well as tissue-specific responses. Understanding the cellular and molecular mechanisms underlying these processes will provide novel avenues leading to the discovery of biomarkers for disease stratification, molecular diagnosis and prognosis, and devising therapeutic strategies against lung cancer. Over 10 years ago, it was suggested that treatments options for NSCLC other than chemotherapy needed to be investigated [254]. So far, only one phase III clinical trial showed survival benefit of combining an anti-angiogenic agent to standard platinum-based chemotherapy in patients with advanced stage NSCLC. Selected groups of patients responded to anti-angiogenic therapies that result in tumor shrinkage and disease stabilization; however, in aggregate, antiangiogenic therapy has not yet had a major clinical impact in most of the trials conducted so far [215]. Many clinical benefits are short-lived; while numerous trials have shown an increase in survival of patients treated with antiangiogenic therapy, the increase for many has been a matter of months [255]. Several possibilities have been suggested to explain why anti-angiogenic trials have not yielded significant benefit in NSCLC. For example, lack of predictive biomarkers continues to be a major hurdle in the selection of adequate patient cohorts that are most likely to benefit. In fact, some studies have alluded to a possible link between antiangiogenic therapy and increased metastasis in multiple tumor types [256, 257].

Immunotherapy has been heralded as a new era of lung cancer therapy. Blocking PD1-PDL1 or CTLA-4 immune checkpoints has resulted in striking and durable responses, with global overall response rates of 20% to 25% as monotherapy in metastatic NSCLC. In order to increase response rates, it has been suggested that identifying patients who might respond to immunotherapy would be particularly useful, as correlations between PD-L1 expression and EGFR mutation, and PD-1 expression and KRAS mutations has been observed (D'Incecco et al. Journal of Thoracic Oncology 2014). Notably, activation of the PD-1 pathway was shown to contribute to immune escape in mutant EGFR-driven lung tumors in mice, and blockade of this escape pathway improved survival [258]. These findings support further investigation of anti-PD-L1 or anti-PD-1 agents in combination with various targeted therapies, including epigenetic therapy. While immune checkpoint inhibitors such as ipilimumab (anti-CTLA-4 antibody) have been approved for the treatment of melanoma, they have yet not been approved for lung cancer. However, several classes of new drugs appear to be active in various ongoing clinical trials, and their impending approval for use in lung cancer is presumed. At present, several new therapeutic agents are being tested in more than 600 clinical trials in patients with advanced NSCLC, and based on early phase data exhibiting potential, some of these new agents have the capacity to translate to phase III trials, and eventually benefit patients.

Acknowledgement We thank Sharell Lee for reading the manuscript.

References

1. Gao D, Mittal V (2009) The role of bone-marrow-derived cells in tumor growth, metastasis initiation and progression. Trends Mol Med 15:333–343
2. Hanahan D, Coussens LM (2012) Accessories to the crime: functions of cells recruited to the tumor microenvironment. Cancer Cell 21:309–322
3. Hanahan D, Weinberg RA (2011) Hallmarks of cancer: the next generation. Cell 144:646–674
4. Joyce JA, Pollard JW (2009) Microenvironmental regulation of metastasis. Nat Rev Cancer 9:239–252
5. Albini A, Sporn MB (2007) The tumour microenvironment as a target for chemoprevention. Nat Rev Cancer 7:139–147
6. DeNardo DG, Brennan DJ, Rexhepaj E, Ruffell B, Shiao SL, Madden SF, Gallagher WM, Wadhwani N, Keil SD, Junaid SA et al (2011) Leukocyte complexity predicts breast cancer survival and functionally regulates response to chemotherapy. Cancer Discov 1:54–67
7. Ebos JM, Kerbel RS (2011) Antiangiogenic therapy: impact on invasion, disease progression, and metastasis. Nat Rev Clin Oncol 8:210–221
8. Gao D, Vahdat LT, Wong S, Chang JC, Mittal V (2012) Microenvironmental regulation of epithelial-mesenchymal transitions in cancer. Cancer Res 72:4883–4889
9. Lee G, Walser TC, Dubinett SM (2009) Chronic inflammation, chronic obstructive pulmonary disease, and lung cancer. Curr Opin Pulm Med 15:303–307
10. Punturieri A, Szabo E, Croxton TL, Shapiro SD, Dubinett SM (2009) Lung cancer and chronic obstructive pulmonary disease: needs and opportunities for integrated research. J Natl Cancer Inst 101:554–559
11. Fridlender ZG, Sun J, Kim S, Kapoor V, Cheng G, Ling L, Worthen GS, Albelda SM (2009) Polarization of tumor-associated neutrophil phenotype by TGF-beta: "N1" versus "N2" TAN. Cancer Cell 16:183–194
12. Mantovani A, Sica A (2010) Macrophages, innate immunity and cancer: balance, tolerance, and diversity. Curr Opin Immunol 22:231–237

13. Orimo A, Gupta PB, Sgroi DC, Arenzana-Seisdedos F, Delaunay T, Naeem R, Carey VJ, Richardson AL, Weinberg RA (2005) Stromal fibroblasts present in invasive human breast carcinomas promote tumor growth and angiogenesis through elevated SDF-1/CXCL12 secretion. Cell 121:335–348
14. Zeng Q, Li S, Chepeha DB, Giordano TJ, Li J, Zhang H, Polverini PJ, Nor J, Kitajewski J, Wang CY (2005) Crosstalk between tumor and endothelial cells promotes tumor angiogenesis by MAPK activation of Notch signaling. Cancer Cell 8:13–23
15. Coussens LM, Werb Z (2002) Inflammation and cancer. Nature 420:860–867
16. Gadea BB, Joyce JA (2006) Tumour-host interactions: implications for developing anti-cancer therapies. Expert Rev Mol Med 8:1–32
17. Joyce JA (2005) Therapeutic targeting of the tumor microenvironment. Cancer Cell 7:513–520
18. Bergers G, Benjamin LE (2003) Angiogenesis: tumorigenesis and the angiogenic switch. Nat Rev Cancer 3:401–410
19. Hanahan D, Folkman J (1996) Patterns and emerging mechanisms of the angiogenic switch during tumorigenesis. Cell 86:353–364
20. Mantovani A, Allavena P, Sica A, Balkwill F (2008) Cancer-related inflammation. Nature 454:436–444
21. Gupta RA, Dubois RN (2001) Colorectal cancer prevention and treatment by inhibition of cyclooxygenase-2. Nat Rev Cancer 1:11–21
22. Rothwell PM, Fowkes FG, Belch JF, Ogawa H, Warlow CP, Meade TW (2011) Effect of daily aspirin on long-term risk of death due to cancer: analysis of individual patient data from randomised trials. Lancet 377:31–41
23. Rothwell PM, Wilson M, Price JF, Belch JF, Meade TW, Mehta Z (2012) Effect of daily aspirin on risk of cancer metastasis: a study of incident cancers during randomised controlled trials. Lancet 379:1591–1601
24. Murdoch C, Muthana M, Coffelt SB, Lewis CE (2008) The role of myeloid cells in the promotion of tumour angiogenesis. Nat Rev Cancer 8:618–631
25. Shojaei F, Wu X, Zhong C, Yu L, Liang XH, Yao J, Blanchard D, Bais C, Peale FV, van Bruggen N et al (2007) Bv8 regulates myeloid-cell-dependent tumour angiogenesis. Nature 450:825–831
26. Kessenbrock K, Plaks V, Werb Z (2010) Matrix metalloproteinases: regulators of the tumor microenvironment. Cell 141:52–67
27. Lewis CE, Pollard JW (2006) Distinct role of macrophages in different tumor microenvironments. Cancer Res 66:605–612
28. Qian B, Deng Y, Im JH, Muschel RJ, Zou Y, Li J, Lang RA, Pollard JW (2009) A distinct macrophage population mediates metastatic breast cancer cell extravasation, establishment and growth. PLoS One 4, e6562
29. Condeelis J, Pollard JW (2006) Macrophages: obligate partners for tumor cell migration, invasion, and metastasis. Cell 124:263–266
30. Coniglio SJ, Eugenin E, Dobrenis K, Stanley ER, West BL, Symons MH, Segall JE (2012) Microglial stimulation of glioblastoma invasion involves epidermal growth factor receptor (EGFR) and colony stimulating factor 1 receptor (CSF-1R) signaling. Mol Med 18:519–527
31. Goswami S, Sahai E, Wyckoff JB, Cammer M, Cox D, Pixley FJ, Stanley ER, Segall JE, Condeelis JS (2005) Macrophages promote the invasion of breast carcinoma cells via a colony-stimulating factor-1/epidermal growth factor paracrine loop. Cancer Res 65:5278–5283
32. Wyckoff J, Wang W, Lin EY, Wang Y, Pixley F, Stanley ER, Graf T, Pollard JW, Segall J, Condeelis J (2004) A paracrine loop between tumor cells and macrophages is required for tumor cell migration in mammary tumors. Cancer Res 64:7022–7029
33. Gocheva V, Zeng W, Ke D, Klimstra D, Reinheckel T, Peters C, Hanahan D, Joyce JA (2006) Distinct roles for cysteine cathepsin genes in multistage tumorigenesis. Genes Dev 20:543–56
34. Shree T, Olson OC, Elie BT, Kester JC, Garfall AL, Simpson K, Bell-McGuinn KM, Zabor EC, Brogi E, Joyce JA (2011) Macrophages and cathepsin proteases blunt chemotherapeutic response in breast cancer. Genes Dev 25:2465–2479

35. Pyonteck SM, Akkari L, Schuhmacher AJ, Bowman RL, Sevenich L, Quail DF, Olson OC, Quick ML, Huse JT, Teijeiro V et al (2013) CSF-1R inhibition alters macrophage polarization and blocks glioma progression. Nat Med 19:1264–1272
36. Balkwill F, Charles KA, Mantovani A (2005) Smoldering and polarized inflammation in the initiation and promotion of malignant disease. Cancer Cell 7:211–217
37. Grivennikov SI, Greten FR, Karin M (2010) Immunity, inflammation, and cancer. Cell 140:883–899
38. Ben-Neriah Y, Karin M (2011) Inflammation meets cancer, with NF-κB as the matchmaker. Nat Immunol 12:715–723
39. Ammirante M, Luo JL, Grivennikov S, Nedospasov S, Karin M (2010) B-cell-derived lymphotoxin promotes castration-resistant prostate cancer. Nature 464:302–305
40. Vakkila J, Lotze MT (2004) Inflammation and necrosis promote tumour growth. Nat Rev Immunol 4:641–648
41. Zitvogel L, Apetoh L, Ghiringhelli F, Kroemer G (2008) Immunological aspects of cancer chemotherapy. Nat Rev Immunol 8:59–73
42. Pardoll DM (2012) The blockade of immune checkpoints in cancer immunotherapy. Nat Rev Cancer 12:252–264
43. Chioda M, Peranzoni E, Desantis G, Papalini F, Falisi E, Solito S, Samantha S, Mandruzzato S, Bronte V (2011) Myeloid cell diversification and complexity: an old concept with new turns in oncology. Cancer Metastasis Rev 30:27–43
44. Gabrilovich DI, Nagaraj S (2009) Myeloid-derived suppressor cells as regulators of the immune system. Nat Rev Immunol 9:162–174
45. Greten TF, Manns MP, Korangy F (2011) Myeloid derived suppressor cells in human diseases. Int Immunopharmacol 11:802–807
46. Serafini P, Borrello I, Bronte V (2006) Myeloid suppressor cells in cancer: recruitment, phenotype, properties, and mechanisms of immune suppression. Semin Cancer Biol 16:53–65
47. Gabitass RF, Annels NE, Stocken DD, Pandha HA, Middleton GW (2011) Elevated myeloid-derived suppressor cells in pancreatic, esophageal and gastric cancer are an independent prognostic factor and are associated with significant elevation of the Th2 cytokine interleukin-13. Cancer Immunol Immunother 60:1419–1430
48. Solito S, Falisi E, Diaz-Montero CM, Doni A, Pinton L, Rosato A, Francescato S, Basso G, Zanovello P, Onicescu G et al (2011) A human promyelocytic-like population is responsible for the immune suppression mediated by myeloid-derived suppressor cells. Blood 118:2254–2265
49. Hoechst B, Voigtlaender T, Ormandy L, Gamrekelashvili J, Zhao F, Wedemeyer H, Lehner F, Manns MP, Greten TF, Korangy F (2009) Myeloid derived suppressor cells inhibit natural killer cells in patients with hepatocellular carcinoma via the NKp30 receptor. Hepatology 50:799–807
50. Talmadge JE, Gabrilovich DI (2013) History of myeloid-derived suppressor cells. Nat Rev Cancer 13:739–752
51. Ostrand-Rosenberg S, Sinha P (2009) Myeloid-derived suppressor cells: linking inflammation and cancer. J Immunol 182:4499–4506
52. Trikha P, Carson WE (2014) Signaling pathways involved in MDSC regulation. Biochim Biophys Acta 1846:55–65
53. Vasquez-Dunddel D, Pan F, Zeng Q, Gorbounov M, Albesiano E, Fu J, Blosser RL, Tam AJ, Bruno T, Zhang H et al (2013) STAT3 regulates arginase-I in myeloid-derived suppressor cells from cancer patients. J Clin Invest 123:1580–1589
54. Movahedi K, Guilliams M, Van den Bossche J, Van den Bergh R, Gysemans C, Beschin A, De Baetselier P, Van Ginderachter JA (2008) Identification of discrete tumor-induced myeloid-derived suppressor cell subpopulations with distinct T cell-suppressive activity. Blood 111:4233–4244
55. Markowitz J, Wesolowski R, Papenfuss T, Brooks TR, Carson WE (2013) Myeloid-derived suppressor cells in breast cancer. Breast Cancer Res Treat 140:13–21
56. Kusmartsev S, Cheng F, Yu B, Nefedova Y, Sotomayor E, Lush R, Gabrilovich D (2003) All-trans-retinoic acid eliminates immature myeloid cells from tumor-bearing mice and improves the effect of vaccination. Cancer Res 63:4441–4449

57. Jemal A, Bray F, Center MM, Ferlay J, Ward E, Forman D (2011) Global cancer statistics. CA Cancer J Clin 61:69–90
58. Herbst RS, Heymach JV, Lippman SM (2008) Lung cancer. N Engl J Med 359:1367–1380
59. Slebos RJ, Kibbelaar RE, Dalesio O, Kooistra A, Stam J, Meijer CJ, Wagenaar SS, Vanderschueren RG, van Zandwijk N, Mooi WJ (1990) K-ras oncogene activation as a prognostic marker in adenocarcinoma of the lung. N Engl J Med 323:561–565
60. Takahashi T, Nau MM, Chiba I, Birrer MJ, Rosenberg RK, Vinocour M, Levitt M, Pass H, Gazdar AF, Minna JD (1989) p53: a frequent target for genetic abnormalities in lung cancer. Science 246:491–494
61. Zochbauer-Muller S, Gazdar AF, Minna JD (2002) Molecular pathogenesis of lung cancer. Annu Rev Physiol 64:681–708
62. Haber DA, Bell DW, Sordella R, Kwak EL, Godin-Heymann N, Sharma SV, Lynch TJ, Settleman J (2005) Molecular targeted therapy of lung cancer: EGFR mutations and response to EGFR inhibitors. Cold Spring Harb Symp Quant Biol 70:419–426
63. Lynch TJ, Bell DW, Sordella R, Gurubhagavatula S, Okimoto RA, Brannigan BW, Harris PL, Haserlat SM, Supko JG, Haluska FG et al (2004) Activating mutations in the epidermal growth factor receptor underlying responsiveness of non-small-cell lung cancer to gefitinib. N Engl J Med 350:2129–2139
64. Sequist LV, Martins RG, Spigel D, Grunberg SM, Spira A, Jänne PA, Joshi VA, McCollum D, Evans TL, Muzikansky A et al (2008) First-line gefitinib in patients with advanced non-small-cell lung cancer harboring somatic EGFR mutations. J Clin Oncol 26:2442–2449
65. Choi YL, Soda M, Yamashita Y, Ueno T, Takashima J, Nakajima T, Yatabe Y, Takeuchi K, Hamada T, Haruta H et al (2010) EML4-ALK mutations in lung cancer that confer resistance to ALK inhibitors. N Engl J Med 363:1734–1739
66. Engelman JA, Zejnullahu K, Mitsudomi T, Song Y, Hyland C, Park JO, Lindeman N, Gale CM, Zhao X, Christensen J et al (2007) MET amplification leads to gefitinib resistance in lung cancer by activating ERBB3 signaling. Science 316:1039–1043
67. Pao W, Miller VA, Politi KA, Riely GJ, Somwar R, Zakowski MF, Kris MG, Varmus H (2005) Acquired resistance of lung adenocarcinomas to gefitinib or erlotinib is associated with a second mutation in the EGFR kinase domain. PLoS Med 2, e73
68. Farmer P, Bonnefoi H, Anderle P, Cameron D, Wirapati P, Becette V, André S, Piccart M, Campone M, Brain E et al (2009) A stroma-related gene signature predicts resistance to neoadjuvant chemotherapy in breast cancer. Nat Med 15:68–74
69. Finak G, Bertos N, Pepin F, Sadekova S, Souleimanova M, Zhao H, Chen H, Omeroglu G, Meterissian S, Omeroglu A et al (2008) Stromal gene expression predicts clinical outcome in breast cancer. Nat Med 14:518–527
70. Chang HY, Sneddon JB, Alizadeh AA, Sood R, West RB, Montgomery K, Chi JT, van de Rijn M, Botstein D, Brown PO (2004) Gene expression signature of fibroblast serum response predicts human cancer progression: similarities between tumors and wounds. PLoS Biol 2, E7
71. Navab R, Strumpf D, Bandarchi B, Zhu CQ, Pintilie M, Ramnarine VR, Ibrahimov E, Radulovich N, Leung L, Barczyk M et al (2011) Prognostic gene-expression signature of carcinoma-associated fibroblasts in non-small cell lung cancer. Proc Natl Acad Sci U S A 108:7160–7165
72. Ito M, Ishii G, Nagai K, Maeda R, Nakano Y, Ochiai A (2012) Prognostic impact of cancer-associated stromal cells in stage I lung adenocarcinoma patients. Chest 142:151–8
73. Nakamura H, Saji H, Ogata A, Hosaka M, Hagiwara M, Saijo T, Kawasaki N, Kato H (2003) cDNA microarray analysis of gene expression in pathologic stage IA nonsmall cell lung carcinomas. Cancer 97:2798–2805
74. Ramaswamy S, Ross KN, Lander ES, Golub TR (2003) A molecular signature of metastasis in primary solid tumors. Nat Genet 33:49–54
75. Ilie M, Long E, Hofman V, Selva E, Bonnetaud C, Boyer J, Vénissac N, Sanfiorenzo C, Ferrua B, Marquette CH et al (2014) Clinical value of circulating endothelial cells and of soluble CD146 levels in patients undergoing surgery for non-small cell lung cancer. Br J Cancer 110:1236–1243

76. Diaz-Montero CM, Salem ML, Nishimura MI, Garrett-Mayer E, Cole DJ, Montero AJ (2009) Increased circulating myeloid-derived suppressor cells correlate with clinical cancer stage, metastatic tumor burden, and doxorubicin-cyclophosphamide chemotherapy. Cancer Immunol Immunother 58:49–59
77. Sharma S, Dubinett S, Salgia R (2012) CD14(+)S100A9(+) myeloid-derived suppressor cells portend decreased survival in patients with advanced lung cancer. Am J Respir Crit Care Med 186:940–941
78. Bellocq A, Antoine M, Flahault A, Philippe C, Crestani B, Bernaudin JF, Mayaud C, Milleron B, Baud L, Cadranel J (1998) Neutrophil alveolitis in bronchioloalveolar carcinoma: induction by tumor-derived interleukin-8 and relation to clinical outcome. Am J Pathol 152:83–92
79. Eck M, Schmausser B, Scheller K, Brändlein S, Müller-Hermelink HK (2003) Pleiotropic effects of CXC chemokines in gastric carcinoma: differences in CXCL8 and CXCL1 expression between diffuse and intestinal types of gastric carcinoma. Clin Exp Immunol 134:508–515
80. Kimura YN, Watari K, Fotovati A, Hosoi F, Yasumoto K, Izumi H, Kohno K, Umezawa K, Iguchi H, Shirouzu K et al (2007) Inflammatory stimuli from macrophages and cancer cells synergistically promote tumor growth and angiogenesis. Cancer Sci 98:2009–2018
81. Al-Shibli K, Al-Saad S, Donnem T, Persson M, Bremnes RM, Busund LT (2009) The prognostic value of intraepithelial and stromal innate immune system cells in non-small cell lung carcinoma. Histopathology 55:301–312
82. Dieu-Nosjean MC, Antoine M, Danel C, Heudes D, Wislez M, Poulot V, Rabbe N, Laurans L, Tartour E, de Chaisemartin L et al (2008) Long-term survival for patients with non-small-cell lung cancer with intratumoral lymphoid structures. J Clin Oncol 26:4410–4417
83. Becker M, Müller CB, De Bastiani MA, Klamt F (2014) The prognostic impact of tumor-associated macrophages and intra-tumoral apoptosis in non-small cell lung cancer. Histol Histopathol 29:21–31
84. Dai F, Liu L, Che G, Yu N, Pu Q, Zhang S, Ma J, Ma L, You Z (2010) The number and microlocalization of tumor-associated immune cells are associated with patient's survival time in non-small cell lung cancer. BMC Cancer 10:220
85. Takanami I, Takeuchi K, Naruke M (2000) Mast cell density is associated with angiogenesis and poor prognosis in pulmonary adenocarcinoma. Cancer 88:2686–2692
86. Al-Shibli KI, Donnem T, Al-Saad S, Persson M, Bremnes RM, Busund LT (2008) Prognostic effect of epithelial and stromal lymphocyte infiltration in non-small cell lung cancer. Clin Cancer Res 14:5220–5227
87. Wakabayashi O, Yamazaki K, Oizumi S, Hommura F, Kinoshita I, Ogura S, Dosaka-Akita H, Nishimura M (2003) CD4+ T cells in cancer stroma, not CD8+ T cells in cancer cell nests, are associated with favorable prognosis in human non-small cell lung cancers. Cancer Sci 94:1003–1009
88. Shimizu K, Nakata M, Hirami Y, Yukawa T, Maeda A, Tanemoto K (2010) Tumor-infiltrating Foxp3+ regulatory T cells are correlated with cyclooxygenase-2 expression and are associated with recurrence in resected non-small cell lung cancer. J Thorac Oncol 5:585–590
89. Edlund K, Lindskog C, Saito A, Berglund A, Pontén F, Göransson-Kultima H, Isaksson A, Jirström K, Planck M, Johansson L et al (2012) CD99 is a novel prognostic stromal marker in non-small cell lung cancer. Int J Cancer 131:2264–2273
90. Lohr M, Edlund K, Botling J, Hammad S, Hellwig B, Othman A, Berglund A, Lambe M, Holmberg L, Ekman S et al (2013) The prognostic relevance of tumour-infiltrating plasma cells and immunoglobulin kappa C indicates an important role of the humoral immune response in non-small cell lung cancer. Cancer Lett 333:222–228
91. Demarchi LM, Reis MM, Palomino SA, Farhat C, Takagaki TY, Beyruti R, Saldiva PH, Capelozzi VL (2000) Prognostic values of stromal proportion and PCNA, Ki-67, and p53 proteins in patients with resected adenocarcinoma of the lung. Mod Pathol 13:511–520
92. Maeshima AM, Niki T, Maeshima A, Yamada T, Kondo H, Matsuno Y (2002) Modified scar grade: a prognostic indicator in small peripheral lung adenocarcinoma. Cancer 95:2546–2554

93. Shimosato Y, Suzuki A, Hashimoto T, Nishiwaki Y, Kodama T, Yoneyama T, Kameya T (1980) Prognostic implications of fibrotic focus (scar) in small peripheral lung cancers. Am J Surg Pathol 4:365–373
94. Augsten M (2014) Cancer-associated fibroblasts as another polarized cell type of the tumor microenvironment. Front Oncol 4:62
95. Madar S, Goldstein I, Rotter V (2013) 'Cancer associated fibroblasts'–more than meets the eye. Trends Mol Med 19:447–453
96. Polanska UM, Orimo A (2013) Carcinoma-associated fibroblasts: non-neoplastic tumour-promoting mesenchymal cells. J Cell Physiol 228:1651–1657
97. Bremnes RM, Dønnem T, Al-Saad S, Al-Shibli K, Andersen S, Sirera R, Camps C, Marinez I, Busund LT (2011) The role of tumor stroma in cancer progression and prognosis: emphasis on carcinoma-associated fibroblasts and non-small cell lung cancer. J Thorac Oncol 6:209–217
98. Direkze NC, Hodivala-Dilke K, Jeffery R, Hunt T, Poulsom R, Oukrif D, Alison MR, Wright NA (2004) Bone marrow contribution to tumor-associated myofibroblasts and fibroblasts. Cancer Res 64:8492–8495
99. Kalluri R, Zeisberg M (2006) Fibroblasts in cancer. Nat Rev Cancer 6:392–401
100. Ostman A, Augsten M (2009) Cancer-associated fibroblasts and tumor growth–bystanders turning into key players. Curr Opin Genet Dev 19:67–73
101. Tripathi M, Billet S, Bhowmick NA (2012) Understanding the role of stromal fibroblasts in cancer progression. Cell Adh Migr 6:231–235
102. Xing F, Saidou J, Watabe K (2010) Cancer associated fibroblasts (CAFs) in tumor microenvironment. Front Biosci 15:166–179
103. Abulaiti A, Shintani Y, Funaki S, Nakagiri T, Inoue M, Sawabata N, Minami M, Okumura M (2013) Interaction between non-small-cell lung cancer cells and fibroblasts via enhancement of TGF-β signaling by IL-6. Lung Cancer 82:204–213
104. Vicent S, Sayles LC, Vaka D, Khatri P, Gevaert O, Chen R, Zheng Y, Gillespie AK, Clarke N, Xu Y et al (2012) Cross-species functional analysis of cancer-associated fibroblasts identifies a critical role for CLCF1 and IL-6 in non-small cell lung cancer in vivo. Cancer Res 72:5744–5756
105. Chen WJ, Ho CC, Chang YL, Chen HY, Lin CA, Ling TY, Yu SL, Yuan SS, Chen YJ, Lin CY et al (2014) Cancer-associated fibroblasts regulate the plasticity of lung cancer stemness via paracrine signalling. Nat Commun 5:3472
106. Shintani Y, Abulaiti A, Kimura T, Funaki S, Nakagiri T, Inoue M, Sawabata N, Minami M, Morii E, Okumura M (2013) Pulmonary fibroblasts induce epithelial mesenchymal transition and some characteristics of stem cells in non-small cell lung cancer. Ann Thorac Surg 96:425–433
107. Wang W, Li Q, Yamada T, Matsumoto K, Matsumoto I, Oda M, Watanabe G, Kayano Y, Nishioka Y, Sone S et al (2009) Crosstalk to stromal fibroblasts induces resistance of lung cancer to epidermal growth factor receptor tyrosine kinase inhibitors. Clin Cancer Res 15:6630–6638
108. Yano S, Yamada T, Takeuchi S, Tachibana K, Minami Y, Yatabe Y, Mitsudomi T, Tanaka H, Kimura T, Kudoh S et al (2011) Hepatocyte growth factor expression in EGFR mutant lung cancer with intrinsic and acquired resistance to tyrosine kinase inhibitors in a Japanese cohort. J Thorac Oncol 6:2011–2017
109. Chaudhri VK, Salzler GG, Dick SA, Buckman MS, Sordella R, Karoly ED, Mohney R, Stiles BM, Elemento O, Altorki NK et al (2013) Metabolic alterations in lung cancer-associated fibroblasts correlated with increased glycolytic metabolism of the tumor. Mol Cancer Res 11:579–592
110. Franses JW, Edelman ER (2011) The evolution of endothelial regulatory paradigms in cancer biology and vascular repair. Cancer Res 71:7339–7344
111. Pober JS, Sessa WC (2007) Evolving functions of endothelial cells in inflammation. Nat Rev Immunol 7:803–815

112. Franses JW, Baker AB, Chitalia VC, Edelman ER (2011) Stromal endothelial cells directly influence cancer progression. Sci Transl Med 3:66ra65
113. Dundar E, Oner U, Peker BC, Metintas M, Isiksoy S, Ak G (2008) The significance and relationship between mast cells and tumour angiogenesis in non-small cell lung carcinoma. J Int Med Res 36:88–95
114. Herbst RS, Onn A, Sandler A (2005) Angiogenesis and lung cancer: prognostic and therapeutic implications. J Clin Oncol 23:3243–3256
115. Hu J, Bianchi F, Ferguson M, Cesario A, Margaritora S, Granone P, Goldstraw P, Tetlow M, Ratcliffe C, Nicholson AG et al (2005) Gene expression signature for angiogenic and nonangiogenic non-small-cell lung cancer. Oncogene 24:1212–1219
116. Offersen BV, Pfeiffer P, Hamilton-Dutoit S, Overgaard J (2001) Patterns of angiogenesis in nonsmall-cell lung carcinoma. Cancer 91:1500–1509
117. Ding BS, Nolan DJ, Guo P, Babazadeh AO, Cao Z, Rosenwaks Z, Crystal RG, Simons M, Sato TN, Worgall S et al (2011) Endothelial-derived angiocrine signals induce and sustain regenerative lung alveolarization. Cell 147:539–553
118. Lee JH, Bhang DH, Beede A, Huang TL, Stripp BR, Bloch KD, Wagers AJ, Tseng YH, Ryeom S, Kim CF (2014) Lung stem cell differentiation in mice directed by endothelial cells via a BMP4-NFATc1-thrombospondin-1 axis. Cell 156:440–455
119. Harris AL (2002) Hypoxia–a key regulatory factor in tumour growth. Nat Rev Cancer 2:38–47
120. Semenza GL (2003) Targeting HIF-1 for cancer therapy. Nat Rev Cancer 3:721–732
121. Li X, Lu Y, Liang K, Pan T, Mendelsohn J, Fan Z (2008) Requirement of hypoxia-inducible factor-1alpha down-regulation in mediating the antitumor activity of the anti-epidermal growth factor receptor monoclonal antibody cetuximab. Mol Cancer Ther 7:1207–1217
122. Minakata K, Takahashi F, Nara T, Hashimoto M, Tajima K, Murakami A, Nurwidya F, Yae S, Koizumi F, Moriyama H et al (2012) Hypoxia induces gefitinib resistance in non-small-cell lung cancer with both mutant and wild-type epidermal growth factor receptors. Cancer Sci 103:1946–1954
123. Murakami A, Takahashi F, Nurwidya F, Kobayashi I, Minakata K, Hashimoto M, Nara T, Kato M, Tajima K, Shimada N et al (2014) Hypoxia increases gefitinib-resistant lung cancer stem cells through the activation of insulin-like growth factor 1 receptor. PLoS One 9, e86459
124. Houghton AM (2013) Mechanistic links between COPD and lung cancer. Nat Rev Cancer 13:233–245
125. Lee JM, Yanagawa J, Peebles KA, Sharma S, Mao JT, Dubinett SM (2008) Inflammation in lung carcinogenesis: new targets for lung cancer chemoprevention and treatment. Crit Rev Oncol Hematol 66:208–217
126. Yao H, Rahman I (2009) Current concepts on the role of inflammation in COPD and lung cancer. Curr Opin Pharmacol 9:375–383
127. Keohavong P, Kahkonen B, Kinchington E, Yin J, Jin J, Liu X, Siegfried JM, DI YP (2011) K-ras mutations in lung tumors from NNK-treated mice with lipopolysaccharide-elicited lung inflammation. Anticancer Res 31:2877–2882
128. Xu X, Padilla MT, Li B, Wells A, Kato K, Tellez C, Belinsky SA, Kim KC, Lin Y (2014) MUC1 in macrophage: contributions to cigarette smoke-induced lung cancer. Cancer Res 74:460–470
129. Murin S, Inciardi J (2001) Cigarette smoking and the risk of pulmonary metastasis from breast cancer. Chest 119:1635–1640
130. Scanlon EF, Suh O, Murthy SM, Mettlin C, Reid SE, Cummings KM (1995) Influence of smoking on the development of lung metastases from breast cancer. Cancer 75:2693–2699
131. Abrams JA, Lee PC, Port JL, Altorki NK, Neugut AI (2008) Cigarette smoking and risk of lung metastasis from esophageal cancer. Cancer Epidemiol Biomarkers Prev 17:2707–2713
132. Murin S, Pinkerton KE, Hubbard NE, Erickson K (2004) The effect of cigarette smoke exposure on pulmonary metastatic disease in a murine model of metastatic breast cancer. Chest 125:1467–1471

133. Das Roy L, Pathangey LB, Tinder TL, Schettini JL, Gruber HE, Mukherjee P (2009) Breast-cancer-associated metastasis is significantly increased in a model of autoimmune arthritis. Breast Cancer Res 11:R56
134. Roy LD, Curry JM, Sahraei M, Besmer DM, Kidiyoor A, Gruber HE, Mukherjee P (2013) Arthritis augments breast cancer metastasis: role of mast cells and SCF/c-Kit signaling. Breast Cancer Res 15:R32
135. Yan L, Cai Q, Xu Y (2013) The ubiquitin-CXCR4 axis plays an important role in acute lung infection-enhanced lung tumor metastasis. Clin Cancer Res 19:4706–4716
136. Jiang M, Xu X, Bi Y, Xu J, Qin C, Han M (2014) Systemic inflammation promotes lung metastasis via E-selectin upregulation in mouse breast cancer model. Cancer Biol Ther 15:789–796
137. Stathopoulos GT, Sherrill TP, Han W, Sadikot RT, Yull FE, Blackwell TS, Fingleton B (2008) Host nuclear factor-kappaB activation potentiates lung cancer metastasis. Mol Cancer Res 6:364–371
138. Said N, Sanchez-Carbayo M, Smith SC, Theodorescu D (2012) RhoGDI2 suppresses lung metastasis in mice by reducing tumor versican expression and macrophage infiltration. J Clin Invest 122:1503–1518
139. Qian BZ, Li J, Zhang H, Kitamura T, Zhang J, Campion LR, Kaiser EA, Snyder LA, Pollard JW (2011) CCL2 recruits inflammatory monocytes to facilitate breast-tumour metastasis. Nature 475:222–225
140. Kim S, Takahashi H, Lin WW, Descargues P, Grivennikov S, Kim Y, Luo JL, Karin M (2009) Carcinoma-produced factors activate myeloid cells through TLR2 to stimulate metastasis. Nature 457:102–106
141. Carlini MJ, De Lorenzo MS, Puricelli L (2011) Cross-talk between tumor cells and the microenvironment at the metastatic niche. Curr Pharm Biotechnol 12:1900–1908
142. Erler JT, Bennewith KL, Cox TR, Lang G, Bird D, Koong A, Le QT, Giaccia AJ (2009) Hypoxia-induced lysyl oxidase is a critical mediator of bone marrow cell recruitment to form the premetastatic niche. Cancer Cell 15:35–44
143. Hiratsuka S, Watanabe A, Aburatani H, Maru Y (2006) Tumour-mediated upregulation of chemoattractants and recruitment of myeloid cells predetermines lung metastasis. Nat Cell Biol 8:1369–1375
144. Kaplan RN, Psaila B, Lyden D (2006) Bone marrow cells in the 'pre-metastatic niche': within bone and beyond. Cancer Metastasis Rev 25:521–529
145. Psaila B, Lyden D (2009) The metastatic niche: adapting the foreign soil. Nat Rev Cancer 9:285–293
146. Hiratsuka S, Watanabe A, Sakurai Y, Akashi-Takamura S, Ishibashi S, Miyake K, Shibuya M, Akira S, Aburatani H, Maru Y (2008) The S100A8-serum amyloid A3-TLR4 paracrine cascade establishes a pre-metastatic phase. Nat Cell Biol 10:1349–1355
147. Creelan BC (2014) Update on immune checkpoint inhibitors in lung cancer. Cancer Control 21:80–89
148. Fisher JP, Heuijerjans J, Yan M, Gustafsson K, Anderson J (2014) γδ T cells for cancer immunotherapy: a systematic review of clinical trials. Oncoimmunology 3:e27572
149. Bonneville M, O'Brien RL, Born WK (2010) Gammadelta T cell effector functions: a blend of innate programming and acquired plasticity. Nat Rev Immunol 10:467–478
150. Kang N, Zhou J, Zhang T, Wang L, Lu F, Cui Y, Cui L, He W (2009) Adoptive immunotherapy of lung cancer with immobilized anti-TCRgammadelta antibody-expanded human gammadelta T-cells in peripheral blood. Cancer Biol Ther 8:1540–1549
151. Nakajima J, Murakawa T, Fukami T, Goto S, Kaneko T, Yoshida Y, Takamoto S, Kakimi K (2010) A phase I study of adoptive immunotherapy for recurrent non-small-cell lung cancer patients with autologous gammadelta T cells. Eur J Cardiothorac Surg 37:1191–1197
152. Kobayashi H, Tanaka Y, Shimmura H, Minato N, Tanabe K (2010) Complete remission of lung metastasis following adoptive immunotherapy using activated autologous gammadelta T-cells in a patient with renal cell carcinoma. Anticancer Res 30:575–579
153. Kusmartsev SA, Kusmartseva IN, Afanasyev SG, Cherdyntseva NV (1998) Immunosuppressive cells in bone marrow of patients with stomach cancer. Adv Exp Med Biol 451:189–194

154. Young MR, Lathers DM (1999) Myeloid progenitor cells mediate immune suppression in patients with head and neck cancers. Int J Immunopharmacol 21:241–252
155. Young MR, Wright MA, Pandit R (1997) Myeloid differentiation treatment to diminish the presence of immune-suppressive CD34+ cells within human head and neck squamous cell carcinomas. J Immunol 159:990–996
156. Srivastava MK, Andersson Å, Zhu L, Harris-White M, Lee JM, Dubinett S, Sharma S (2012) Myeloid suppressor cells and immune modulation in lung cancer. Immunotherapy 4:291–304
157. Srivastava MK, Zhu L, Harris-White M, Kar UK, Kar U, Huang M, Johnson MF, Lee JM, Elashoff D, Strieter R et al (2012) Myeloid suppressor cell depletion augments antitumor activity in lung cancer. PLoS One 7, e40677
158. Nagaraj S, Youn JI, Weber H, Iclozan C, Lu L, Cotter MJ, Meyer C, Becerra CR, Fishman M, Antonia S et al (2010) Anti-inflammatory triterpenoid blocks immune suppressive function of MDSCs and improves immune response in cancer. Clin Cancer Res 16:1812–1823
159. Huang A, Zhang B, Wang B, Zhang F, Fan KX, Guo YJ (2013) Increased CD14(+)HLA-DR (-/low) myeloid-derived suppressor cells correlate with extrathoracic metastasis and poor response to chemotherapy in non-small cell lung cancer patients. Cancer Immunol Immunother 62:1439–1451
160. Paget S (1989) The distribution of secondary growths in cancer of the breast. 1889. Cancer Metastasis Rev 8:98–101
161. Kaplan RN, Riba RD, Zacharoulis S, Bramley AH, Vincent L, Costa C, MacDonald DD, Jin DK, Shido K, Kerns SA et al (2005) VEGFR1-positive haematopoietic bone marrow progenitors initiate the pre-metastatic niche. Nature 438:820–827
162. Chang J, Erler J (2014) Hypoxia-mediated metastasis. Adv Exp Med Biol 772:55–81
163. Erler JT, Bennewith KL, Nicolau M, Dornhöfer N, Kong C, Le QT, Chi JT, Jeffrey SS, Giaccia AJ (2006) Lysyl oxidase is essential for hypoxia-induced metastasis. Nature 440:1222–1226
164. Malanchi I, Santamaria-Martínez A, Susanto E, Peng H, Lehr HA, Delaloye JF, Huelsken J (2012) Interactions between cancer stem cells and their niche govern metastatic colonization. Nature 481:85–89
165. Oskarsson T, Acharyya S, Zhang XH, Vanharanta S, Tavazoie SF, Morris PG, Downey RJ, Manova-Todorova K, Brogi E, Massagué J (2011) Breast cancer cells produce tenascin C as a metastatic niche component to colonize the lungs. Nat Med 17:867–874
166. Gao D, Joshi N, Choi H, Ryu S, Hahn M, Catena R, Sadik H, Argani P, Wagner P, Vahdat LT et al (2012) Myeloid progenitor cells in the premetastatic lung promote metastases by inducing mesenchymal to epithelial transition. Cancer Res 72:1384–1394
167. Gao D, Nolan DJ, Mellick AS, Bambino K, McDonnell K, Mittal V (2008) Endothelial progenitor cells control the angiogenic switch in mouse lung metastasis. Science 319:195–198
168. Stefanovic S, Schuetz F, Sohn C, Beckhove P, Domschke C (2013) Bone marrow microenvironment in cancer patients: immunological aspects and clinical implications. Cancer Metastasis Rev 32:163–178
169. Catena R, Bhattacharya N, El Rayes T, Wang S, Choi H, Gao D, Ryu S, Joshi N, Bielenberg D, Lee SB et al (2013) Bone marrow-derived gr1+ cells can generate a metastasis-resistant microenvironment via induced secretion of thrombospondin-1. Cancer Discov 3:578–589
170. Junttila MR, de Sauvage FJ (2013) Influence of tumour micro-environment heterogeneity on therapeutic response. Nature 501:346–354
171. Meads MB, Gatenby RA, Dalton WS (2009) Environment-mediated drug resistance: a major contributor to minimal residual disease. Nat Rev Cancer 9:665–674
172. Paull T, Cortez D, Bowers B, Elledge S, Gellert M (2001) Direct DNA binding by Brca1. Proc Natl Acad Sci U S A 98:6086–6091
173. Ye Q, Hu Y, Zhong H, Nye A, Belmont A, Li R (2001) BRCA1-induced large-scale chromatin unfolding and allele-specific effects of cancer-predisposing mutations. J Cell Biol 155:911–921
174. Xu X, Wagner K, Larson D, Weaver Z, Li C, Ried T, Hennighausen L, Wynshaw-Boris A, Deng C (1999) Conditional mutation of Brca1 in mammary epithelial cells results in blunted ductal morphogenesis and tumour formation. Nat Genet 22:37–43
175. Thakur S, Croce C (1999) Positive regulation of the BRCA1 promoter. J Biol Chem 274:8837–8843

176. Xu C, Brown M, Chambers J, Griffiths B, Nicolai H, Solomon E (1995) Distinct transcription start sites generate two forms of BRCA1 mRNA. Hum Mol Genet 4:2259–2264
177. Xu C-F, Chambers J, Solomon E (1997) Complex regulation of the BRCA1 gene. J Biol Chem 272:20994–20997
178. Dimitrov S, Matouskova E, Forejt J (2001) Expression of BRCA1, NBR1 and NBR2 genes in human breast cancer cells. Folia Biol 47:120–127
179. Gudas J, Li T, Nguyen H, Jensen D, Rauscher F, Cowan K (1996) Cell cycle regulation of BRCA1 messenger RNA in human breast epithelial cells. Cell Growth Differ 7:717–723
180. Spillman M, Bowcock A (1996) BRCA1 and BRCA2 mRNA levels are coordinately elevated in human breast cancer cells in response to estrogen. Oncogene 13:1639–1645
181. Suen T, Goss P (1999) Transcription of BRCA1 is dependent on the formation of a specific protein-DNA complex on the minimal BRCA1 Bi-directional promoter. J Biol Chem 274:31297–31304
182. Romagnolo D, Annab L, Thompson T, Risinger J, Terry L, Barrett J, Afshari C (1998) Estrogen upregulation of BRCA1 expression with no effect on localization. Mol Carcinog 22:102–109
183. Atlas E, Stramwasser M, Whiskin K, Mueller C (2000) GA-binding protein alpha/beta is a critical regulator of the BRCA1 promoter. Oncogene 19:1933–1940
184. Marquis S, Rajan J, Wynshaw-Boris A, Xu J, Yin G, Abel K, Weber B, Chodosh L (1995) The developmental pattern of Brca1 expression implies a role in differentiation of the breast and other tissues. Nat Genet 11:17–26
185. Welcsh P, Lee M, Gonzalez-Hernandez R, Black D, Mahadevappa M, Swisher E, Warrington J, King M (2002) BRCA1 transcriptionally regulates genes involved in breast tumorigenesis. Proc Natl Acad Sci U S A 99:7560–7565
186. Hennighausen L, Robinson G (1998) Think globally, act locally: the making of a mouse mammary gland. Genes Dev 12:449–455
187. Blackshear P, Goldsworthy S, Foley J, McAllister K, Bennett L, Collins N, Bunch D, Brown P, Wiseman R, Davis B (1998) Brca1 and Brca2 expression patterns in mitotic and meiotic cells of mice. Oncogene 16:61–68
188. Rajan J, Marquis S, Gardner H, Chodosh L (1997) Developmental expression of Brca2 colocalizes with Brca1 and is associated with proliferation and differentiation in multiple tissues. Dev Biol 184:385–401
189. Du S, Barcellos-Hoff MH (2013) Biologically augmenting radiation therapy by inhibiting TGFβ actions in carcinomas. Semin Radiat Oncol 23:242–251
190. Vignard J, Mirey G, Salles B (2013) Ionizing-radiation induced DNA double-strand breaks: a direct and indirect lighting up. Radiother Oncol 108:362–369
191. Borges FT, Melo SA, Özdemir BC, Kato N, Revuelta I, Miller CA, Gattone VH, LeBleu VS, Kalluri R (2013) TGF-β1–containing exosomes from injured epithelial cells activate fibroblasts to initiate tissue regenerative responses and fibrosis. J Am Soc Nephrol 24:385–392
192. Kioi M, Vogel H, Schultz G, Hoffman RM, Harsh GR, Brown JM (2010) Inhibition of vasculogenesis, but not angiogenesis, prevents the recurrence of glioblastoma after irradiation in mice. J Clin Invest 120:694–705
193. Barcellos-Hoff MH, Park C, Wright EG (2005) Radiation and the microenvironment—tumorigenesis and therapy. Nat Rev Cancer 5:867–875
194. Begg AC, Stewart FA, Vens C (2011) Strategies to improve radiotherapy with targeted drugs. Nat Cancer Rev 11:239–253
195. Erickson AC, Barcellos-Hoff MH (2003) The not-so innocent bystander: microenvironment as a target of cancer therapy. Expert Opin Ther Targets 7:71–88
196. Hasegawa Y, Takanashi S, Kanehira Y, Tsushima T, Imai T, Okumura K (2001) Transforming growth factor-beta1 level correlates with angiogenesis, tumor progression, and prognosis in patients with nonsmall cell lung carcinoma. Cancer 91:964–971
197. Goldstraw P, Ball D, Jett JR, Le Chevalier T, Lim E, Nicholson AG, Shepherd FA (2011) Non-small-cell lung cancer. Lancet 378:1727–1740
198. Jarvis E, Kirk J, Clarke C (1998) Loss of nuclear BRCA1 expression in breast cancers is associated with a highly proliferative tumor phenotype. Cancer Genet Cytogenet 101:109–115

199. Akhurst RJ, Hata A (2012) Targeting the TGF[beta] signalling pathway in disease. Nat Rev Drug Discov 11:790–811
200. Mengxian Z, Kleber S, Roehrich M, Timke C, Han N, Tuettenberg J, Martin-Villalba A, Debus J, Peschke P, Wirkner U et al (2011) Blockade of TGF-beta signaling by the TGF{beta} R-I kinase Inhibitor LY2109761 enhances radiation response and prolongs survival in glioblastoma. Cancer Res 71:155–67
201. Zhang M, Herion TW, Timke C, Han N, Hauser K, Weber KJ, Peschke P, Wirkner U, Lahn M, Huber PE (2011) Trimodal glioblastoma treatment consisting of concurrent radiotherapy, temozolomide, and the novel TGF-β receptor I kinase inhibitor LY2109761. Neoplasia 13:537–549
202. Peñuelas S, Anido J, Prieto-Sánchez RM, Folch G, Barba I, Cuartas I, García-Dorado D, Poca MA, Sahuquillo J, Baselga J et al (2009) TGF-[beta] increases glioma-initiating cell self-renewal through the induction of LIF in human glioblastoma. Cancer Cell 15:315–327
203. Barcellos-Hoff MH, Akhurst RJ (2010) Transforming growth factor-beta in breast cancer: too much, too late. Breast Cancer Res Treat 11:202–208
204. Kirshner J, Jobling MF, Pajares MJ, Ravani SA, Glick A, Lavin M, Koslov S, Shiloh Y, Barcellos-Hoff MH (2006) Inhibition of TGFb1 signaling attenuates ATM activity in response to genotoxic stress. Cancer Res 66:10861–10868
205. Bouquet SF, Pal A, Pilones KA, Demaria S, Hann B, Akhurst RJ, Babb JS, Lonning SM, DeWyngaert JK, Formenti S et al (2011) Transforming growth factor β1 inhibition increases the radiosensitivity of breast cancer cells in vitro and promotes tumor control by radiation in vivo. Clin Cancer Res 17:6754–6765
206. Taylor J, Lymboura M, Pace P, A'hern R, Desai A, Shousha S, Coombes R, Ali S (1998) An important role for BRCA1 in breast cancer progression is indicated by its loss in a large proportion of non-familial breast cancers. Int J Cancer 79:334–342
207. Jones LP, Li M, Halama ED, Ma Y, Lubet R, Grubbs CJ, Deng CX, Rosen EM, Furth PA (2005) Promotion of mammary cancer development by tamoxifen in a mouse model of Brca1-mutation-related breast cancer. Oncogene 24:3554–3562
208. Barcellos-Hoff MH, Lyden D, Wang TC (2013) The evolution of the cancer niche during multistage carcinogenesis. Nat Rev Cancer 13:511–518
209. Formenti SC, Demaria S (2009) Systemic effects of local radiotherapy. Lancet Oncol 10:718–726
210. Yang L, DeBusk LM, Fukuda K, Fingleton B, Green-Jarvis B, Shyr Y, Matrisian LM, Carbone DP, Lin PC (2004) Expansion of myeloid immune suppressor Gr+ CD11b+ cells in tumor-bearing host directly promotes tumor angiogenesis. Cancer Cell 6:409–421
211. Shojaei F, Wu X, Malik AK, Zhong C, Baldwin ME, Schanz S, Fuh G, Gerber HP, Ferrara N (2007) Tumor refractoriness to anti-VEGF treatment is mediated by CD11b+ Gr1+ myeloid cells. Nat Biotechnol 25:911–920
212. Shaked Y, Ciarrocchi A, Franco M, Lee CR, Man S, Cheung AM, Hicklin DJ, Chaplin D, Foster FS, Benezra R et al (2006) Therapy-induced acute recruitment of circulating endothelial progenitor cells to tumors. Science 313:1785–1787
213. Jemal A, Tiwari RC, Murray T, Ghafoor A, Samuels A, Ward E, Feuer EJ, Thun MJ (2004) Cancer statistics, 2004. CA Cancer J Clin 54:8–29
214. Blumenschein GR (2012) Developmental antiangiogenic agents for the treatment of non-small cell lung cancer (NSCLC). Invest New Drugs 30:1802–1811
215. Korpanty G, Smyth E, Carney DN (2011) Update on anti-angiogenic therapy in non-small cell lung cancer: are we making progress? J Thorac Dis 3:19–29
216. Herbst RS (2008) Bevacizumab/chemotherapy in non-small-cell lung cancer: looking for a few good men? Clin Lung Cancer 9:75–76
217. Planchard D (2011) Bevacizumab in non-small-cell lung cancer: a review. Expert Rev Anticancer Ther 11:1163–1179
218. Sandler A, Gray R, Perry MC, Brahmer J, Schiller JH, Dowlati A, Lilenbaum R, Johnson DH (2006) Paclitaxel-carboplatin alone or with bevacizumab for non-small-cell lung cancer. N Engl J Med 355:2542–2550

219. Reck M, von Pawel J, Zatloukal P, Ramlau R, Gorbounova V, Hirsh V, Leighl N, Mezger J, Archer V, Moore N et al (2009) Phase III trial of cisplatin plus gemcitabine with either placebo or bevacizumab as first-line therapy for nonsquamous non-small-cell lung cancer: AVAil. J Clin Oncol 27:1227–1234
220. Huang J, Frischer JS, Serur A, Kadenhe A, Yokoi A, McCrudden KW, New T, O'Toole K, Zabski S, Rudge JS et al (2003) Regression of established tumors and metastases by potent vascular endothelial growth factor blockade. Proc Natl Acad Sci U S A 100:7785–7790
221. Neal JW, Wakelee HA (2013) Aflibercept in lung cancer. Expert Opin Biol Ther 13:115–120
222. Blumenschein GR, Kabbinavar F, Menon H, Mok TS, Stephenson J, Beck JT, Lakshmaiah K, Reckamp K, Hei YJ, Kracht K et al (2011) A phase II, multicenter, open-label randomized study of motesanib or bevacizumab in combination with paclitaxel and carboplatin for advanced nonsquamous non-small-cell lung cancer. Ann Oncol 22:2057–2067
223. Das M, Wakelee H (2012) Anti-angiogenic agents in Non-Small-Cell Lung Cancer (NSCLC): a perspective on the MONET1 (Motesanib NSCLC Efficacy and Tolerability) study. J Thorac Dis 4:558–561
224. Scagliotti GV, Vynnychenko I, Park K, Ichinose Y, Kubota K, Blackhall F, Pirker R, Galiulin R, Ciuleanu TE, Sydorenko O et al (2012) International, randomized, placebo-controlled, double-blind phase III study of motesanib plus carboplatin/paclitaxel in patients with advanced nonsquamous non-small-cell lung cancer: MONET1. J Clin Oncol 30:2829–2836
225. Paz-Ares LG, Biesma B, Heigener D, von Pawel J, Eisen T, Bennouna J, Zhang L, Liao M, Sun Y, Gans S et al (2012) Phase III, randomized, double-blind, placebo-controlled trial of gemcitabine/cisplatin alone or with sorafenib for the first-line treatment of advanced, nonsquamous non-small-cell lung cancer. J Clin Oncol 30:3084–3092
226. Reck M, Kaiser R, Mellemgaard A, Douillard JY, Orlov S, Krzakowski M, von Pawel J, Gottfried M, Bondarenko I, Liao M et al (2014) Docetaxel plus nintedanib versus docetaxel plus placebo in patients with previously treated non-small-cell lung cancer (LUME-Lung 1): a phase 3, double-blind, randomised controlled trial. Lancet Oncol 15:143–155
227. Lara PN, Douillard JY, Nakagawa K, von Pawel J, McKeage MJ, Albert I, Losonczy G, Reck M, Heo DS, Fan X et al (2011) Randomized phase III placebo-controlled trial of carboplatin and paclitaxel with or without the vascular disrupting agent vadimezan (ASA404) in advanced non-small-cell lung cancer. J Clin Oncol 29:2965–2971
228. McKeage MJ, Reck M, Jameson MB, Rosenthal MA, Gibbs D, Mainwaring PN, Freitag L, Sullivan R, Von Pawel J (2009) Phase II study of ASA404 (vadimezan, 5,6-dimethylxanthenone-4-acetic acid/DMXAA) 1800mg/m(2) combined with carboplatin and paclitaxel in previously untreated advanced non-small cell lung cancer. Lung Cancer 65:192–197
229. McKeage MJ, Von Pawel J, Reck M, Jameson MB, Rosenthal MA, Sullivan R, Gibbs D, Mainwaring PN, Serke M, Lafitte JJ et al (2008) Randomised phase II study of ASA404 combined with carboplatin and paclitaxel in previously untreated advanced non-small cell lung cancer. Br J Cancer 99:2006–2012
230. Aggarwal C, Somaiah N, Simon G (2012) Antiangiogenic agents in the management of non-small cell lung cancer: where do we stand now and where are we headed? Cancer Biol Ther 13:247–263
231. Wang D, Dubois RN (2006) Prostaglandins and cancer. Gut 55:115–122
232. Wall RJ, Shyr Y, Smalley W (2007) Nonsteroidal anti-inflammatory drugs and lung cancer risk: a population-based case control study. J Thorac Oncol 2:109–114
233. McCormack VA, Hung RJ, Brenner DR, Bickeböller H, Rosenberger A, Muscat JE, Lazarus P, Tjønneland A, Friis S, Christiani DC et al (2011) Aspirin and NSAID use and lung cancer risk: a pooled analysis in the International Lung Cancer Consortium (ILCCO). Cancer Causes Control 22:1709–1720
234. Edelman MJ, Hodgson L, Wang X, Kratzke RA, Vokes EE (2012) Cyclooxygenase-2 (COX-2) as a predictive marker for the use of COX-2 inhibitors in advanced non-small-cell lung cancer. J Clin Oncol 30:2019–2020; author reply 2020

235. Drazen JM (2005) COX-2 inhibitors–a lesson in unexpected problems. N Engl J Med 352:1131–1132
236. Daniluk J, Liu Y, Deng D, Chu J, Huang H, Gaiser S, Cruz-Monserrate Z, Wang H, Ji B, Logsdon CD (2012) An NF-κB pathway-mediated positive feedback loop amplifies Ras activity to pathological levels in mice. J Clin Invest 122:1519–1528
237. Xia Y, Yeddula N, Leblanc M, Ke E, Zhang Y, Oldfield E, Shaw RJ, Verma IM (2012) Reduced cell proliferation by IKK2 depletion in a mouse lung-cancer model. Nat Cell Biol 14:257–265
238. Langer CJ (2015) Emerging immunotherapies in the treatment of non-small cell lung cancer (NSCLC): the role of immune checkpoint inhibitors. Am J Clin Oncol 38:422–30
239. Callahan MK, Wolchok JD, Allison JP (2010) Anti-CTLA-4 antibody therapy: immune monitoring during clinical development of a novel immunotherapy. Semin Oncol 37:473–484
240. Wolchok JD, Hoos A, O'Day S, Weber JS, Hamid O, Lebbé C, Maio M, Binder M, Bohnsack O, Nichol G et al (2009) Guidelines for the evaluation of immune therapy activity in solid tumors: immune-related response criteria. Clin Cancer Res 15:7412–7420
241. Drilon A, Rekhtman N, Ladanyi M, Paik P (2012) Squamous-cell carcinomas of the lung: emerging biology, controversies, and the promise of targeted therapy. Lancet Oncol 13:e418–426
242. Konishi J, Yamazaki K, Azuma M, Kinoshita I, Dosaka-Akita H, Nishimura M (2004) B7-H1 expression on non-small cell lung cancer cells and its relationship with tumor-infiltrating lymphocytes and their PD-1 expression. Clin Cancer Res 10:5094–5100
243. Mu CY, Huang JA, Chen Y, Chen C, Zhang XG (2011) High expression of PD-L1 in lung cancer may contribute to poor prognosis and tumor cells immune escape through suppressing tumor infiltrating dendritic cells maturation. Med Oncol 28:682–688
244. Brahmer JR (2014) Immune checkpoint blockade: the hope for immunotherapy as a treatment of lung cancer? Semin Oncol 41:126–132
245. Sznol M, Chen L (2013) Antagonist antibodies to PD-1 and B7-H1 (PD-L1) in the treatment of advanced human cancer. Clin Cancer Res 19:1021–1034
246. Zhang Y, Huang S, Gong D, Qin Y, Shen Q (2010) Programmed death-1 upregulation is correlated with dysfunction of tumor-infiltrating CD8+ T lymphocytes in human non-small cell lung cancer. Cell Mol Immunol 7:389–395
247. Forde PM, Kelly RJ, Brahmer JR (2014) New strategies in lung cancer: translating immunotherapy into clinical practice. Clin Cancer Res 20:1067–1073
248. Lynch TJ, Bondarenko I, Luft A, Serwatowski P, Barlesi F, Chacko R, Sebastian M, Neal J, Lu H, Cuillerot JM et al (2012) Ipilimumab in combination with paclitaxel and carboplatin as first-line treatment in stage IIIB/IV non-small-cell lung cancer: results from a randomized, double-blind, multicenter phase II study. J Clin Oncol 30:2046–2054
249. Iwama S, De Remigis A, Callahan MK, Slovin SF, Wolchok JD, Caturegli P (2014) Pituitary expression of ctla-4 mediates hypophysitis secondary to administration of ctla-4 blocking antibody. Sci Transl Med 6:230ra245
250. Brahmer JR, Tykodi SS, Chow LQ, Hwu WJ, Topalian SL, Hwu P, Drake CG, Camacho LH, Kauh J, Odunsi K et al (2012) Safety and activity of anti-PD-L1 antibody in patients with advanced cancer. N Engl J Med 366:2455–2465
251. Al Omar S, Middleton D, Marshall E, Porter D, Xinarianos G, Raji O, Field JK, Christmas SE (2010) Associations between genes for killer immunoglobulin-like receptors and their ligands in patients with solid tumors. Hum Immunol 71:976–981
252. Diaz-Montero CM, Finke J, Montero AJ (2014) Myeloid-derived suppressor cells in cancer: therapeutic, predictive, and prognostic implications. Semin Oncol 41:174–184
253. Iclozan C, Antonia S, Chiappori A, Chen DT, Gabrilovich D (2013) Therapeutic regulation of myeloid-derived suppressor cells and immune response to cancer vaccine in patients with extensive stage small cell lung cancer. Cancer Immunol Immunother 62:909–918
254. Carney DN (2002) Lung cancer–time to move on from chemotherapy. N Engl J Med 346:126–128

255. Kerbel RS (2008) Tumor angiogenesis. N Engl J Med 358:2039–2049
256. Ebos JM, Lee CR, Cruz-Munoz W, Bjarnason GA, Christensen JG, Kerbel RS (2009) Accelerated metastasis after short-term treatment with a potent inhibitor of tumor angiogenesis. Cancer Cell 15:232–239
257. Paez-Ribes M, Allen E, Hudock J, Takeda T, Okuyama H, Vinals F, Inoue M, Bergers G, Hanahan D, Casanovas O (2009) Antiangiogenic therapy elicits malignant progression of tumors to increased local invasion and distant metastasis. Cancer Cell 15:220–231
258. Akbay EA, Koyama S, Carretero J, Altabef A, Tchaicha JH, Christensen CL, Mikse OR, Cherniack AD, Beauchamp EM, Pugh TJ et al (2013) Activation of the PD-1 pathway contributes to immune escape in EGFR-driven lung tumors. Cancer Discov 3:1355–1363

Epigenetics in Personalized Management of Lung Cancer

Aamir Ahmad

Abstract In last several years, the focus on the origin and progression of human cancers has shifted from genetic to epigenetic regulation, with particular attention to methylation and acetylation events that have profound effect on the eventual expression of oncogenes and the suppression of tumor suppressors. A few drugs targeting these epigenetic changes have already been approved for treatment, albeit not for lung cancer. With the recent advances in the push towards personalized therapy, questions have been asked about the possible targeting of epigenetic events for personalized lung cancer therapy. Some progress has been made but a lot needs to be done. In this chapter, a succinct review of these topics is provided.

Keywords Epigenetics • Methylation • Acetylation • DNMT • HDAC inhibitors

1 Introduction

Lung cancer is a deadly disease that affects millions of lives worldwide. It is the leading cause of cancer-related deaths [1] and the rate of incidence is only predicted to go up in coming decades [2]. A number of targeted therapies have been evaluated to fight lung cancer, primarily targeting the various signaling pathways [2], and the results are far from satisfactory. In recent years, epigenetic events have gained attention based on the many reports that support a crucial role of these events in tumor progression.

Although the concept of epigenetics was first introduced by Waddington more than 70 years back in the year 1939 [3], it was not until about 30 years back when the first connection between epigenetics and cancer was noted in the year 1983 when lower DNA methylation and 5-methylcytosine levels were observed in human tumors, compared to normal tissues [4, 5]. A number of studies have emerged in the recent years that advocate the importance of epigenetics in the management of

A. Ahmad (✉)
Karmanos Cancer Institute, Wayne State University, Detroit, MI 48201, USA
e-mail: ahmada@karmanos.org

A. Ahmad, S.M. Gadgeel (eds.), *Lung Cancer and Personalized Medicine: Novel Therapies and Clinical Management*, Advances in Experimental Medicine and Biology 890, DOI 10.1007/978-3-319-24932-2_6

human cancers [6–9]. Epigenetics has been studied in the context of tumor progression [10], drug resistance, cancer stem cells (CSCs) [11–13], epithelial-mesenchymal transition (EMT) [14, 15] as well as the microRNAs (miRNAs) [16, 17]. There is also an indication for the use of nutraceuticals to bring about epigenetic changes, leading to improved cancer therapy [18, 19]. A number of studies have focused on epigenetics in lung cancer [20–23] which gives us enough information to ponder on how to use this information for an efficient clinical management of lung cancer patients.

Towards the advancement of personalized therapy, it is important to identify gene(s) or a gene signature that may pre-dispose individual patients to poor prognosis. For the early stage non-small cell lung cancer (NSCLC) patients, curative surgery is the primary strategy. A majority of these patients with resected cancer do well but about 30 % patients exhibit relapse and ultimately succumb to this deadly disease [24]. With this problem in mind, Harris and his coworkers at NCI worked on identifying a genetic signature that can help prognosis of NSCLC patients at particular risk of relapse and progression. In an initial report [25], four genes—BRCA1, HIF1A, DLC1 and XPO1 were identified as the gene signature associated with prognosis. The study involved cohorts from different geographical locations—US, Japan and Norway. As relevant to discussion on personalized medicine, this work suggests that stage I NSCLC patients undergoing curative surgery should further be tested for these four genes and, based on the test results, be monitored on a regular basis or appropriately recommended for adjuvant chemotherapy.

In a follow-up study on the four gene cluster above, a more robust meta-analysis was recently reported [24]. A total of 12 publicly available cohorts were selected for the analysis with 1069 stage I lung cancer patients. Geographical locations represented in this study were—US, Japan, Norway, Sweden, France and South Korea. The major finding of this analysis was that the patients identified as ‘high risk’, based on the expression of four gene signature, had worse overall survival. Since the patient cohorts had wide diversity in race and ethnicity, the results seem to be robust enough to be applied to almost any populations. One interesting observation from this study was that the gene signature was found to be prognostic only for adenocarcinoma. When the analysis was extended to squamous cell carcinoma, no prognostic value of this four gene cluster was observed. Regardless, these studies have helped identify a cluster of four genes that can help fine tune the post-operative management of a subset of early stage lung cancer patients which is a critical step towards personalized medicine.

2 Epigenetics: Promises and Challenges

A number of concepts have emerged in the last decade or so, such as targeting EMT or the CSCs or the miRNAs but nothing very concrete has come out with regards to targeted therapies. In contrast, epigenetics is blessed to have been evaluated/targeted in clinics through the use of several drugs that effectively target methylation and histone acetylation [8]. Of all the different types of epigenetic changes, methylation and acetylation are the ones that have been studied in detail, with the aim of pharmacological intervention. Methylation is controlled by methyltransferases that increase methylation and the demethylases that decrease methylation. Acetylation is controlled by acetyl transferases that add acetyl groups (acetylation) and the deacetylases that remove acetyl groups (deacetylation). Acetylation generally leads to activation while deacetylation causes gene silencing [26]. Inhibitors of all these enzymes are being tested as anticancer therapies. This is ironical in a way, and exemplifies our evolving knowledge in the field. For example, inhibitors of histone deacetylases (HDACs), also called HDAC inhibitors, are one class of inhibitors that have gained a lot of attention with regards to their promise in anticancer therapy [27–29]. This is based on the concept that acetylation of genes is generally associated with reduced metastasis and reduced aggressiveness of cancers, and, therefore, deacteylation leads to increased metastasis and aggressiveness. It is thus conceived that inhibitors of deacetylases can work as anticancer agents by helping increase the acetylation of genes. While this concept has been tested well, through HDAC inhibitors such as trichostatin A and suberoylanilide hydroxamic acid (SAHA), it is interesting to mention that even the inhibitors of histone acetyltransferases (HATs), referred to as HAT inhibitors, have been proposed as promising anticancer agents [30, 31]. HDAC inhibitor trichostatin A has shown promise against small cell lung cancer [32] while HDAC inhibitors entinostat [26], CG200745 [33] have shown promise against NSCLC. In a study performed in prostate cancer model [34], we reported that HDAC inhibitors induced EMT and also enriched the CSC markers. This study indicated that HDAC inhibition might actually be counterproductive and may increase the cancer aggressiveness. While this may provide rationale for the mostly disappointing results with HDAC inhibitors in clinics, it also makes a case for more detailed studies on understanding the precise balance of acetylation and deacetylation in human genome.

An interesting aspect about epigenetic changes is that these alterations are reversible [35]. This is in contrast to genetic changes which are not. Being reversible, epigenetic changes present unique opportunity as therapeutic targets that can potentially be modulated in clinical settings. A case has also been made for combining epigenetic drugs to make a broader impact but this mostly comes at a cost—increased toxicity and off-target effects. Studies to combat this are in progress and there are early indications that novel drugs with pleiotropic effects against DNMTs and HDACs might be the way to go [36].

3 Methylation

Methylation is one of the better studied epigenetic event [37]. It was the first identified epigenetic mark [38]. In the methylation of DNA, a methyl group is transferred to the cytosine nucleotide within the DNA. The most vulnerable sites for such methylation are the CpG islands i.e. cytosines that are immediately followed by guanines. Increased methylation (hypermethylation) leads to silencing of genes and, conversely, reduced methylation (hypomethylation) results in increased expression of genes. In a bioinformatics study that aimed to predict lung cancer, methylation of CpG islands was found to be the most important feature that influenced the predictive power [39] and methylation of CpG island has been proposed as a biomarker for early detection of lung cancers [40]. As mentioned above, methyltransferases add methyl groups while demethylases remove methyl groups. Thus, there is a dynamic process in place where methylation and demethylation events are synchronized to bring about the silencing and expression of genes, as needed. The main reason methylation is connected to gene silencing is because methylation makes genes inaccessible to cellular transcriptional machinery. Recently, DNA methylation patterns have been proposed as predictors of breast cancer [41] which makes it a valid assumption that similar predictors might be possible for lung cancer as well.

Three methyltransferases particularly involved in a bulk of methyl transfers are DNMT1 (DNA MethylTransferase-1), DNMT3A and DNMT3B. These DNMTs are attractive targets for drugs that affect methylation. A number of DNMT inhibitors are known, and some of them have been approved by FDA for treatment of specific cancers. Examples are 5-azacytidine and decitabine. EZH2 is another methyltransferase that adds methyl groups to its target histone H3 leading to suppression of tumor suppressors, which, in turn, leads to tumor progression and metastasis. Consequently, targeting of EZH2 in cancer therapy has been advocated [42–44]. EZH2 expression has been linked to acquisition of cancer stem cell properties and aggressive phenotype [45], thus validating its targeting for the treatment of human cancers. In NSCLC model, inhibition of epigenetic activity of EZH2 has been demonstrated to sensitize BRG1 and EGFR mutant lung cancers to inhibitors of topoisomerase II [46]. KMT1E/SETDB1 is yet another methyltransferase that methylates histone H3 and silences several genes. However, in contrast to EZH2, it is a tumor suppressor [47] that inhibits invasive and metastatic potential of lung cancer cells when over-expressed, and is significantly down-regulated in highly metastatic lung cancer cells. So, right here, we notice a conflict where one methyltransferase is oncogenic while the other one is a tumor-suppressor. EZH2 is comparatively more widely studied methyltransferase and we need to wait on more reports on KMT1E/SETDB1 to be able to make more sense of targeting these particular methyltransferases for the personalized treatment of lung cancers.

In addition to methylation of DNA, epigenetic changes also include methylation of histones wherein methyl group is transferred to individual amino acids in the histone proteins, for example, methylation of lysine 9 or lysine 27 in the histone H3 leading to H3K9me2/3 and H3K27me3 respectively. These methylations also lead to gene repression. There is also evidence of methylation leading to gene activation, such as the one seen in H3K4me3 [48]. While inhibitors of DNMTs were the first off the block, inhibitors of histone methyltransferases (HMTs) are also now being evaluated against many cancers [49].

Personalized treatment of lung cancer patients involving targeting of methylation, thus, comes across as a valid approach. In a cell line based study [50] that involved generation of highly aggressive lung cancer cells in vivo, a comparison of methylation status of parental vs. the derivative highly metastatic cells revealed significant changes in the DNA methylation. Inhibition of DNMT, by azacytidine, reversed the metastatic phenotype, thus confirming the important role of DNA methylation in the metastatic potential in a lung cancer model.

4 Hypomethylation

As a proof that reduced methylation, or 'hypomethylation', causes over-expression, it has been reported that oncogenic KCNN4's promoter is hypomethylated and, therefore, KCNN4 is over-expressed in aggressive NSCLC cells [51] which also makes it a strong predictor for poor prognosis. Hypomethylation was also found prevalent in tumors, compared to adjacent non-malignant lung tissues, in a study that looked at lung cancers in non-smokers [52]. Tumors were found to be typically hypomethylated which would suggest over-expression of many oncogenes. Such differential methylation was particularly concentrated at CpG sites, although non-CpG sites were also found to be differentially methylated. ELMO3 (engulfment and cell motility 3) is another oncogene that was found to be hypomethylated, consistent with its over-expression in primary tumors from patients with distant metastases [53]. As suggested by these recent reports, it is evident that a role of reduced methylation, leading to induced expression of oncogenes, is increasingly being realized. From the perspective of personalized therapy, hypomethylation will need to be countered with increased rate of methylation, or the use of inhibitors that can target demethylases. This is rather a novel area of research as most of the focus has been on the inhibitors of methyltransferases. With the expansion of our knowledge on this subject, it would be interesting to evaluate findings with inhibitors of demethylases.

5 Hypermethylation

Hypermethylation is a more widely studied epigenetic event. As discussed by Barrow and Michels [54], there is evidence for hypermethylation of specific genes that can potentially be used for early diagnosis of lung cancer or for the identification of individuals at particular high risk. For example, methylation of three genes (*CDKN2A/p16*, *DAPK*, and *RASSF1A*) in sputum, conferred a significant increase in risk (OR > 1.5), particularly in smokers [55]. To test if such hypermethylation can be an early predictive event, analyses of sputum collected 18 or 19–72 months prior to diagnosis were performed. In samples collected within 18 months of diagnosis, a 6.5-fold increase in the risk of lung cancer was observed in individuals with hypermethylation of at least three genes from a six-gene panel (*CDKN2A/p16*, *DAPK*, *RASSF1A*, *GATA5*, *MGMT* and *PAX5 β*). However, 36 % controls also had similar hypermethylation. In samples collected 19–72 months before diagnosis, hypermethylation of just one gene (*CDKN2A/p16*) conferred an 80 % increased risk of developing cancer. Further, another study reported hypermethylation of *CDKN2A/p16* and *RASSF1A* in only 1 of 18 sputum samples [56], thus putting a question mark on the utility of *CDKN2A/p16* and *RASSF1A* hypermethylation as biomarkers. A meta-analysis of 18 studies did identify hypermethylation of *CDKN2A/p16* as predictive of reduced disease-free survival [57]. Combined, it is evident that more detailed studies are needed to establish a role of hypermethylation of select genes as markers for lung cancer.

Multiple reports have found a connection between hypermethylation and reduced expression/silencing of genes. For example, β-catenin [58], CDH13 [59] and MARVELD1 [60] were reported to be epigenetically silenced through hypermethylation in lung cancers. Liu *et al.* reported hypermethylation of tumor suppressor TMEM196 [61] which was consistent with its reduced expression leading to aggressive lung cancer. Hypermethylation was found in close to two-thirds primary lung tumors and correlated with shortened survival, poor differentiation and pathological stage. Such hypermethylation of CpG islands has been linked to prognosis in stage I lung adenocarcinoma in an independent study [62]. In another example of hypermethylation-mediated suppression, NPTX1 was found to be hypermethylated at its promoter in lung cancer cells [63]. Hypermethylation was also observed in neoplastic human lung specimens, which correlated negatively with the mRNA levels of NPTX1. The overall survival time was significantly reduced in patients that harbored hypermethylated NPTX1. Li *et al.* [64] found evidence of hypermethylation of SOX1 in two-thirds of human lung cancer specimens which contrasted with increased methylation in just a quarter of adjacent normal lung tissues. As expected, methylation inversely correlated with SOX1 expression in NSCLC cells. Interestingly, an association between smoking and promoter hypermethylation has also been observed [65].

6 Epigenetics in Drug Resistance of Lung Cancers

Resistance to standard therapies is a major clinical problem. In recent years, some evidence has emerged that establishes a connection between epigenetic events and resistance to therapies. As an example, reduced methylation and resulting over-expression of MEOX2 correlated with chemoresistance in lung cancer patients [66]. HDAC inhibitors SAHA and ST3595 were found to significantly reduce the aggressive phenotype of cisplatin-resistant NSCLC cells A549 and H460 [67]. This was attributed to the ability of HDAC inhibitors to up-regulate tumor suppressor KiSS1. In a study that used paired cell lines—parental and doxorubicin resistant lung cancer cells A549, a number of epigenetic markers were found to be differentially expressed [68]. These included reduced levels of HDACs, DNMT and acetylated histones in the resistant cells, relative to parental cells. Trichostatin A and 5-aza-2′-deoxycytidine, the epigenetic modifiers re-sensitized resistant cells to doxorubicin, thus validating an important role of epigenetic modifications in the acquisition of drug resistance in lung cancer cells. Epigenetic changes can modulate sensitivity to docetaxel as well because DNA methylation and resulting suppression of tumor-suppressor DKK3 (Dickkopf-related protein 3) has been linked to docetaxel resistance in NSCLC cells [69].

Although these reports are indicative of a role of epigenetic changes in drug resistance, and also point to the possibility of developing a personalized plan for the effective reversal of epigenetic changes for the successful 're-sensitization' to available therapies, it is important to note that the information on the subject is still evolving and more robust studies need to be planned. This notion is highlighted by a recent study that observed no-to-minimal utility of using epigenetic drugs as sensitization agents in different models representing NSCLCs [70].

7 Epigenetic Epidemiology

Another interesting concept that can be exploited in relation to personalized therapy of lung cancer is the study of epigenetic epidemiology [54]. This is a study of correlations between epigenetic variations and the risk of cancer within populations. The central concept is that population-wide analyses can help identify epigenetic changes that can predict either the onset of particular cancers or even resistance to therapies. For example, in lung cancer, tobacco smoke and air pollution are known risk factors that can influence DNA methylation. There is evidence of hypomethylation of *F2RL3*, *AHRR* and two intergenic regions smokers' blood, compared to non-smokers [71, 72]. *AHRR* stood out as a gene that significantly hypomethylated. It was interesting to note that hypomethylation could be detected in former smokers, albeit at a lesser degree, which is suggestive of a possible use of this gene as long-term marker of exposure [54]. Air pollution can also influence hypomethylation, as evident by hypomethylation of LINE-1 elements in leukocytes when exposed to black carbon and $PM_{2.5}$ [73]. Since tobacco smoke and air pollution represent high risk factors for lung cancers, understanding how they affect the epigenome will be important for early diagnosis of the disease. Such studies with broader populations can potentially yield some interesting results but are also prone to inconclusive findings, given the heterogeneity among individuals. They might also not be relevant to personalized therapy just because of the wider appeal, as opposed to focus on an individual patient.

8 Personalized Epigenetic Therapy: A Reality Check

As discussed in the preceding sections, we are slowly but surely realizing the big impact that epigenetic events seem to have on the onset, progression and outcome of lung cancers. However, it is still too premature to imagine a patient on a therapeutic path, based on that patient's individual epigenome. There are many challenges that need to be overcome. The first and foremost is the mapping of patient's epigenome and the need to decipher all the unique epigenetic signatures that the patient presents. As might be evident from the discussion here, methylation and acetylation represent two better understood epigenetic events. However, there are several more epigenetic events that have although been recognized, such as ubiquitination, phosphorylation, sumoylation etc., but not necessarily studied in relatively detail. Many methodologies are emerging that have enabled high throughput analyses, again mostly focused on methylation and acetylation, but they do have associated economic barriers. Even when we go beyond this challenge, the next and even more formidable hurdle is the lack of targeted therapies to reverse the epigenetic changes for effective enforcement of personalized therapy. This is something that will only get better with more detailed studies. Clearly this area of cancer research is still in its infancy. Data from mostly in vitro studies is emerging with some encouraging validations in lung tumor specimens. The missing connection between these preclinical studies and the future clinical trials is the lack of appropriate in vivo models, although there seems to be some progress on that front too [74]. In an effort to make targeting of epigenetic events a part of personalized therapy, the next few years will be crucial. We will hopefully see more mechanism-based studies that will help establish clear marker sets that can eventually be tested as predictors or biomarkers.

9 Conclusions and Perspective

Enormous advances in last few years, like for example the next-generation DNA sequencing have aided in the evaluation of epigenetic events that accompany diseases, including cancer. We have seen an exponential increase in the research publications on the topic of epigenetics in cancer in recent years. By all indications, this area of research is not going to slow down. Several epigenetic therapies have been approved by FDA [75] and many more are in the pipeline. These advances, particularly in clinical trials, only verify the big potential of epigenetics in current cancer research because we clearly do not have a final word on how the epigenetic events are finely tuned, and, more importantly, how can they be manipulated by therapeutic interventions for the benefit of patients in clinics. While 'modifying' epigenome, it is important to recognize that epigenetic changes are rather global and are inherently associated with off-target effects, and the resulting toxicity. A tight regulation of epigenetic events can be achieved by targeting epigenetic enzymes to specific loci through the use of DNA-binding proteins such as zinc finger proteins (ZFPs), transcription activator-like effectors (TALEs) and clustered regularly interspaced short palindromic repeats (CRISPRs) [49]. This is an interesting concept and results from pre-clinical and clinical studies will be eagerly awaited.

References

1. Siegel RL, Miller KD, Jemal A (2015) Cancer statistics, 2015. CA Cancer J Clin 65(1):5–29
2. Arcaro A (2015) Targeted therapies for small cell lung cancer: where do we stand? Crit Rev Oncol Hematol 95:133–264
3. Esteller M (2008) Epigenetics in cancer. N Engl J Med 358(11):1148–1159
4. Feinberg AP, Vogelstein B (1983) Hypomethylation distinguishes genes of some human cancers from their normal counterparts. Nature 301(5895):89–92
5. Gama-Sosa MA, Slagel VA, Trewyn RW, Oxenhandler R, Kuo KC, Gehrke CW et al (1983) The 5-methylcytosine content of DNA from human tumors. Nucleic Acids Res 11(19):6883–6894
6. Steenbergen RD, Snijders PJ, Heideman DA, Meijer CJ (2014) Clinical implications of (epi) genetic changes in HPV-induced cervical precancerous lesions. Nat Rev Cancer 14(6):395–405
7. Choi JD, Lee JS (2013) Interplay between epigenetics and genetics in cancer. Genomics Inform 11(4):164–173
8. Campbell RM, Tummino PJ (2014) Cancer epigenetics drug discovery and development: the challenge of hitting the mark. J Clin Invest 124(1):64–69
9. Heyn H, Esteller M (2012) DNA methylation profiling in the clinic: applications and challenges. Nat Rev Genet 13(10):679–692
10. Li J, Jin H, Wang X (2014) Epigenetic biomarkers: potential applications in gastrointestinal cancers. ISRN Gastroenterol 2014:464015
11. Shukla S, Meeran SM (2014) Epigenetics of cancer stem cells: pathways and therapeutics. Biochim Biophys Acta 1840(12):3494–3502
12. Ohnishi K, Semi K, Yamada Y (2014) Epigenetic regulation leading to induced pluripotency drives cancer development in vivo. Biochem Biophys Res Commun 455:10–15
13. Easwaran H, Tsai HC, Baylin SB (2014) Cancer epigenetics: tumor heterogeneity, plasticity of stem-like states, and drug resistance. Mol Cell 54(5):716–727
14. Tam WL, Weinberg RA (2013) The epigenetics of epithelial-mesenchymal plasticity in cancer. Nat Med 19(11):1438–1449
15. Wang Y, Shang Y (2013) Epigenetic control of epithelial-to-mesenchymal transition and cancer metastasis. Exp Cell Res 319(2):160–169
16. Liu X, Chen X, Yu X, Tao Y, Bode AM, Dong Z et al (2013) Regulation of microRNAs by epigenetics and their interplay involved in cancer. J Exp Clin Cancer Res 32:96
17. Baer C, Claus R, Plass C (2013) Genome-wide epigenetic regulation of miRNAs in cancer. Cancer Res 73(2):473–477
18. Ahmad A, Li Y, Bao B, Kong D, Sarkar FH (2014) Epigenetic regulation of miRNA-cancer stem cells nexus by nutraceuticals. Mol Nutr Food Res 58(1):79–86
19. Miceli M, Bontempo P, Nebbioso A, Altucci L (2014) Natural compounds in epigenetics: a current view. Food Chem Toxicol 73c:71–83
20. Langevin SM, Kratzke RA, Kelsey KT (2014) Epigenetics of lung cancer. Transl Res 165:74–90
21. Jakopovic M, Thomas A, Balasubramaniam S, Schrump D, Giaccone G, Bates SE (2013) Targeting the epigenome in lung cancer: expanding approaches to epigenetic therapy. Front Oncol 3:261
22. Vandermeers F, Neelature Sriramareddy S, Costa C, Hubaux R, Cosse JP, Willems L (2013) The role of epigenetics in malignant pleural mesothelioma. Lung Cancer 81(3):311–318
23. Balgkouranidou I, Liloglou T, Lianidou ES (2013) Lung cancer epigenetics: emerging biomarkers. Biomark Med 7(1):49–58
24. Okayama H, Schetter AJ, Ishigame T, Robles A, Kohno T, Yokota J et al (2014) The expression of four genes as a prognostic classifier for stage I lung adenocarcinoma in 12 independent cohorts. Cancer Epidemiol Biomarkers Prev 23:2884–2894

25. Akagi I, Okayama H, Schetter AJ, Robles AI, Kohno T, Bowman ED et al (2013) Combination of protein coding and noncoding gene expression as a robust prognostic classifier in stage I lung adenocarcinoma. Cancer Res 73(13):3821–3832
26. Ruiz R, Raez LE, Rolfo C (2015) Entinostat (SNDX-275) for the treatment of non-small cell lung cancer. Expert Opin Investig Drugs 24:1101–1109
27. Falkenberg KJ, Johnstone RW (2014) Histone deacetylases and their inhibitors in cancer, neurological diseases and immune disorders. Nat Rev Drug Discov 13(9):673–691
28. Heerboth S, Lapinska K, Snyder N, Leary M, Rollinson S, Sarkar S (2014) Use of epigenetic drugs in disease: an overview. Genet Epigenet 6:9–19
29. Mottamal M, Zheng S, Huang TL, Wang G (2015) Histone deacetylase inhibitors in clinical studies as templates for new anticancer agents. Molecules 20(3):3898–3941
30. Dekker FJ, Haisma HJ (2009) Histone acetyl transferases as emerging drug targets. Drug Discov Today 14(19–20):942–948
31. Manzo F, Tambaro FP, Mai A, Altucci L (2009) Histone acetyltransferase inhibitors and preclinical studies. Expert Opin Ther Pat 19(6):761–774
32. Platta CS, Greenblatt DY, Kunnimalaiyaan M, Chen H (2007) The HDAC inhibitor trichostatin A inhibits growth of small cell lung cancer cells. J Surg Res 142(2):219–226
33. Chun SM, Lee JY, Choi J, Lee JH, Hwang JJ, Kim CS et al (2015) Epigenetic modulation with HDAC inhibitor CG200745 induces anti-proliferation in non-small cell lung cancer cells. PLoS One 10(3), e0119379
34. Kong D, Ahmad A, Bao B, Li Y, Banerjee S, Sarkar FH (2012) Histone deacetylase inhibitors induce epithelial-to-mesenchymal transition in prostate cancer cells. PLoS One 7(9), e45045
35. Miozzo M, Vaira V, Sirchia SM (2015) Epigenetic alterations in cancer and personalized cancer treatment. Future Oncol 11(2):333–348
36. Shukla S, Khan S, Kumar S, Sinha S, Farhan M, Bora HK et al (2015) Cucurbitacin B alters the expression of tumor-related genes by epigenetic modifications in NSCLC and inhibits NNK-induced lung tumorigenesis. Cancer Prev Res (Phila) 8(6):552–562
37. Tang J, Xiong Y, Zhou HH, Chen XP (2014) DNA methylation and personalized medicine. J Clin Pharm Ther 39(6):621–627
38. Clark SJ, Statham A, Stirzaker C, Molloy PL, Frommer M (2006) DNA methylation: bisulphite modification and analysis. Nat Protoc 1(5):2353–2364
39. Li J, Ching T, Huang S, Garmire LX (2015) Using epigenomics data to predict gene expression in lung cancer. BMC Bioinf 16(suppl 5):S10
40. Kim Y, Kim DH (2015) CpG island hypermethylation as a biomarker for the early detection of lung cancer. Methods Mol Biol 1238:141–171
41. Khakpour G, Pooladi A, Izadi P, Noruzinia M, Tavakkoly Bazzaz J (2015) DNA methylation as a promising landscape: a simple blood test for breast cancer prediction. Tumour Biol 36:4905–4912
42. Volkel P, Dupret B, Le Bourhis X, Angrand PO (2015) Diverse involvement of EZH2 in cancer epigenetics. Am J Transl Res 7(2):175–193
43. McCabe MT, Creasy CL (2014) EZH2 as a potential target in cancer therapy. Epigenomics 6(3):341–351
44. Kondo Y (2014) Targeting histone methyltransferase EZH2 as cancer treatment. J Biochem 156(5):249–257
45. Kong D, Heath E, Chen W, Cher ML, Powell I, Heilbrun L et al (2012) Loss of let-7 up-regulates EZH2 in prostate cancer consistent with the acquisition of cancer stem cell signatures that are attenuated by BR-DIM. PLoS One 7(3), e33729
46. Fillmore CM, Xu C, Desai PT, Berry JM, Rowbotham SP, Lin YJ et al (2015) EZH2 inhibition sensitizes BRG1 and EGFR mutant lung tumours to TopoII inhibitors. Nature 520(7546):239–242
47. Wu PC, Lu JW, Yang JY, Lin IH, Ou DL, Lin YH et al (2014) H3K9 histone methyltransferase, KMT1E/SETDB1, cooperates with the SMAD2/3 pathway to suppress lung cancer metastasis. Cancer Res 74(24):7333–7343
48. Barski A, Cuddapah S, Cui K, Roh TY, Schones DE, Wang Z et al (2007) High-resolution profiling of histone methylations in the human genome. Cell 129(4):823–837

49. Falahi F, Sgro A, Blancafort P (2015) Epigenome engineering in cancer: fairytale or a realistic path to the clinic? Front Oncol 5:22
50. Dai SP, Xie C, Ding N, Zhang YJ, Han L, Han YW (2015) Targeted inhibition of genome-wide DNA methylation analysis in epigenetically modulated phenotypes in lung cancer. Med Oncol 32(6):615
51. Bulk E, Ay AS, Hammadi M, Ouadid-Ahidouch H, Schelhaas S, Hascher A et al (2015) Epigenetic dysregulation of K 3.1 channels induces poor prognosis in lung cancer. Int J Cancer 137:1306–1317
52. Mansfield AS, Wang L, Cunningham JM, Jen J, Kolbert CP, Sun Z et al (2015) DNA methylation and RNA expression profiles in lung adenocarcinomas of never-smokers. Cancer Genet 208(5):253–260
53. Soes S, Daugaard IL, Sorensen BS, Carus A, Mattheisen M, Alsner J et al (2014) Hypomethylation and increased expression of the putative oncogene ELMO3 are associated with lung cancer development and metastases formation. Oncoscience 1(5):367–374
54. Barrow TM, Michels KB (2014) Epigenetic epidemiology of cancer. Biochem Biophys Res Commun 455:70–83
55. Belinsky SA, Liechty KC, Gentry FD, Wolf HJ, Rogers J, Vu K et al (2006) Promoter hypermethylation of multiple genes in sputum precedes lung cancer incidence in a high-risk cohort. Cancer Res 66(6):3338–3344
56. Cirincione R, Lintas C, Conte D, Mariani L, Roz L, Vignola AM et al (2006) Methylation profile in tumor and sputum samples of lung cancer patients detected by spiral computed tomography: a nested case-control study. Int J Cancer 118(5):1248–1253
57. Lou-Qian Z, Rong Y, Ming L, Xin Y, Feng J, Lin X (2013) The prognostic value of epigenetic silencing of p16 gene in NSCLC patients: a systematic review and meta-analysis. PLoS One 8(1), e54970
58. Miao Y, Wang L, Zhang X, Xu X, Jiang G, Fan C et al (2014) Promoter methylation-mediated silencing of beta-catenin enhances invasiveness of non-small cell lung cancer and predicts adverse prognosis. PLoS One 9(11), e112258
59. Xue R, Yang C, Zhao F, Li D (2014) Prognostic significance of CDH13 hypermethylation and mRNA in NSCLC. Onco Targets Ther 7:1987–1996
60. Shi M, Wang S, Yao Y, Li Y, Zhang H, Han F et al (2014) Biological and clinical significance of epigenetic silencing of MARVELD1 gene in lung cancer. Sci Rep 4:7545
61. Liu WB, Han F, Jiang X, Chen HQ, Zhao H, Liu Y et al (2015) TMEM196 acts as a novel functional tumour suppressor inactivated by DNA methylation and is a potential prognostic biomarker in lung cancer. Oncotarget 6:21225–21239
62. Rhee YY, Lee TH, Song YS, Wen X, Kim H, Jheon S et al (2015) Prognostic significance of promoter CpG island hypermethylation and repetitive DNA hypomethylation in stage I lung adenocarcinoma. Virchows Arch 466(6):675–683
63. Zhou C, Qin Y, Xie Z, Zhang J, Yang M, Li S et al (2015) NPTX1 is a novel epigenetic regulation gene and associated with prognosis in lung cancer. Biochem Biophys Res Commun 458(2):381–386
64. Li N, Li S (2015) Epigenetic inactivation of SOX1 promotes cell migration in lung cancer. Tumour Biol 36:4603–4610
65. Li W, Deng J, Wang SS, Ma L, Pei J, Zeng XX et al (2014) Association of methylation of the RAR-beta gene with cigarette smoking in non-small cell lung cancer with Southern-Central Chinese population. Asian Pac J Cancer Prev 15(24):10937–10941
66. Avila-Moreno F, Armas-Lopez L, Alvarez-Moran AM, Lopez-Bujanda Z, Ortiz-Quintero B, Hidalgo-Miranda A et al (2014) Overexpression of MEOX2 and TWIST1 is associated with H3K27me3 levels and determines lung cancer chemoresistance and prognosis. PLoS One 9(12), e114104
67. Zuco V, Cassinelli G, Cossa G, Gatti L, Favini E, Tortoreto M et al (2015) Targeting the invasive phenotype of cisplatin-resistant non-small cell lung cancer cells by a novel histone deacetylase inhibitor. Biochem Pharmacol 94(2):79–90

68. El-Awady RA, Herzi F, Al-Tunaiji H, Saleh EM, Abdel-Wahab AH, Al Homssi A et al (2015) Epigenetics and miRNA as predictive markers and targets for lung cancer chemotherapy. Cancer Biol Ther 16:1056–1070
69. Tao L, Huang G, Chen Y, Chen L (2015) DNA methylation of DKK3 modulates docetaxel chemoresistance in human nonsmall cell lung cancer cell. Cancer Biother Radiopharm 30(2):100–106
70. Vendetti FP, Topper M, Huang P, Dobromilskaya I, Easwaran H, Wrangle J et al (2015) Evaluation of azacitidine and entinostat as sensitization agents to cytotoxic chemotherapy in preclinical models of non-small cell lung cancer. Oncotarget 6(1):56–70
71. Shenker NS, Polidoro S, van Veldhoven K, Sacerdote C, Ricceri F, Birrell MA et al (2013) Epigenome-wide association study in the European Prospective Investigation into Cancer and Nutrition (EPIC-Turin) identifies novel genetic loci associated with smoking. Hum Mol Genet 22(5):843–851
72. Shenker NS, Ueland PM, Polidoro S, van Veldhoven K, Ricceri F, Brown R et al (2013) DNA methylation as a long-term biomarker of exposure to tobacco smoke. Epidemiology 24(5):712–716
73. Baccarelli A, Wright RO, Bollati V, Tarantini L, Litonjua AA, Suh HH et al (2009) Rapid DNA methylation changes after exposure to traffic particles. Am J Respir Crit Care Med 179(7):572–578
74. Belinsky SA (2015) Unmasking the lung cancer epigenome. Annu Rev Physiol 77:453–474
75. Hamm CA, Costa FF (2015) Epigenomes as therapeutic targets. Pharmacol Ther 151:72–86

Next-Generation Sequencing and Applications to the Diagnosis and Treatment of Lung Cancer

Kristina M. Kruglyak, Erick Lin, and Frank S. Ong

Abstract Cancer is a genetic disease characterized by uncontrolled growth of abnormal cells. Over time, somatic mutations accumulate in the cells of an individual due to replication errors, chromosome segregation errors, or DNA damage. When not caught by traditional mechanisms, these somatic mutations can lead to cellular proliferation, the hallmark of cancer. Lung cancer is the leading cause of cancer-related mortality in the United States, accounting for approximately 160,000 deaths annually. Five year survival rates for lung cancer remain low (<50 %) for all stages, with even worse prognosis (<15 %) in late stage cases. Technological advances, including advances in next-generation sequencing (NGS), offer the vision of personalized medicine or precision oncology, wherein an individual's treatment can be based on his or her individual molecular profile, rather than on historical population-based medicine. Towards this end, NGS has already been used to identify new biomarker candidates for the early diagnosis of lung cancer and is increasingly used to guide personalized treatment decisions. In this review we will provide a high-level overview of NGS technology and summarize its application to the diagnosis and treatment of lung cancer. We will also describe how NGS can drive advances that bring us closer to precision oncology and discuss some of the technical challenges that will need to be overcome in order to realize this ultimate goal.

Keywords Next-generation sequencing • Cancer • Lung cancer • Precision oncology • Personalized medicine

K.M. Kruglyak, Ph.D.
Oncology, Illumina, Inc., San Diego, CA, USA

E. Lin, M.D., Ph.D.
Medical Affairs, Ambry Genetics, Inc., Aliso Viejo, CA, USA

F.S. Ong, M.D. (✉)
Medical Affairs and Clinical Development, NantHealth, LLC, Culver City, CA, USA
e-mail: frank.ong@nanthealth.com

A. Ahmad, S.M. Gadgeel (eds.), *Lung Cancer and Personalized Medicine: Novel Therapies and Clinical Management*, Advances in Experimental Medicine and Biology 890, DOI 10.1007/978-3-319-24932-2_7

1 Introduction

Cancer is characterized by uncontrolled growth of abnormal cells. While this fact has long been understood based on the presence of tumors in cancer patients, the understanding that these abnormal cells are unique at a genetic level has only arrived relatively recently [1]. Cancer is a genetic disease: over time, somatic mutations accumulate in the cells of an individual, due to replication errors [2], chromosome segregation errors, or DNA damage [3], and are not caught by traditional cellular mechanisms. When one of these somatic mutations confers a growth or survival advantage to the particular population of cells, by promoting cellular division or by inhibiting apoptosis, this clonal population proliferates and manifests as cancer.

Today more than 13.7 million Americans have a history of cancer. Furthermore, cancer is the second most common cause of death in the United States after heart disease. In terms of cancer-related mortality, lung cancer accounts for approximately 1.4 million deaths per year worldwide and approximately 160,000 deaths per year in the United States [ACS1 & 2]. To put this into perspective, in the US, lung cancer deaths account for approximately 27 % of all US cancer deaths which is more than colon, prostate and breast cancer deaths combined. For diagnosis, lung cancers are classified into two main histological types, small cell lung cancer (SCLC) and non-small cell lung cancer (NSCLC), that are based on the appearance of the neoplastic cells under a microscope. SCLC accounts for approximately 15 % of bronchogenic carcinomas while NSCLC accounts for the remaining 85 % of bronchogenic carcinomas. Regardless of histologic subtype, both SCLC and NSCLC have high mortality rates with survival rates that correlate directly with the stage of the lung cancer. For example, data from the National Cancer Institute's Surveillance, Epidemiology, and End Results (SEER) database, reveals that the 5-year survival rate of NSCLC as a function of stage are Stage IA (49 %), Stage IIA (30 %), Stage IIIA (14 %) and Stage IV (1 %). For SCLC, the 5-year survival rates based on stage are Stage I (30 %), Stage II (19 %), Stage III (8 %) and Stage IV (2 %).

The extremely high mortality rate of lung cancers can be attributed to several reasons. First, both SCLC and NSCLC tend to be caught at a late stage when treatments are less likely to be effective [4]. Second, even when caught early, treatments for lung cancer have a lower success rate than other cancer types such as breast [5]. Third, and perhaps most critically, the mutation burden of lung cancer patients with a history of smoking tends be higher than in patients with "age-related" cancers [6]. This last factor plays a crucial role in oncogenesis because as the number of somatic mutations increases, so too does the number of driver mutations—those mutations that confer a selective advantage to the tumor cell. As a consequence, the probability of identifying a single driver mutation with a corresponding single drug appropriate for that specific mutation is very low for most cancer patients. In the clinical scenario of cancers with high mutation burdens due to the accumulation of multiple causative or "driver" mutations, clinical oncologists only have a very limited armament of targeted therapies available to treat cancer patients.

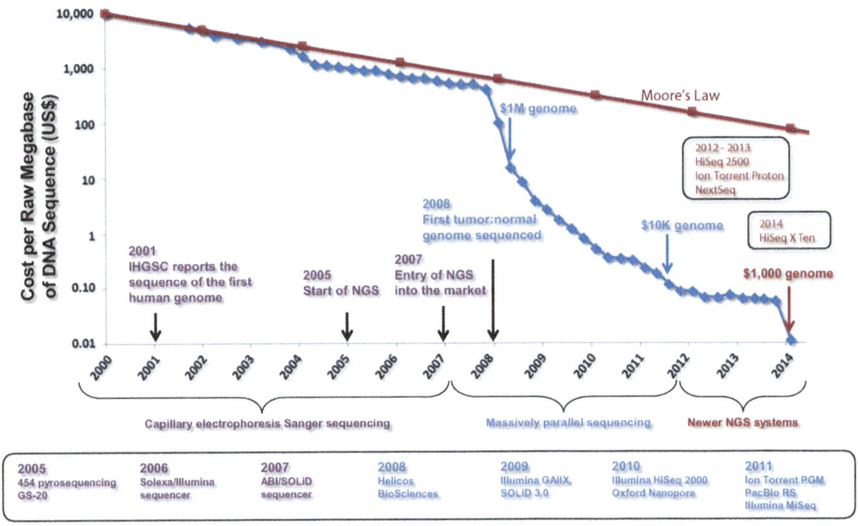

Fig. 1 The cost of DNA sequencing has decreased faster than Moore's Law since the introduction of NGS technologies. Landmark events are indicated by arrows on the timeline. The cost to sequence a full human genome has been driven to $1000 with the introduction of the Illumina HiSeqX instrument. Adapted from: MacConaill LE. Existing and emerging technologies for tumor genomic profiling. *Journal of Clinical Oncology*, 31(15), 1815–1824 (2013)

However, with the advent of next-generation sequencing (NGS), the promises of early detection and molecularly precise diagnosis for many cancers have given patients and clinicians new hope for targeted, personalized treatment and improved outcomes. The throughput and cost of NGS has reached the point where a whole human genome can be sequenced for less than $1000 [7] (Fig. 1). Targeted assays such as whole exome sequencing (WES) or multi-gene panels have become commonplace in the clinical research setting, and the performance of these assays combined with their cost are gradually displacing Sanger sequencing [8–12]. In the area of lung cancer, NGS has been used to identify promising biomarker candidates for early diagnosis, to detect the causative mutations in clinical cases, and to guide targeted treatment decisions [13–17].

2 General Applications of NGS

At the time of the completion of the first rough draft from the Human Genome Project in 2000, the cost to sequence a single human genome was approximately $3 billion and required years of dedicated work [18]. Today, genomic sequencing assays are ubiquitous in research, and the number of applications of NGS has grown correspondingly. NGS assays can be broadly separated into whether they are seeking to

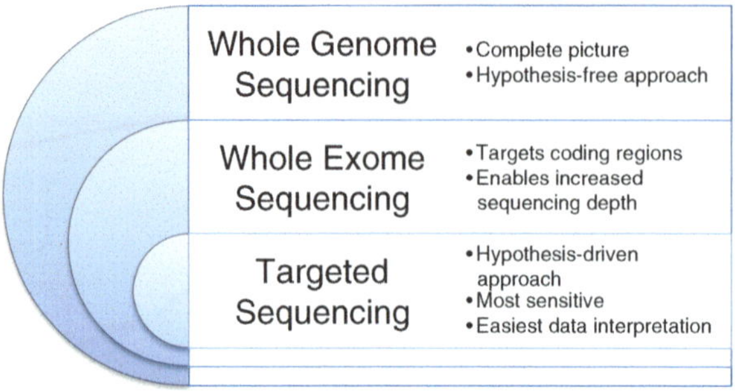

Fig. 2 Clinical NGS assays range from whole genome sequencing (WGS) to whole exome sequencing (WES) to targeted sequencing. WGS offers a hypothesis-free approach to identify somatic variants across the whole genome, though typical sequencing depth is below 100×. WES profiles the protein-coding region of the genome, which enables increased sequencing depth. Targeted sequencing assays focus on specific genes, regions, or variants in the genome that are known to be associated with the condition of interest. Targeted sequencing assays can provide a hypothesis-driven approach and allow for extremely high sequencing depth, which in turn improves the sensitivity of variant detection

decipher the genotype or the phenotype of a sample. Genotypic assays—aka DNA sequencing—differ as to the level of comprehensiveness they seek, ranging from focused assays that target only a handful of genes, to whole exome sequencing (WES), which targets the entire set of protein-encoding exons, to whole genome sequencing (WGS) (Fig. 2). Phenotypic assays comprise a broader spectrum of options, reflective of the fact that phenotype can manifest itself in many ways. Phenotypic changes that can be queried with NGS include a variety of epigenetic modifications of DNA that regulate gene expression and gene expression itself. We shall return to discuss some of these phenotypic assays in more detail after first discussing some of the considerations in selecting DNA sequencing assays.

WGS, WES, and targeted sequencing broadly fall into the category of DNA re-sequencing, meaning that DNA is sequenced, and the approaches differ in whether an entire genome, exome, or smaller sub-region is sequenced. The sequencing assay remains the same irrespective of the targeted area; the targeting process is addressed during sample preparation. The key factors in deciding which approach to take include: budget, the degree of exploration one wishes to engage in, and sample abundance and purity. Because targeted sequencing uses less reagents, computer time, data storage, and expert analysis, it is less expensive per sample than WGS. Given this, one of the chief benefits of targeted sequencing is that it is inexpensive enough to permit sequencing with great depth, that is, with many independent reads through a given region. By deeply sampling the regions of interest as shown in Fig. 3, one can discover mutations present even in the face of the two key sources of signal dilution in a cancer sample: contamination of the tumor specimen with normal cells and clonal heterogeneity. The notion of heterogeneity is particularly important in a disease such as lung cancer, where the mutation burden is high, even compared to other malignancies [19]. If one's purpose is simply to

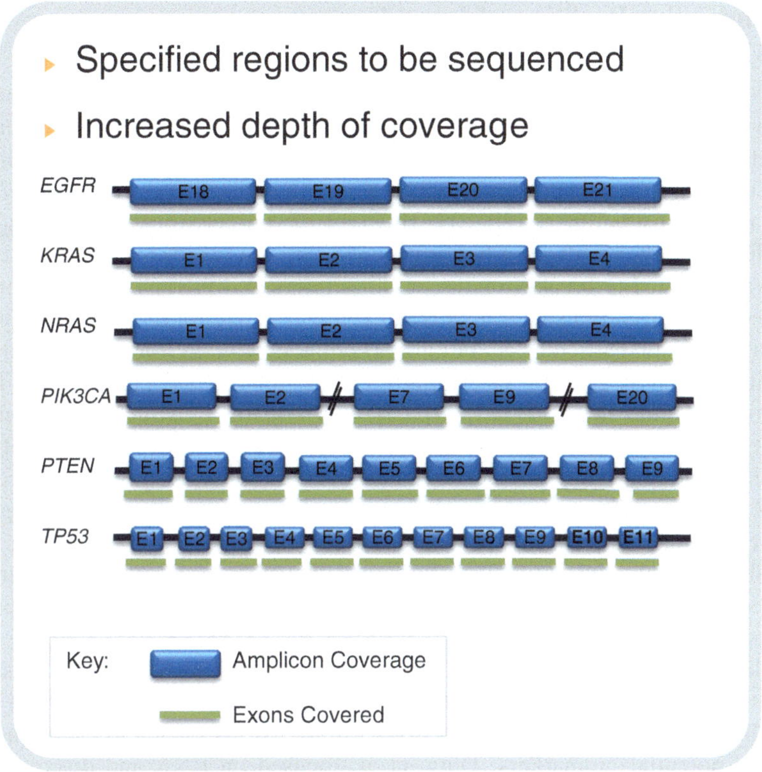

Fig. 3 Targeted sequencing assays allow the user to define custom content related to the condition of interest. In the case of lung cancer, a targeted sequencing panel may include specific exons of the genes *EGFR*, *KRAS*, *NRAS*, *PIK3CA*, *PTEN*, and *TP53*. By selectively targeting regions that have higher relevance to the condition of interest, the targeted regions can be sequenced to high depth, which in turn allows for high sensitivity

determine if a set of samples has mutations in a defined set of genes or hotspots (e.g., all exons of genes implicated in causing SCLC), then a narrow net can be cast, and targeted approaches are appropriate. The primary reason for performing was is to be comprehensive.

The most common phenotypic assay, RNA-Sequencing (RNA-Seq), analyzes RNA as opposed to DNA. RNA-Seq experiments are used to study the transcriptome of an organism, which, as a necessary intermediate of protein expression, and can be linked to phenotype, including disease state. Bisulfite sequencing is an application used to study the patterns of cytosine methylation in the genome that control the transcription of nearby genes to RNA. Similarly, NGS can be used to probe other aspects of epigenetic state, including chromatin-bound portions of DNA and those bound by particular transcription factors. Thus, like RNA-seq, bisulfite sequencing can be used as a readout of biological states linked to disease. All of these experimental techniques have been applied towards the understanding of lung cancer, with the goal of ultimately improving patient outcomes.

3 Molecular Profiling of Lung Cancer

Lung cancer has classically been defined as either SCLC or NSCLC based on the relative size of tumor cells under a microscope. These classes may be further subcategorized based on the genetic signatures present in each, especially in cases of tobacco-associated lung cancer, where G-to-T transversions in the *TP53* gene are a robust hallmark [20, 21]. This type of sub-classification points to the specific pathways involved in tumor progression; as a result, research into these pathways has led to breakthroughs in mutation-guided therapy for lung cancer. Many drugs currently used to treat NSCLC are effective for use only in a subset of patients with particular mutations. Treatment with *EGFR* tyrosine kinase inhibitors, such as gefitinib or erlotinib, is used for NSCLC patients who have somatic mutations in *EGFR* [22, 23]. Crizotinib treatment, which acts to inhibit *ALK* tyrosine kinase, is similarly prescribed for patients with fusions involving the *ALK* gene (e.g., *EML4-ALK*) [24]. However, these targeted therapies are not 100 % effective. Recent work has demonstrated that even within the same gene, different mutations may have different transcriptional effects [25], which may contribute to this sub-optimal performance. In such cases, it is important to understand the entire pathway, as mutations upstream may also be appropriate targets for therapy.

Other research has focused on identifying those cancers with high metastatic potential, with the goal of improving early detection rates for this important subset. This work has successfully employed a range of experimental techniques to identify potential biomarkers. Ding, et al. focused on RNA and discovered a single nucleotide variant (SNV) within the microRNA miRNA-502 that was associated with longer survival in SCLC patients [26]. Qian et al. performed bisulfite sequencing of NSCLC cell lines with low and high metastatic potential, and found +58CpG methylation in the latter group, which may affect metastatic potential through down-regulation of E-cadherin [27]. Most recently, Zhao, et al. performed WGS and WGS on both tumor tissue and adjacent normal tissue from ten patients with Stage I lung cancer. In addition to the well-known *EGFR* mutations, they also identified recurrent somatic variation in *BCHE* and *TP53*, which may serve as both biomarkers for early detection and new avenues for targeted treatments [28].

These examples illustrate the relative ease with which discoveries can be made in an important disease with the advent of sequencing-based methods. Additionally, as population-scale sequencing projects become more commonplace and the data from these experiments are made public, it will become easier for researchers to mine existing data rather than perform additional sequencing experiments (e.g., through resources such as the Cancer Genome Atlas or Sequence Read Archive). The widespread availability of "big data" may lead to the democratizing of medical breakthroughs, and perhaps speed up the pace of discovery and innovation.

4 Outstanding Technical Challenges

While NGS in its various forms have clearly contributed significantly to the understanding of cancer, many outstanding issues remain that NGS is currently not able to address. Though cancer is a genetic disease, the heterogeneity among the cells in a single tumor is astounding, making detection of low-level mutations difficult [29, 30]. Tumors are known to vary in terms of their mutational load; that is, secondary tumors are not genetically identical to the primary tumor from which they originate [29]. This fact is one possible explanation why the rate of relapse is so high in patients whose cancer has metastasized to a secondary location. Traditional treatments involve surgery to remove the primary tumor followed by one or more rounds of chemotherapy and/or radiation in order to destroy any traces of the cancer missed by the surgical extraction. Ideally, the preferred chemotherapy should be selected based on the specific genetic characteristics of that patient's cancer. For example, if one patient's cancer is driven by a mutation in *PTEN*, the selected treatment should not be the same as if his cancer were driven by a mutation in *KRAS*. In the former case *PTEN* acts as a tumor suppressor, and one possible goal of treatment would thus be to activate the corresponding pathway that the mutation presumably down-regulated. In the latter case, *KRAS* acts as an oncogene, and the goal of treatment would thus be to de-activate the pathway that was up-regulated in the cancer cells. While this makes intuitive sense, tumor heterogeneity makes such one-size-fit-all ideas impractical. A primary tumor, through driven by a mutation in a tumor suppressor gene, may give rise to secondary tumors, undetectable at the time of surgery, that additionally have mutations in one or more oncogenes [29]. Thus adjuvant chemotherapy will confer temporary remission, but only until the secondary population is detectable by clinical tests. Such circumstances are unfortunately all too common in cancer treatment.

Other technical difficulties persist as well. Because of tumor heterogeneity, some authors have recommended sequencing both primary and secondary tumors in order to understand the range of somatic mutations present [31–34]. Even in the case of a single primary tumor, some authors have proposed sequencing from multiple areas [35, 36]. In many cancers, but especially in the case of lung cancer, this requirement poses difficulties as the biopsy is both a painful procedure for the patient and can be technically challenging for interventional radiologists to perform based on tumor location(s) [30]. Additionally, requiring continuous biopsies in order to monitor the effect of treatment is not feasible long-term. One promising alternative to taking biopsies and sequencing tumors is to sequence circulating tumor DNA (ctDNA) via non-invasive blood draws [37, 38]. Though still being evaluated for feasibility, ctDNA has the potential to make cancer detection a standard laboratory assay.

Another issue relating to the clinical presentation of cancer is the fact that there are many disease subtypes that are not currently differentiable to the oncologist. In fact, each presentation of cancer in an individual is effectively unique. For example, in colorectal cancer, two subtypes exist: hypermutated and non-hypermutated.

In the former case, the genetic signature is marked by microsatellite instability; in the latter case, the genetic signature is differentiated by mutation of the *TP53* and *APC* genes. In non-hypermutated colorectal cancer, 60 % of patients have a mutation in *TP53*, while only 20 % of patients with the non-hypermutated form have such mutations [39]. One can envision future work further classifying non-hypermutated cancers into finer subtypes to guide treatment decisions. Ultimately however, this goal of increased granularity must give way to the view of cancer as an individual disease rather than as a disease to be treated based on population-level patterns and outcome statistics.

To eventually reach this goal, and also because of genetic heterogeneity, researchers are required to sequence a large number of samples in order to identify mutations that are of lower frequency in the general population [40]. The requisite number is magnified when one considers that the manifestation of subtypes may vary significantly based on population. For example, activating mutations of EGFR in NSLC tumors, have been found to be approximately tenfold higher in a Japanese NSLC population compared to a US population, which is consistent with previously observed population differences in response to EGFR inhibitors [22]. Thus, when performing genomic analysis for the purpose of biomarker discovery, it can be important to sample different populations to ensure that findings are broadly applicable. Accessing a large number of samples for research purposes is also hampered by basic sample collection difficulties, especially in the case of lung cancer, where the tumor is not easily accessible for biopsy, and the biopsy process itself is difficult and painful for the patient. It is clearly preferable to avoid multiple biopsies, but for the purposes of research, it is of extreme importance to understand the manner in which a tumor population changes over time and based on treatment. It would therefore be preferable for researchers to have access to a "liquid biopsy" based on blood, urine, or saliva, assuming that the tumor signature was detectable from such sources. Currently however, limitations in our knowledge of the stability and predictive value of circulating nucleic acids restricts their widespread use, though a large amount of work is being performed to reach this goal [41–44].

5 Outstanding Bioinformatics Challenges

All of the outstanding challenges listed above represent facets of the presentation of cancer that make its study difficult from a practical point of view; however, they also represent hurdles for the analysis of genetic data in general, specifically from the standpoint of downstream bioinformatics. When reviewing NGS data, tumor heterogeneity manifests itself as low-level somatic variants that are seen in only a small number of sequencing reads. For rare variants, identification may be difficult or impossible because they may not be differentiable from errors due to instrument noise [45]. For example, if the genome is sequenced to a mean depth of 100, then a variant present at a level of 1 % would be expected to appear in only one read. Currently, sequencing accuracy is very high, generally reported at 99.9 % or above for the majority of bases [46]. However, this implies that one base per thousand sequenced will be in error. At a depth of 100, this means that 300 billion bases will be sequenced across the genome, and therefore, that one in ten positions (or 300 million bases across the genome) will have a single read reporting an alternate base. Clearly, a cancer signature does not encompass 300 million sites, so a 1 % somatic frequency is effectively impossible to differentiate from noise. By contrast, a 5 % somatic frequency is much more unique, and setting such a threshold (or increasing sequencing depth) would reduce the number of false positive calls substantially.

A related bioinformatics challenge is the identification of variants beyond the well-studied SNVs and small indels. Complex variant types such as copy number variants (CNVs; loss or gain of one or more copies of a region of the genome), structural variants (SVs; include duplications, inversions, and translocations), and epigenetic variations all pose difficulties in detection and are therefore associated with higher error rates [47–51]. Both CNVs and SVs are more difficult to detect using the current generation of variant callers. In the case of CNVs, the variant will manifest as slightly higher or lower coverage on average in the particular CNV region compared to the remainder of the genome [48]. In the case of SVs, one read of a paired-end sequencing experiment will align to one part of the genome, and the other read will align to a different part of the genome [50].

Regardless of the variant type, once a set of variants is identified from a cancer sample, a further challenge is to classify each as driver vs. passenger [31, 34]. Current methods that are utilized in the clinical research setting for such classification are generally based on calculation of risk scores, such as SIFT or PolyPhen [52, 53]; determination of the protein coding effect of each mutation, either sense, missense, or nonsense; or identification within a relevant database, such as dbSNP, COSMIC, OMIM, or HapMap [54–57]. All of these methods are largely qualitative in nature, and the result of such methods is not a final classification of each variant, but rather a ranking of the identified variants according to likelihood of pathogenicity. Some pipelines endeavor to identify drivers vs. passengers at the gene level rather than at the variant level, with the rationale that many variants within a single gene are more likely to affect its function and are thus related to cancer progression [19, 58–60]. Many studies have been published across cancer types that identify risk genes rather than specific variants; however, more recently, prominent groups have raised concern with this method, since as sample size increases, the significant results balloons and is dominated by false positives [19]. After noting many published studies that implausibly identified olfactory receptors as risk genes for a wide range of cancers, Lawrence, et al. developed MutSigCV, which accounts for the mutational heterogeneity of cancer when evaluating candidate genes [19]. Related tools to identify driver variants and genes have been developed by other groups and are well-summarized by Gonzalez-Perez et al. [61].

6 Present and Future of NGS-Based Cancer Assays

Perhaps some of the most serious challenges to the realization of personalized medicine are not technical, but rather those related to institutional adoption and barriers related to the workflow in the practice of medicine. Until NGS-based assays and

WGS are reimbursed by insurance carriers, the hurdle to widespread adoption is impossibly high. Even after a majority of carriers and providers adopt this technology, incorporation of NGS results into a patient's EHR is a daunting proposition [62–66]. In a review of six CSER sites that are incorporating WGS and WES into the EHR, Tarczy-Hornoch et al. reported that development across sites was independent and non-standardized [67]. Workflows varied widely, and in all cases, the final output was a human-readable, PDF report that was attached to the EHR, with only three sites additionally providing a machine-readable version of identified variants. Progress in institutional implementation is generally much slower than the pace of development, so it is important that this issue is addressed quickly and collaboratively by healthcare networks and EHR vendors [62], ideally with input from the NGS community.

Though challenges exist, NGS in clinical oncology has already achieved more than most could have predicted. WGS is now part of the physician-patient discussion when evaluating options around cancer treatment, a state that was unimaginable even a few years ago. NGS has the potential to transform all aspects of cancer treatment: detection, treatment decision, and various monitoring aspects. As more biomarkers are associated with specific forms of cancer and therapies, it will be easier to design targeted assays that effectively act as "cancer screens" and can be applied quickly and cheaply to an entire at-risk population, comparable to today's blood panel tests. Notably, as the cost of WGS decreases, it will be most effective to sequence the entire genome, and then bioinformatically report only those variants or genes requested by the treating physician, perhaps with guidance from medical standards setting organizations. Such a non-invasive, broad screening option will increase the rate of early detection across all cancer types, ideally allowing treatments to begin prior to metastasis. Those treatments will also be guided by the results from WGS. As described above, chemotherapy tailored to an individual's mutational spectrum will have a much greater success rate than a general therapy that may not target the specific driver mutations of that individual. After a treatment option is chosen, NGS methods can be used to monitor the efficacy of that treatment over a specific period of time. For example, if a patient's lung cancer is shown to be dominated by a specific mutation in *EGFR*, then regular targeted screenings for this variant can show the success or failure of the chosen treatment in near to real-time.

If the promise of ctDNA bears out, a ctDNA-based NGS-assay following surgery will perhaps be used to identify whether the surgery was successful in removing the entirety of the tumor. The half-life of circulating DNA in the blood is less than half an hour [68], meaning that within 4 h of surgery, less than 1 % of ctDNA would remain in the blood if the surgery were successful. Thus, if the assay were administered one day following surgery and was able to detect any level of the variant in question, it would indicate that the surgical procedure was not complete. Similar screens administered quarterly will also serve as the best option for monitoring recurrence. Even today, with ctDNA methods in their infancy, NGS assays have been shown to be more sensitive compared to traditional imaging technologies used to monitor recurrence [38]. Eventually, NGS-based option will become the norm across the entire spectrum of cancer-related clinical procedures. The hope is that this will allow cancer to be considered a chronic disease; that is, a condition to be monitored and managed, rather than as a serious, acute condition as it is considered today.

7 Conclusion

We have presented a broad overview of the inroads that NGS has made and continues to make in the field of oncology, specifically lung cancer. Though we are only at the beginning of the era of personalized medicine, NGS is a powerful technology that has the potential to make even more major contributions to this field in terms of biological understanding and clinical treatments. Several other aspects unique to NGS, especially in terms of clinical applications, have not been discussed here, specifically, legal and ethical implications of incidental findings, the evolving concept of privacy in the context of inherited conditions, and general considerations related to the size of NGS data and its storage when WGS testing becomes routine. For a thorough discussion of these topics, we refer to Jackson et al. [69], Presidential Commission et al. [70], and Ury [65], respectively.

References

1. Stratton MR, Campbell PJ, Futreal PA (2009) The cancer genome. Nature 458:719–724
2. Peña-Diaz J et al (2012) Noncanonical mismatch repair as a source of genomic instability in human cells. Mol Cell 47:669–680
3. Pfeifer GP (2010) Environmental exposures and mutational patterns of cancer genomes. Genome Med 2:54
4. Heuvers ME, Wisnivesky J, Stricker BH, Aerts JG (2012) Generalizabliity of results from the National Lung Screening Trial. Eur J Epidemiol 27:669–672
5. National Lung Screening Trial Research Team et al (2011) Reduced lung-cancer mortality with low-dose computed tomographic screening. N Engl J Med 365:395–409
6. Alexandrov LB et al (2013) Signatures of mutational processes in human cancer. Nature 500:415–421
7. Winnick E (2014) Illumina launches two new platforms at JP Morgan Conference; claims $1,000 genome. GenomeWeb 2014. http://www.genomeweb.com/sequencing/illumina-launches-two-new-platforms-jp-morgan-conference-claims-1000-genome. Accessed 27 Jan 2014
8. Adams MD et al (2012) Global mutational profiling of formalin-fixed human colon cancers from a pathology archive. Mod Pathol 25:1599–1608
9. Rehm HL (2013) Disease-targeted sequencing: a cornerstone in the clinic. Nat Rev Genet 14:295–300
10. Park JY, Kricka LJ, Fortina P (2013) Next-generation sequencing in the clinic. Nat Biotechnol 31:990–992
11. Strom SP et al (2014) Assessing the necessity of confirmatory testing for exome-sequencing results in a clinical molecular diagnostics laboratory. Genet Med 16(7):510–515
12. Grosu DS et al (2014) Clinical investigational studies for validation of the first next-generation sequencing *in vitro* diagnostic for cystic fibrosis testing. Expert Rev Mol Diagn 14(5): 605–622

13. Karnes HE, Duncavage EJ, Bernadt CT (2013) Targeted next-generation sequencing using fine-needle aspirates from adenocarcinomas of the lung. Cancer Cytopathol 122(2):104–113
14. Chen Y, Shi JX, Pan XF, Feng J, Zhao H (2013) Identification of candidate genes for lung cancer somatic mutation test kits. Genet Mol Biol 36:455–464
15. Wu K, Huang RS, House L, Cho WC (2013) Next-generation sequencing for lung cancer. Future Oncol 9:1323–1336
16. Tuononen K et al (2013) Comparison of targeted next-generation sequencing (NGS) and real-time PCR in the detection of EGFR, KRAS, and BRAF mutation on formalin-fixed, paraffin-embedded tumor material of non-small cell lung carcinoma—superiority of NGS. Genes Chromosomes Cancer 52:503–511
17. Buttitta F et al (2013) Effective assessment of egfr mutation status in bronchoalveolar lavage and pleural fluids by next-generation sequencing. Clin Cancer Res 19:691–698
18. Evans JP (2010) The human genome project at 10 years: a teachable moment. Genet Med 12:477
19. Lawrence MS et al (2013) Mutational heterogeneity in cancer and the search for new cancer-associated genes. Nature 499:214–218
20. Hainaut P, Pfeifer GP (2001) Patterns of p53 G→T transversions in lung cancers reflect the primary mutagenic signature of DNA-damage by tobacco smoke. Carcinogenesis 22:367–374
21. Pfeifer GP, Besaratinia A (2009) Mutational spectra of human cancer. Hum Genet 125:493–506
22. Paez JG et al (2004) *EGFR* mutations in lung cancer: correlation with clinical response to gefitibin therapy. Science 304:1497–1500
23. Pao W et al (2004) EGF receptor gene mutations are common in lung cancers from "never smokers" and are associated with sensitivity of tumors to gefitinib and erlotinib. Proc Natl Acad Sci U S A 101:13306–13311
24. Kwak EL et al (2010) Anaplastic lymphoma kinase inhibition in non-small-cell lung cancer. N Engl J Med 363:1693–1703
25. Choi K, Creighton CJ, Stivers D, Fujimoto N, Kurie JM (2007) Transcriptional profiling of non-small cell lung cancer cells activating *EGFR* somatic mutations. PLoS One 11, e1226
26. Ding C, Li R, Peng J, Guo Z (2012) A polymorphism at the miR-502 binding site in the 3′ untranslated region of the SET8 gene is associated with the outcome of small-cell lung cancer. Exp Ther Med 3:689–692
27. Qian Q et al (2014) Methylated +58CpG site decreases DCN mRNA expression and enhances TGF-β/Smad signaling in NSCLC cells with high metastatic potential. Int J Oncol 44:874–882
28. Zhao Y et al (2014) Identification of somatic alterations in stage I lung adenocarcinomas by next-generation sequencing. Genes Chromosomes Cancer 53(4):289–298
29. Vogelstein B et al (2013) Cancer genome landscapes. Science 339:1546–1558
30. Thomas A, Rajan A, Lopez-Chavez A, Wang Y, Giaccone G (2013) From targets to targeted therapies and molecular profiling in non-small cell lung carcinoma. Ann Oncol 24:577–585
31. Zhang J et al (2013) Exome profiling of primary, metastatic and recurrent ovarian carcinomas in a BRCA1-positive patient. BMC Cancer 13:146
32. Vignot S et al (2013) Next-generation sequencing reveals high concordance of recurrent somatic alterations between primary tumor and metastases from patients with non-small-cell lung cancer. J Clin Oncol 31:2167–2172
33. De Mattow-Arruda L et al (2013) Establishing the origin of metastatic deposits in the setting of multiple primary malignancies: the role of massively parallel sequencing. Mol Oncol 8(1):150–158
34. Zhang J et al (2013) Identifying driver mutations from sequencing data of heterogeneous tumors in the era of personalized genome sequencing. Brief Bioinform 15(2):244–255
35. Kismidou V et al (2013) Tumor heterogeneity revealed by KRAS, BRAF, and PIK3CA pyro-sequencing: KRAS and PIK3CA intratumour mutation profile differences and their therapeutic implications. Hum Mutat 35(3):329–340

36. Ni X et al (2013) Reproducible copy number variation patterns among single circulating tumor cells of lung cancer patients. Proc Natl Acad Sci U S A 110:1083–1088
37. Lecomte T, Ceze N, Dorval E, Laurent-Luig P (2010) Circulating free tumor DNA and colorectal cancer. Gasteoenterol Clin Biol 34:662–681
38. Dawson SJ et al (2013) Analysis of circulating tumor DNA to monitor metastatic breast cancer. N Engl J Med 368:1199–1209
39. The Cancer Genome Atlas Network (2013) Comprehensive molecular characterization of human colon and rectal cancer. Nature 487(7407):330–337
40. The Cancer Genome Atlas Research Network (2013) The cancer genome atlas pan-cancer analysis project. Nat Gen 45:1113–1120
41. Pantel K, Alix-Panabieres C (2013) Real-time liquid biopsy in cancer patients: fact or fiction? Cancer Res 73:6384–6388
42. Schwarzenback H (2013) Circulating nucleic acids as biomarkers in breast cancer. Breast Cancer Res 15:211
43. Crowley E, Di Nicolantonio F, Loupakis F, Bardelli A (2013) Liquid biopsy: monitoring cancer-genetics in the blood. Nat Rev Clin Oncol 10:472–484
44. Heitzer E et al (2013) Complex tumor genomes inferred from single circulating tumor cells by array-CGH and next-generation sequencing. Cancer Res 73:2965–2975
45. Kim SY, Speed TP (2013) Comparing somatic variant callers: beyond Venn diagrams. BMC Bioinformatics 10:189
46. Harismendy O, Ng PC, Strausberg RL, Wang X, Stockwell TB, Beeson KY, Schork NJ, Murray SS, Topol EJ, Levy S, Frazer KA. Evaluation of next generation sequencing platforms for population targeted sequencing studies. Genome Biol. 2009;10(3):R32. doi: 10.1186/gb-2009-10-3-r32. Epub 2009 Mar 27. PMID: 19327155
47. Ivahkno S et al (2010) CNAseg—a novel framework for identification of copy number changes in cancer from second-generation sequencing data. Bioinformatics 26:3051–3058
48. Xie C, Tammi MT (2009) CNV-seq, a new method to detect copy number variation using high-throughput sequencing. BMC Bioinformatics 10:80
49. Escaramís G et al (2013) PeSV-Fisher: identification of somatic and non-somatic structural variants using next generation sequencing data. PLoS One 8, e63377
50. Chen K et al (2009) BreakDancer: an algorithm for high-resolution mapping of genomic structural variation. Nat Methods 6:677–681
51. Chan KC et al (2013) Noninvasive detection of cancer-associated genome-wide hypomethylation and copy number aberrations by plasma DNA bisulfite sequencing. Proc Natl Acad Sci U S A 110:18761–18768
52. Ng PC, Henikoff S (2003) SIFT: predicting amino acid changes that affect protein function. Nucl Acids Res 31:3812–3814
53. Adzhubei IA et al (2010) A method and server for predicting damaging missense mutations. Nat Methods 7:248–249
54. Sherry ST, Ward M, Sirotkin K (1999) DbSNP-database for single nucleotide polymorphisms and other classes of minor genetic variation. Genome Res 9:677–679
55. Bamford S et al (2004) The COSMIC (catalogue of somatic mutations in cancer) database and website. Br J Cancer 91:355–358
56. Hamosh A, Scott AF, Amberger J, Valle D, McKusick VA (2000) Online Mendelian Inheritance in Man (OMIM). Hum Mutat 15:57–61
57. International HapMap Consortium (2003) The International HapMap project. Nature 426:789–796
58. Gonzalez-Perez A, Lopez-Bigas N (2012) Functional impact bias reveals cancer drivers. Nucl Acids Res 40, e169
59. Hodis E et al (2012) A landscape of driver mutations in melanoma. Cell 150:251–263
60. Reimand J, Bader GD (2013) Systematic analysis of somatic mutations in phosphorylation signaling predicts novel cancer drivers. Mol Sys Biol 9:637
61. Gonzalez-Perez A et al (2013) Computational approaches to identify functional genetic variants in cancer genomes. Nat Methods 10:723–729

62. Hartzler A et al (2013) Stakeholder engagement: a key component of integrating genomic information into electronic health records. Genet Med 15:792–801
63. Gottesman O et al (2013) The Electronic Medical Records and Genomics (eMERGE) Network: past, present, and future. Genet Med 15:761–771
64. Kho AN et al (2013) Practical challenges in integrating genomic data into the electronic health record. Genet Med 15:772–778
65. Ury AG (2013) Storing and interpreting genomic information in widely deployed electronic health record systems. Genet Med 15:779–785
66. Hazin R et al (2013) Ethical, legal, and social implications of incorporating genomic information into electronic health records. Genet Med 15:810–816
67. Tarczy-Hornoch P et al (2013) A survey of informatics approaches to whole-exome and whole-genome clinical reporting in the electronic health record. Genet Med 15:824–832
68. Lo YM et al (1999) Rapid clearance of fetal DNA from maternal plasma. Am J Hum Genet 64:218–224
69. Jackson L, Goldsmith L, O'Connor A, Skirton H (2012) Incidental findings in genetic research and clinical diagnostic tests: a systematic review. Am J Med Genet A 158A:3159–3167
70. Presidential Commission for the Study of Bioethical Issues (2012) Privacy and progress in whole genome sequencing. Presidential Commission for the Study of Bioethical Issues 2012. Washington, DC. http://bioethics.gov/sites/default/files/PrivacyProgress508_1.pdf. Accessed 27 Jan 2014

Nanomedicine for Treatment of Lung Cancer

Sajid Hussain

Abstract Lung cancer is the second most common cancer and the primary cause of cancer-related death in both men and women in the United States and rest of the world. Due to diagnosis at an advanced stage, it is associated with a high mortality in a majority of patients. In recent years, enormous advances have occurred in the development and application of nanotechnology in the detection, diagnosis, and therapy of cancer. This progress has led to the development of the emerging field of "cancer nanomedicine." Nanoparticle-based therapeutic systems have gained immense popularity due to their bioavailability, in vivo stability, intestinal absorption, solubility, sustained and targeted delivery, and therapeutic effectiveness of several anticancer agents. Currently, a plethora of nanocarrier formulations are utilized including lipid-based, polymeric and branched polymeric, metal-based, magnetic, and mesoporous silica. In lung cancer, nanoparticle-based therapeutics is paving the way in the diagnosis, imaging, screening, and treatment of primary and metastatic tumors. The application and expansion of novel nanocarriers for drug delivery is an exciting and challenging research filed, in particular for the delivery of emerging cancer therapies. Some of the current progress and challenges in nanoparticle-based drug delivery systems for lung cancer treatment are discussed.

Keywords Nanoparticle • Drug delivery • Polymer conjugates • Therapy • Lung cancer

Abbreviations

DACHPt	(1,2-diaminocyclohexane) platinum(II)
EGF	Epithelial growth factor
EPR	Enhanced permeability and retention effect
GPs	Gelatin nanoparticles

S. Hussain, Ph.D. (✉)
NCI-designated Cancer Center, Sanford Burnham Prebys Medical Discovery Institute, 10901 N. Torrey Pines Rd, La Jolla, CA 92037, USA
e-mail: shussain@sbpdiscovery.org

A. Ahmad, S.M. Gadgeel (eds.), *Lung Cancer and Personalized Medicine: Novel Therapies and Clinical Management*, Advances in Experimental Medicine and Biology 890, DOI 10.1007/978-3-319-24932-2_8

MSNs	Mesoporous silica nanoparticles
MTD	Maximum tolerated dose
MTX	Methotrexate
NSCLC	Non-small-cell lung carcinoma
PCL	Poly (ε-caprolactone)
PEG	Polyethylene glycol
PLA	Poly(D,L-lactic acid)
PLGA	Poly(D,L-lactic-co-glycolic acid)
PTX	Paclitaxel
RES	Reticuloendothelial system
SAR	Structure-activity relationship
SCLC	Small-cell lung carcinoma
SPIO	Superparamagnetic iron oxide

1 Background

Lung cancer is the second most common cancer in both men and women worldwide. It accounts for about 14 % of all new cancers with a dismal 5-year survival rate of only 15 % [1]. Recent data suggests that lung cancer is likely to overtake breast cancer as the main cause of cancer death among European women by the middle of this decade [2]. According to The American Cancer Society, an estimated 220,000 new cases of lung cancer has been diagnosed in the United States in 2013 (118,080 in men and 110,110 in women) of which 85 % of the cases are classified as non-small-cell lung carcinoma (NSCLC) [1], while the remaining cases are diagnosed as small-cell lung carcinoma (SCLC). Genetic and environmental factors, as well as their interaction, influence the risk of developing lung cancer. Although smoking is the main cause of lung cancer, risk also is increased by exposure to secondhand smoke; environmental exposures, such as radon, workplace toxins (e.g., asbestos, arsenic), and air pollution. Recent data suggest that the hazard ratios for lung cancer mortality are staggering: 17.8 for female smokers and 14.6 for male smokers [3].

Depending on the type of malignancy and stage at the time of diagnosis, lung cancer treatment often involves a combination of surgery, chemotherapy, and/or radiation therapy. However, due to the deficiency in early-stage diagnostics, most lung cancers are only detected at advanced stages, with local tumor invasion or distant metastasis and are not suitable for surgery. Therefore, a systemic chemotherapy treatment modality that addresses the majority of lung cancers is currently the mainstay of advanced lung cancer treatment regimens, aimed at extending survival and improving quality of life [3]. Standard first-line chemotherapy regimens for lung cancer include platinum-based drugs such as cisplatin and carboplatin. However, platinum-based chemotherapy is riddled with dose-limiting side effects including nephro- and cardiotoxicity, anemia, intestinal injury, and peripheral neuropathy as well as less serious symptoms of uneasiness, nausea, and fatigue [4]. To mitigate many of these untoward effects, platinum drugs are used in combination with other anticancer agents resulting in increased therapeutic effectiveness and reduced dosage of each individual drug required to produce an observable therapeutic response. The recommended treatment for patients with advanced NSCLCs involves systemic platinum-based chemotherapy (e.g., cisplatin, oxaliplatin) combined with taxens (such as Paclitaxel or Docetaxel) or Gemcitabine [5]. However, the main problem associated with current therapies is their low efficacy due to unspecific toxicity to normal tissues, which precludes the use of curative doses. Additionally, the hydrophobic nature of the majority of the cancer chemotherapeutics makes them poorly water soluble and therefore limits their administration at high doses [6]. Thus, the unmet medical need is for more effective anticancer agents, especially for strategies that focus toxicity to tumor cells and away from normal tissues. This has led to development of methods to improve tumor-targeted delivery of chemotherapeutics that will result in increased drug efficacy with improved pharmacological properties and minimal toxicity to normal tissues remain a priority in cancer therapy.

2 Nanoparticle Drug Delivery for Lung Cancer Therapy

One highly efficient way of delivering drugs to diseased sites is encapsulation of anticancer agents in nanocarriers. The major clinical advantage of nanocarrier-based strategies over free drugs is specific delivery of large amounts of chemotherapeutic agents by favorably altering their pharmacokinetic properties, resulting in increased tumor localization, improved antitumor effects, and decreased nonspecific toxicities [7–9]. In recent years, various nanoparticle formulations including liposomes and polymers, which are designed to efficiently deliver anticancer drugs and nucleic acids such as DNA & siRNA to metastatic lung cells and bear the potential to become candidates for the next-generation therapy for advanced-stage lung cancer [10, 11]. Typically, nanocarrier-based approaches include a carrier, a targeting moiety that is bound to the carrier via specific conjugation chemistry, and a drug. Carriers may be composed of lipids, polymeric nanoparticles, inorganic nanoparticles, or dendrimers. Targeting moieties may include high affinity ligands, antibodies and nucleic acids, and they may be conjugated to the carriers utilizing a variety of chemistries.

2.1 Lipid-Based Nanoparticles

The major classes of lipid-based nanoparticles for drug delivery applications are liposomes and micelles. Liposomes are vesicles composed of a phospholipid bilayer commonly used to deliver chemotherapeutic drugs. Hydrophobic agents are incorporated in the lipid bilayer and hydrophilic drugs are encapsulated in the inner aqueous core. The physical structure of lipid-based nanocarriers primarily defined by its phospholipids composition, which determines the chemophysical features, such as size, shape, curvature, and charge [12]. Varying the lipid compositions and reducing the number of lipid bilayers changes the surface charge, reduces the size of the liposomes to nanometer scale with the aim to prolong their in vivo circulation time and enhance tumor localization. Lipid-based nanocarriers have become a favorable platform for delivery of anticancer drugs mainly due to their non-toxic, biodegradable, and biocompatible nature [10, 13]. Particularly promising are liposomes containing surface-grafted lipid derivatives conjugated with polyethylene glycol (PEG) [8, 14]. These sterically stabilized liposomes (also called "Stealth" liposomes) have long circulation times in the blood as a consequence of reduced uptake by the reticuloendothelial system (RES) [7, 9]. A variety of chemotherapeutic agents, such as doxorubicin and vincristine, have been encapsulated in PEGylated liposomes and validated in preclinical models in vitro and in vivo [8, 15–17]. PEGylated liposomes achieve a higher drug load in tumors due to a passive targeting process, which exploits the "enhanced permeability and retention effect" (EPR), resulting from increased vascular permeability inherent to many solid tumors [14, 18]. PEGylated liposomal doxorubicin (Doxil/Caelyx) has been approved for use in acquired immunodeficiency syndrome–related Kaposi's sarcoma, and refractory ovarian and breast cancers, and several other liposomal anticancer agents are currently under clinical investigation (http://clinicaltrials.gov).

Lipid-based nanoparticles represent a promising delivery system for drugs and genes for the treatment of lung cancer. For the last two decades, cisplatin is the drug of choice for the treatment of NSCLC. Furthermore, only three platinates—cisplatin, carboplatin, and oxaliplatin— have been successfully used in the clinics [19]. However, cisplatin is implicated in the development of nephrotoxicity in 20 % of patients receiving high doses [4] . In order to reduce the systemic toxicity of cisplatin and improve therapeutic efficacy, Lipoplatin, a liposomally encapsulated cisplatin was developed for various cancer indications, including non-small cell lung cancer and pancreatic cancer [20]. Furthermore, these researchers also demonstrated Lipoplatin exceed the size cutoff for clearance by the kidney [21] and therefore exhibited limited cisplatin-associated nephrotoxicity compared to standard therapy [22]. Exciting and promising data were announced from a randomized Phase III study on Lipoplatin™ in the treatment of non-squamous non-small cell lung cancer (NSCLC). This study used Lipoplatin in combination with paclitaxel as first line treatment against non-squamous NSCLC and compared response rates and toxicities to a similar group of patients treated with cisplatin plus paclitaxel. This study has demonstrated statistically significant increase in tumor response rate in the Lipoplatin arm (59.22 %) versus the cisplatin arm (42.42 %) while also reducing most major toxicities of cisplatin, especially nephrotoxicity [22].

Taxanes are another class of the most widely used anticancer drugs [23]. However, the hydrophobic structure of a typical taxane molecule such as paclitaxel (PTX), a diterpenoid centered around a bulky and fused taxane ring with multiple hydrophobic substitutions limits its solubility. Historically, it was formulated using Cremophor EL to enhance its solubility in physiological fluids. However, this resulted in hypersensitivity reactions and associated with serious side effects complicating its systemic delivery and efficacy [24]. In order to circumvent this problem, liposomal-paclitaxel formulations were developed to enhance therapeutic efficacy. It has been demonstrated in both pre-clinical animal models and human clinical trials that liposomal-paclitaxel formulations significantly increase a maximum tolerated dose (MTD) of PTX which outperform that for Taxol®. Liposomal PTX formulations are in various stages of clinical trials. LEP-ETU (NeoPharm) and EndoTAG®-1 (Medigene) have reached the phase II of the clinical trials. Lipusu® (Luye Pharma Group) has already been commercialized [25] in China. In 2010, a phase I clinical trial in China assessing liposomal paclitaxel in combination with cisplatin as first-line chemotherapy for patients with advanced NSCLC with regional lymph-node metastasis [26].

Another class of lipid-based nanoparticles are micelles which are self-assemblies of block copolymers that have gained increasing popularity as tumor-targetable nanocarriers since they were first used as drug vehicles in the late 1980s [27–29]. These micelles, which are several tens of nanometers in size and have a characteristic core shell structure consisting of a drug-loaded hydrophobic core and poly(ethylene glycol) (PEG) hydrophilic shell, are long-lived in the bloodstream and effectively accumulate in solid tumors after intravenous injection [30]. The critical features of polymeric micelles for their function as drug vehicles, including size, drug loading and release, and specific binding to the target cells, can be modulated by engineering the constituent block copolymers. At present, micelle formulations incorporating doxorubicin, paclitaxel, SN-38, cisplatin, and (1,2-diaminocyclohexane) platinum(II) (DACHPt) are undergoing clinical trials [30] and four of these have advanced to Phase II studies [31, 32]. These clinical studies have revealed that polymeric micelles reduce side effects from the incorporated drugs and are effective against various intractable tumors, such as lung cancer and triple-negative breast cancers [33], indicating their clinical potential.

Recently, increasing attention has also been paid to another potentially useful property of nanocarriers to achieve subcellular drug targeting [30]. Subcellular drug targeting of nanomedicine could enhance the pharmacological activity of the loaded drugs through improved subcellular drug distribution [34]. Drug vehicles designed to release active drugs in acidic organelles, such as the endosome and lysosome, can circumvent recognition by the drug efflux pump (for example, P-glycoprotein) through internalization by endocytosis, thus overcoming multidrug resistance in cancer cells [35, 36]. This approach is particularly appealing for platinum agents such as cisplatin and oxaliplatin which can be engineered by harnessing a structure-activity relationship (SAR). Employing such a strategy, a novel nanoplatinate was designed inspired by the mechanisms underlying cisplatin bioactivation. This novel lipid-based platinum (Pt) complex self-assembled into a nanoparticle, which releases cisplatin in a pH-dependent manner. The nanoparticles exhibited significantly improved antitumor efficacy in terms of tumor growth delay in breast and lung cancers, and resulted in reduced systemic and nephrotoxicity [37].

2.2 *Polymer Conjugates as Nanocarriers*

Polymeric nanoparticles are synthesized from polymers. Polymer-based nanomedicine, an arena that entails the use of polymeric NPs, polymer micelles, dendrimers, polymersomes, polyplexes, polymer–lipid hybrid systems, and polymer–drug/protein conjugates for improvement in efficacy of cancer therapeutics, has been widely explored. Biodegradable polymers such as poly(D,L-lactic acid) (PLA), poly(D,L-lactic-co-glycolic acid) (PLGA), and poly (ε-caprolactone) (PCL), polycaprolactone, and poly-alkyl-cyanoacrylates, gelatin, albumin, chitosan, and their copolymers diblocked or multiblocked with poly(ethylene glycol) (PEG) have been commonly used to form polymeric nanoparticles (NPs) to encapsulate a variety of therapeutic compounds. These include polymeric micelles, capsules, colloids, dendrimers, etc. [38]. Polymeric NPs can be formulated by self-assembly of block copolymers consisting of two or more polymer chains with different hydrophobicity. Drug release rates from the polymeric NPs can be controlled by modifying polymer chemical and physical properties.

Polymer nanoparticles have been shown to enhance the chemo- and radio-therapeutic efficacy of anticancer agents [39]. Abraxane, an FDA-approved albumin-based nanoparticle carrying paclitaxel, is indicated for first-line treatment of locally advanced or metastatic NSCLC in combination with carboplatin in patients who are not candidates for curative surgery or radiation therapy [39]. Polyethylene glycol- (PEG-) modified polylactic acid nanoparticles loaded with taxanes have significantly improved the efficacy of chemoradiation therapy in both in vitro and in an A549 lung tumor xenograft model [40]. Other research groups have developed a cremophor free nanoformulation of paclitaxel and cisplatin using block copolymers of PEG and polylactic acid for the treatment of lung cancer [41]. One such polymeric NP is Genexol-PM, a PLGA-b-methoxyPEG NP encapsulating paclitaxel, which has received regulatory approval in South Korea for clinical use and is currently undergoing phase II clinical trials for a number of cancer indications, including patients with advanced NSCLC, in the United States [38]. Results are awaited for a phase II trial of Genexol-PM and Gemcitabine in patients with metastatic lung cancer (http://clinicaltrials.gov/show/NCT01770795). PEG–poly-glutamic acid block copolymer micelles loaded with cisplatin demonstrated remarkably prolonged blood circulation and accumulation in solid tumors (Lewis lung carcinoma cells) about 20-fold higher than free cisplatin. The micellar system was found to confer both sufficient stability to ensure prolonged circulation in the bloodstream and sustained drug release kinetics upon accumulation at the delivery site. Treatment with micelles led to complete tumor regression with no significant body weight loss, whereas free drug treatment resulted in tumor survivals and approximately 20 % of body weight loss at the equivalent dose [41]. Polymer nanoparticles have been extensively used in studies aimed at delivering targeted chemotherapeutics to lung cancer. Gelatin nanoparticles (GPs) were grafted with biotinylated epithelial growth factor (EGF) molecules for targeting lung cancer. These nanocarriers demonstrated increased cellular uptake on A549 lung adenocarcinoma cells in vitro and in vivo aerosol administration to cancerous lung in a mouse model [42].

Dendrimers are synthetic, repeatedly branched polymeric macromolecules having numerous extensions from central core, resulting in a tree-like structure. The structure of dendrimers and modifiable surface functionality allow for either encapsulation/conjugation of therapeutic agent, in the core or on the surface, making them attractive carriers for anticancer therapeutics [43]. Poly(glycerol-succinic acid) dendrimers were explored as potential carriers for camptothecin [44]. The anticancer activity of the camptothecin-encapsulated dendrimer formulation was examined using human breast adenocarcinoma (MCF-7), colorectal adenocarcinoma (HT-29), non-small-cell lung carcinoma (NCI-H460), and glioblastoma (SF-268) [45]. A recent study illustrated the use of dendrimer-targeting peptide conjugates as a carrier for drugs towards NSCLC. These dendrimer-peptide conjugates when administered to a lung tumor-bearing athymic mouse model were efficiently taken up by the cancer cells demonstrating their potential as a drug carrier for the treatment of lung cancer [46]. In a related study, a newly designed PEGylated dendrimer nanoparticle showed promising application as an aerosol-inhaled drug delivery modality. The smaller dendrimer particles are reported to enter the blood stream via inhalation while larger particles are sequestered in the lung for an extended period of time. In the future, this method of controlled drug delivery to the lungs could provide an alternative to injectable drug systems [46, 47].

2.3 Other Nanoparticle Systems

Recent years have seen tremendous progress in the design and study of metal-based nanomaterials of gold and silver, geared towards biological and biomedical applications. Most notable among these being the noble metal gold nanoparticles where the surface-plasmon resonance-enhanced optical properties of colloidal gold nanoparticles directed towards recent biomedical applications with an emphasis on diagnosis and therapy of cancer, including lung cancer [48, 49]. Recently, gold nanoparticles have also successfully been tested as sensors for discriminating and classifying different lung cancer histologies. The sensor was able to distinguish between normal and cancerous cells, SCLCand NSCLC, and between two subtypes of NSCLCs [50]. Gold nanoparticle conjugates of methotrexate (MTX), a drug with high water solubility and low tumor retention, have shown high tumor retention and enhanced therapeutic efficacy in a Lewis lung carcinoma mouse model [51].

Magnetic nanoparticles have been extensively investigated and applied in diagnosis and treatment of various cancers. Theranostic nanoparticles concurrently facilitate imaging and delivery of therapeutic agents. Magnetic hyperthermia is a noninvasive therapeutic approach for lung cancer that entails the heat-induced ablation of desired tumor tissue. When subjected to alternating currents the magnetic material, such as superparamagnetic iron oxide (SPIO), nanoparticles generate sublethal heat that causes local tissue damage. In one study, the tumor-targeted SPIO nanoparticles were highly effective in the hyperthermic destruction and inhibition of tumor growth in a mouse model of NSCLC [52].

Mesoporous silica nanoparticles (MSNs) have been increasingly used in anticancer drug delivery research due to their dynamic capacity for drug loading, controlled drug release property, and multifunctional ability. The first report on in vivo applicability of Mesoporous silica nanoparticles (MSNs) was published by the Mou group in 2008 [53]. Multifunctional mesoporous silica nanoparticles have been used for intracellular labeling and animal magnetic resonance imaging studies. Human lung cancer cells primarily take up MSNs by endocytosis [54]. A tumor targeted MSN-based drug delivery system was developed for inhalation treatment of lung cancer. The system was capable of effectively delivering inside cancer cells anticancer drugs (doxorubicin and cisplatin) combined with two types of siRNA targeted to MRP1 and BCL2 mRNA for suppression of pump and non-pump cellular resistance in NSLC, respectively. Targeting of MSN to cancer cells was achieved by the conjugation of LHRH peptide on the surface of MSN via poly(ethylene glycol) spacer [55].

3 Challenges and Future Perspective

The past decade has witnessed tremendous growth and development of drug delivery technology utilizing nanoparticle systems. Nanocarriers have emerged as an important treatment modality for therapeutic intervention in clinical oncology. Different types of nanocarriers have established excellent therapeutic potential at both preclinical and clinical development stages. Some of the challenges being faced in the nanomedicine area are the bridging of rapidly developing novel ideas and translating them into clinical practice. Towards this end, safety of nanocarriers is an important consideration which needs to be assessed before proceeding to clinical study. One of the hurdles is in synthesizing nanoparticle drug delivery systems having appropriate properties such as size and charge to carry effective drug/gene payload, and ability to target to the right place. Non-uniform size distribution, undefined structure/shape, poor biocompatibility, and improper surface chemistry are possible risk factors in the biological environment. For highly effective drug delivery to the lungs using nanotechnology, it is crucial for these delivery systems to overcome a number of obstacles including immune reaction, rate of clearance from circulation, efficiency in targeting, and ability to cross biological barriers in order for these nanoparticle systems to enter the clinics. Understanding the mechanism of action and the biological behavior of nanoparticles is imperative to achieve the highest drug delivery efficiency. Identification of physicochemical parameters are absolutely critical in determining the particle-particle interaction within a biological environment, aggregation tendencies, adsorption of proteins on nanoparticle surface, and intracellular trafficking of nanoparticles are some of the important considerations to keep in mind.

From the regulatory stand point, nanoparticle-based therapy must overcome the same hurdles faced by any new drug: optimal design of components and properties, reproducible manufacturing processes, robust assay development and analytical methods for sufficient characterization, favorable pharmacology and toxicity profiles, and demonstration of safety and efficacy in clinical trials. Unlike standard drugs which are composed of a single active agent, nanoparticles are complex in nature with multiple active components that can affect the pharmacokinetics and pharmacodynamics. Such complexity necessitates the need for regulatory agencies to develop an exhaustive list of tests and a streamlined approval process to proactively address the emergence of new products based on new technologies and facilitate nanomedicine delivery to the clinic.

In conclusion, nanoparticle-based medicine has infinite potential with novel applications continuously being developed for use in cancer diagnosis, detection, imaging, and treatment. The ability of nanoparticles to be tailored for a personalized medicine strategy makes them ideal vehicles for the treatment of lung cancer. Going forward, the development of different strategies to selectively deliver drugs to lung tumors and lung metastases is dependent on understanding the tumor biology, tumor microenvironment, and the interaction between the tumor cells and the nanoparticles. Particulate nanocarriers and polymer conjugates have increased the arsenal of drugs available to oncologists. These are currently based on passive tissue targeting, mainly by the enhanced permeation and retention (EPR) [18], and not active cellular targeting. New strategies utilizing a specific cell surface receptor as a way to target these nanocarriers into lung tumors or lung metastases are showing great promise and need to be scaled up to be able for translation into the clinic. In addition, new class of drugs, from the RNA family, including small interfering RNAs, microRNAs mimic, or anti-miRs, could effectively be used to modulate the function of specific gene or family of genes and are expected to be the next generation of pathway-specific medicine [11]. It is expected that the ongoing research efforts in nanomedicine will continue to lead towards safe, efficient, and feasible drug delivery and highly sensitive and improved imaging agents for diagnostic and disease monitoring applications.

References

1. Ramalingam SS, Owonikoko TK, Khuri FR (2011) Lung cancer: new biological insights and recent therapeutic advances. CA Cancer J Clin 61(2):91–112
2. Malvezzi M, Bertuccio P, Levi F, La Vecchia C, Negri E (2013) European cancer mortality predictions for the year 2013. Ann Oncol 24(3):792–800
3. Yano T, Okamoto T, Fukuyama S, Maehara Y (2014) Therapeutic strategy for postoperative recurrence in patients with non-small cell lung cancer. World J Clin Oncol 5(5):1048–1054
4. Yao X, Panichpisal K, Kurtzman N, Nugent K (2007) Cisplatin nephrotoxicity: a review. Am J Med Sci 334(2):115–124
5. Carnio S, Novello S, Mele T, Levra MG, Scagliotti GV (2014) Extending survival of stage IV non-small cell lung cancer. Semin Oncol 41(1):69–92
6. Lu J, Liong M, Zink JI, Tamanoi F (2007) Mesoporous silica nanoparticles as a delivery system for hydrophobic anticancer drugs. Small 3(8):1341–1346
7. Allen TM, Cullis PR (2004) Drug delivery systems: entering the mainstream. Science 303(5665):1818–1822
8. Hussain S, Pluckthun A, Allen TM, Zangemeister-Wittke U (2007) Antitumor activity of an epithelial cell adhesion molecule targeted nanovesicular drug delivery system. Mol Cancer Ther 6(11):3019–3027
9. Torchilin VP (2005) Recent advances with liposomes as pharmaceutical carriers. Nat Rev Drug Discov 4(2):145–160
10. Landesman-Milo D, Peer D (2012) Altering the immune response with lipid-based nanoparticles. J Control Release 161(2):600–608
11. Landesman-Milo D, Ramishetti S, Peer D (2015) Nanomedicine as an emerging platform for metastatic lung cancer therapy. Cancer Metastasis Rev 34(2):291–301

12. Drummond DC, Meyer O, Hong K, Kirpotin DB, Papahadjopoulos D (1999) Optimizing liposomes for delivery of chemotherapeutic agents to solid tumors. Pharmacol Rev 51(4):691–743
13. Peer D et al (2007) Nanocarriers as an emerging platform for cancer therapy. Nat Nanotechnol 2(12):751–760
14. Allen TM, Hansen C, Martin F, Redemann C, Yau-Young A (1991) Liposomes containing synthetic lipid derivatives of poly(ethylene glycol) show prolonged circulation half-lives in vivo. Biochim Biophys Acta 1066(1):29–36
15. Sapra P, Allen TM (2004) Improved outcome when B-cell lymphoma is treated with combinations of immunoliposomal anticancer drugs targeted to both the CD19 and CD20 epitopes. Clin Cancer Res 10(7):2530–2537
16. Park JW et al (2002) Anti-HER2 immunoliposomes: enhanced efficacy attributable to targeted delivery. Clin Cancer Res 8(4):1172–1181
17. Hussain S, Pluckthun A, Allen TM, Zangemeister-Wittke U (2006) Chemosensitization of carcinoma cells using epithelial cell adhesion molecule-targeted liposomal antisense against bcl-2/bcl-xL. Mol Cancer Ther 5(12):3170–3180
18. Matsumura Y, Maeda H (1986) A new concept for macromolecular therapeutics in cancer chemotherapy: mechanism of tumoritropic accumulation of proteins and the antitumor agent smancs. Cancer Res 46(12 Pt 1):6387–6392
19. Kelland L (2007) The resurgence of platinum-based cancer chemotherapy. Nat Rev Cancer 7(8):573–584
20. Boulikas T (2004) Low toxicity and anticancer activity of a novel liposomal cisplatin (Lipoplatin) in mouse xenografts. Oncol Rep 12(1):3–12
21. Choi HS et al (2007) Renal clearance of quantum dots. Nat Biotechnol 25(10):1165–1170
22. Stathopoulos GP et al (2011) Comparison of liposomal cisplatin versus cisplatin in non-squamous cell non-small-cell lung cancer. Cancer Chemother Pharmacol 68(4):945–950
23. Bedard PL, Di Leo A, Piccart-Gebhart MJ (2010) Taxanes: optimizing adjuvant chemotherapy for early-stage breast cancer. *Nature reviews*. Clin Oncol 7(1):22–36
24. Zhang Z, Mei L, Feng SS (2013) Paclitaxel drug delivery systems. Expert Opin Drug Deliv 10(3):325–340
25. Koudelka S, Turanek J (2012) Liposomal paclitaxel formulations. J Control Release 163(3):322–334
26. Wang X et al (2010) A phase I clinical and pharmacokinetic study of paclitaxel liposome infused in non-small cell lung cancer patients with malignant pleural effusions. Eur J Cancer 46(8):1474–1480
27. Nishiyama N, Kataoka K (2006) Current state, achievements, and future prospects of polymeric micelles as nanocarriers for drug and gene delivery. Pharmacol Ther 112(3):630–648
28. Yokoyama M et al (1990) Characterization and anticancer activity of the micelle-forming polymeric anticancer drug adriamycin-conjugated poly(ethylene glycol)-poly(aspartic acid) block copolymer. Cancer Res 50(6):1693–1700
29. Kabanov AV, Batrakova EV, Miller DW (2003) Pluronic block copolymers as modulators of drug efflux transporter activity in the blood-brain barrier. Adv Drug Deliv Rev 55(1):151–164
30. Murakami M et al (2011) Improving drug potency and efficacy by nanocarrier-mediated subcellular targeting. Sci Transl Med 3(64):64ra62
31. Matsumura Y et al (2004) Phase I clinical trial and pharmacokinetic evaluation of NK911, a micelle-encapsulated doxorubicin. Br J Cancer 91(10):1775–1781
32. Hamaguchi T et al (2010) Phase I study of NK012, a novel SN-38-incorporating micellar nanoparticle, in adult patients with solid tumors. Clin Cancer Res 16(20):5058–5066
33. Dent R et al (2007) Triple-negative breast cancer: clinical features and patterns of recurrence. Clin Cancer Res 13(15 Pt 1):4429–4434
34. Hubbell JA (2003) Materials science. Enhancing drug function. Science 300(5619):595–596
35. Cho K, Wang X, Nie S, Chen ZG, Shin DM (2008) Therapeutic nanoparticles for drug delivery in cancer. Clin Cancer Res 14(5):1310–1316

36. Kim D, Lee ES, Oh KT, Gao ZG, Bae YH (2008) Doxorubicin-loaded polymeric micelle overcomes multidrug resistance of cancer by double-targeting folate receptor and early endosomal pH. Small 4(11):2043–2050
37. Paraskar AS et al (2010) Harnessing structure-activity relationship to engineer a cisplatin nanoparticle for enhanced antitumor efficacy. Proc Natl Acad Sci U S A 107(28): 12435–12440
38. Chan JM, Valencia PM, Zhang L, Langer R, Farokhzad OC (2010) Polymeric nanoparticles for drug delivery. Methods Mol Biol 624:163–175
39. Wang AZ et al (2010) ChemoRad nanoparticles: a novel multifunctional nanoparticle platform for targeted delivery of concurrent chemoradiation. Nanomedicine (Lond) 5(3):361–368
40. Jung J et al (2012) Polymeric nanoparticles containing taxanes enhance chemoradiotherapeutic efficacy in non-small cell lung cancer. Int J Radiat Oncol Biol Phys 84(1):e77–e83
41. Nishiyama N et al (2003) Novel cisplatin-incorporated polymeric micelles can eradicate solid tumors in mice. Cancer Res 63(24):8977–8983
42. Tseng CL, Su WY, Yen KC, Yang KC, Lin FH (2009) The use of biotinylated-EGF-modified gelatin nanoparticle carrier to enhance cisplatin accumulation in cancerous lungs via inhalation. Biomaterials 30(20):3476–3485
43. Bharali DJ, Khalil M, Gurbuz M, Simone TM, Mousa SA (2009) Nanoparticles and cancer therapy: a concise review with emphasis on dendrimers. Int J Nanomedicine 4:1–7
44. Morgan MT et al (2003) Dendritic molecular capsules for hydrophobic compounds. J Am Chem Soc 125(50):15485–15489
45. Morgan MT et al (2006) Dendrimer-encapsulated camptothecins: increased solubility, cellular uptake, and cellular retention affords enhanced anticancer activity in vitro. Cancer Res 66(24):11913–11921
46. Liu J et al (2011) Novel peptide-dendrimer conjugates as drug carriers for targeting nonsmall cell lung cancer. Int J Nanomedicine 6:59–69
47. Ryan GM et al (2013) Pulmonary administration of PEGylated polylysine dendrimers: absorption from the lung versus retention within the lung is highly size-dependent. Mol Pharm 10(8):2986–2995
48. Kao HW et al (2014) Biological characterization of cetuximab-conjugated gold nanoparticles in a tumor animal model. Nanotechnology 25(29):295102
49. Huang X, Jain PK, El-Sayed IH, El-Sayed MA (2007) Gold nanoparticles: interesting optical properties and recent applications in cancer diagnostics and therapy. Nanomedicine (Lond) 2(5):681–693
50. Barash O et al (2012) Classification of lung cancer histology by gold nanoparticle sensors. Nanomedicine 8(5):580–589
51. Chen YH et al (2007) Methotrexate conjugated to gold nanoparticles inhibits tumor growth in a syngeneic lung tumor model. Mol Pharm 4(5):713–722
52. Sadhukha T, Wiedmann TS, Panyam J (2013) Inhalable magnetic nanoparticles for targeted hyperthermia in lung cancer therapy. Biomaterials 34(21):5163–5171
53. Wu SH et al (2008) Multifunctional mesoporous silica nanoparticles for intracellular labeling and animal magnetic resonance imaging studies. Chembiochem 9(1):53–57
54. Sun W et al (2008) Endocytosis of a single mesoporous silica nanoparticle into a human lung cancer cell observed by differential interference contrast microscopy. Anal Bioanal Chem 391(6):2119–2125
55. Taratula O, Garbuzenko OB, Chen AM, Minko T (2011) Innovative strategy for treatment of lung cancer: targeted nanotechnology-based inhalation co-delivery of anticancer drugs and siRNA. J Drug Target 19(10):900–914

Personalized Therapy of Small Cell Lung Cancer

Bryan J. Schneider and Gregory P. Kalemkerian

Abstract Small cell lung cancer (SCLC) is an aggressive, poorly differentiated neuroendocrine carcinoma with distinct clinical, pathological and molecular characteristics. Despite robust responses to initial chemotherapy and radiation, the prognosis of patients with SCLC remains poor with an overall 5-year survival rate of less than 10 %. Despite the fact that numerous molecularly targeted approaches have thus far failed to demonstrate clinical utility in SCLC, further advances will rely on better definition of the biological pathways that drive survival, proliferation and metastasis. Recent next-generation, molecular profiling studies have identified many new therapeutic targets in SCLC, as well as extreme genomic instability which explains the high degree of resistance. A wide variety of anti-angiogenic agents, growth factor inhibitors, pro-apoptotic agents, and epigenetic modulators have been evaluated in SCLC and many studies of these strategies are on-going. Perhaps the most promising approaches involve agents targeting cancer stem cell pathways and immunomodulatory drugs that interfere with the PD1 and CTLA-4 pathways. SCLC offers many barriers to the development of successful therapy, including limited tumor samples, inadequate preclinical models, high mutational burden, and aggressive tumor growth which impairs functional status and hampers enrollment on clinical trials.

Keywords Lung cancer • Small cell • Targeted therapy • Immunotherapy • Genetic profiling

B.J. Schneider, M.D.
Division of Hematology/Oncology, University of Michigan, C411 Med Inn—SPC 5848, 1500 E. Medical Center Dr., Ann Arbor, MI 48109-5848, USA
e-mail: bryansch@umich.edu

G.P. Kalemkerian, M.D. (✉)
Division of Hematology/Oncology, University of Michigan, C350 Med Inn—SPC 5848, 1500 E. Medical Center Dr., Ann Arbor, MI 48109-5848, USA
e-mail: kalemker@umich.edu

A. Ahmad, S.M. Gadgeel (eds.), *Lung Cancer and Personalized Medicine: Novel Therapies and Clinical Management*, Advances in Experimental Medicine and Biology 890, DOI 10.1007/978-3-319-24932-2_9

1 Introduction

Small cell lung cancer (SCLC) is an aggressive, poorly differentiated neuroendocrine carcinoma with clinical, pathological and molecular characteristics that are distinct from non-small cell lung cancer (NSCLC). Clinically, SCLC is notable for rapid growth, early metastatic spread, and initial responsiveness to cytotoxic chemotherapy and radiation. The primary cause of SCLC is tobacco smoking, and, of all the histologic types of lung cancer, SCLC and squamous cell carcinoma have the strongest correlations with tobacco use, with well over 95 % of patients being current or former smokers [1]. Few other occupational and environmental carcinogens have been linked to SCLC, but chloromethyl ethers, used in chemical manufacturing, and high levels of radon exposure, as reported in uranium miners, have both been associated with a specific increase in the incidence of SCLC [2].

Both the overall incidence of SCLC and the proportional incidence as a percentage of all lung cancer cases have been declining over the past two decades. The incidence rate of SCLC peaked in the late 1980s and has since been declining in parallel with the decreasing prevalence of tobacco smoking in the United States [3, 4]. The male-to-female incidence ratio has also fallen sharply, from 2.6-to-1 in 1973 to 1-to-1 in 2002, due to a marked decline in incidence in men coupled with a steady rise in incidence in women [4]. In the late 1980s, the proportional incidence of SCLC peaked at 17–20 % of all lung cancer cases, but by 2002, SCLC accounted for only 13–15 % of all cases [3, 4]. Despite its declining incidence, SCLC remains a major public health problem, ranking as the sixth most common cause of cancer-related death in the United States [5].

The Veterans' Administration Lung Group classification scheme is routinely used to stage SCLC [6]. Limited-stage (LS) is defined as tumor confined to one hemithorax, with or without regional lymph node involvement, which can be safely encompassed in a tolerable radiotherapy port. Extensive-stage (ES) is defined as disease that has spread beyond this point, including malignant pleural effusion and hematogenous metastases. Two-thirds of patients have ES-SCLC at initial diagnosis [4]. Recently, the IASLC has proposed that the newly revised TNM staging system for NSCLC should also be applied to SCLC since the T and N descriptors, as well as the overall stage I–IV groupings, are discriminatory for survival [7, 8]. However, the degree of distinction between stage categories is smaller than that noted for NSCLC and it is unlikely that the application of TNM staging will substantially alter clinical decision-making, since all of the clinical trials on which current treatment is based utilized the VA staging scheme.

2 Current Therapy for SCLC

The management of SCLC is complicated by the aggressiveness of the disease. Most patients present with symptoms of bulky intrathoracic disease and/or widespread metastases that cause significant debility. Due to the high prevalence of tobacco use, many patients also have substantial co-morbidities that contribute to their impaired performance status and limit the delivery of optimal treatment. These factors also make it challenging to enroll patients with SCLC onto appropriate clinical trials.

LS-SCLC is a potentially curable disease in which recent progress has mainly been made through advances in the use of radiotherapy. Two meta-analyses have demonstrated that the addition of definitive thoracic radiation to chemotherapy significantly improves overall survival in patients with LS-SCLC [9, 10]. Further studies have shown that early thoracic radiotherapy resulted in a greater overall survival benefit than late radiotherapy [11]. Although a large, randomized trial reported an added improvement in survival with hyperfractionated, twice daily, thoracic radiotherapy, this strategy remains controversial and confirmatory studies are on-going [12]. Up to 60 % of patients with SCLC will develop brain metastases during the course of their illness. A meta-analysis of randomized trials evaluating prophylactic cranial irradiation (PCI) reported a significant decrease in the incidence of brain metastases and a 5.4 % increase in 3-year overall survival [13]. At present, the standard-of-care for patients with LS-SCLC consists of 4–6 cycles of cisplatin and etoposide plus early, concurrent thoracic radiotherapy. PCI is recommended for those achieving a good response to initial therapy. With such treatment, objective response is noted in 90 % of patients with long-term survival in 25 %.

ES-SCLC remains an incurable disease in which the mainstay of treatment is platinum-based, two-drug chemotherapy, such as cisplatin or carboplatin plus etoposide, with the goal of palliating symptoms and prolonging survival. This treatment yields an objective response in 60–70 % of patients with up to 10 % having a complete radiographic response. Patients who attain a good response are considered for PCI based on the demonstration of improved survival even in those with extensive-stage disease [14]. Although chemotherapy does significantly improve quality-of-life and prolong survival for patients with ES-SCLC, relapse is inevitable, and only 5 % of patients remain alive 2 years after the initial diagnosis. Numerous chemotherapy-based strategies, including dose-intensification, weekly administration, three- or four-drug regimens, high-dose consolidation, alternating or sequential non-cross-resistant regimens, and maintenance therapy, have failed to improve survival, and several of these approaches have resulted in excessive toxicity [15].

Single-agent chemotherapy is the standard treatment for patients with relapsed SCLC. While response rates are generally higher with combination therapy, overall survival is not improved, and the toxicity of combination regimens is problematic [16]. The benefits of subsequent therapy are strongly impacted by the duration of response to initial treatment, with lower response rates noted in patients who relapse within 2–3 months of initial therapy. Despite the relatively poor responses and short survival associated with second-line chemotherapy, a randomized trial comparing oral topotecan to best supportive care did demonstrate significantly better overall survival in patients receiving chemotherapy (median, 26 vs. 14 weeks; $p=0.01$) [17].

It is unlikely that empiric chemotherapy will lead to further significant improvements in outcome in patients with SCLC. The overall survival of patients with SCLC has changed little since the advent of active chemotherapy regimens in the 1970s [18].

Between 1973 and 2002, the 2-year survival rate for patients with LS-SCLC improved from 15 to 22 %, but there was little change for those with ES-SCLC (3.4 to 5.6 %) [3]. Future advances will rely on efforts to better understand the underlying biology of SCLC and to identify molecular targets that drive survival, proliferation and metastasis. In addition, we must improve and broaden our clinical research infrastructure to optimize enrollment onto rational clinical trials.

3 Identification of Therapeutic Targets

3.1 Early Studies

Over the past 40 years, our understanding of the biologic basis of SCLC has grown exponentially and has led to the identification of a wide variety of rational putative targets for therapeutic interventions that have subsequently been evaluated in both preclinical and clinical studies. The study of the molecular underpinnings of SCLC has been greatly enhanced by the work of the NCI-Navy Medical Oncology Branch with their development of over 100 SCLC cell lines in the 1970s and 1980s [19]. Most of these cell lines were developed from metastatic sites, commonly bone marrow, pleural fluid or lymph nodes, with only 10 % arising from samples of the primary tumor. This effort, along with the rapid advancement of cytogenetic and molecular biological techniques, allowed the description of various genetic derangements and other molecular drivers of SCLC growth [20].

Initial cytogenetic studies in SCLC identified numerous non-random chromosomal aberrations, including loss of heterozygosity at 3p, 13q and 17p. Deletions on 3p14-23 are the most common cytogenetic abnormalities noted in SCLC [21]. Although this region contains several oncogenic genes of interest (*VHL*, *RARβ*, c-*RAF*, c-*ErbA*), the role of 3p deletion in the pathogenesis of SCLC remains undefined. In contrast, deletions of 13q and 17p clearly pointed to the involvement of the tumor suppressor genes *RB1* and *p53*, respectively, the two most ubiquitous oncogenic derangements in SCLC [22, 23]. Early studies also led to the identification of frequent dysregulation of proto-oncogenes, including c-*myc*, L-*myc* and N-*myc*, and, in notable contrast to NSCLC, the complete absence of mutations in *RAS* genes [24].

The extensive work on cell line development highlighted the importance of growth factors in the propagation of SCLC cells. As neuroendocrine-derived cells, SCLC can produce and secrete a host of peptide growth factors, many of which act through autocrine pathways to enhance tumor growth [25]. The recognition of these autocrine growth pathways suggested rational targets to inhibit SCLC growth and led to the first clinical trial of targeted therapy in SCLC, the use of an anti-gastrin-releasing peptide (GRP) antibody in patients with relapsed SCLC [26].

Despite the availability of many cell lines, the identification of actionable molecular targets and the development of targeted therapy in SCLC have been hampered by the limited availability of primary tumor tissue. Very few patients with SCLC undergo surgical resection and in most patients the diagnosis is made by cytological analysis or small biopsies. Nonetheless, in the past few years, the pace at which potential targets for anti-cancer therapy are being identified has accelerated at lightning speed due to the streamlining of sequencing and expression array technology.

3.2 Recent Developments

Several reports have recently been published on the application of advanced, next-generation molecular techniques for the identification of therapeutic targets and predictive biomarkers in SCLC. One of the most striking findings of these studies is the extreme genomic instability exhibited by SCLC tumors, likely due to the prolonged, high-dose exposure to tobacco carcinogens in most patients. Two studies have reported protein-altering mutation frequencies of 5.5 and 7.5 per megabase using exomic sequencing techniques, among the highest rates reported in any type of cancer [27, 28]. Utilizing exomic, transcriptome, and genomic sequencing, along with SNP array analysis, in subsets of 63 primary SCLCs, Peifer et al. confirmed the near ubiquity of *TP53* and *RB1* mutations (>90 %) and identified numerous other common aberrations, including mutations in the histone-modifiers *CREBBP*, *MLL*, and *EP300* (18 %), *MYC*-family gene amplification (16 %), *PTEN* deletion (10 %), and *FGFR1* amplification (6 %) [27]. They also reported mutations in a novel, putative, tumor suppressor gene, *SLIT2*, which is involved in regulation of neural cell migration, in 10 % of tumors. Rudin et al. analyzed subsets of 56 SCLC tumors by the same techniques and reported similar findings, with frequent derangements in *TP53, RB1, PIK3CA, CDKN2A, PTEN* and several chromatin-modifier genes [28]. Abnormalities were also commonly noted in genes involved in DNA repair and cell cycle checkpoint regulation. Interestingly, numerous genes involved in the regulation of "stem-cell" characteristics were affected, including mutations in components of the NOTCH and Hedgehog pathways, and amplification of *SOX2*, a mediator of stem-cell self-renewal, in 27 % of SCLC tumors [28].

Byers et al. took a different approach to target discovery, evaluating the proteomic differences between SCLC and NSCLC cell lines [29]. They identified relative over-expression of the cell cycle regulator, EZH2, and the DNA-repair mediator, PARP1, in SCLC, and demonstrated that siRNA knockdown of EZH2 or PARP1 led to growth inhibition. In addition, PARP inhibition with AZD2881 and AG014699 resulted in growth inhibition and sensitization to the standard chemotherapeutic agents, cisplatin and etoposide, in SCLC cell lines [29]. In order to evaluate the predictive nature of putative therapeutic targets, Sos et al. exposed 44 molecularly characterized SCLC cell lines to 267 inhibitor compounds with potential clinical relevance [30]. Of note, 95 % of the cell lines were derived from patients with ES-SCLC, which is in contrast to the aforementioned studies utilizing primary tumors in which the majority of samples were obtained from patients with LS-SCLC. This difference in stage of disease likely accounts for some of the discrepancies in findings, such as the much higher rate of *MYC* amplification found in the cell lines (44 % vs. 16 %) [27, 30]. Among the many genetic abnormalities identified, several stood out as potential predictive biomarkers. PTEN loss was associated with the activity of HSP inhibitors, but interestingly, not with that of PI3K inhibitors, and FGFR1 amplification partially correlated with the activity of FGFR inhibitors. One of the strongest associations was that of *c-MYC,* but not *L-MYC* or *N-MYC,* amplification with aurora B kinase inhibitor activity [30].

The challenge of obtaining adequate tissue to perform complex genetic analyses remains a major hurdle to the clinical implementation of personalized medicine in patients with lung cancer. One strategy for overcoming this obstacle is to isolate peripheral blood circulating tumor cells (CTCs) which could then undergo molecular characterization. Hou et al. obtained serial blood samples from 97 patients with SCLC, 68 % of whom had extensive-stage disease [31]. CTCs were defined as cells that were positive for EpCam, cytokeratin, and DAPI, but negative for CD45. At the pre-treatment baseline, CTCs were identified in 85 % of patients with a median of 24 cells/7.5 ml (range, 0–44,896). After one cycle of standard chemotherapy, 81 % of patients exhibited a decline in CTCs with a median of 1 cell/7.5 ml (range 0–2960). Poor prognosis was associated with a higher number of CTCs at baseline and a lack of decline with treatment. Most importantly, in many patients the CTCs could be molecularly characterized by flow cytometry and immunohistochemistry [31]. Although, the low number of CTCs identified at baseline in most patients raises concerns about the clinical generalizability of this strategy, emerging technologies such as single-cell genomic analysis, may allow broader molecular classification that is required for optimal implementation of personalized treatments.

It is now clear that the technology exists for rapid and broad characterization of the molecular drivers in cancer cells. In SCLC and other cancers with high mutational burdens brought on by excessive carcinogen exposure, the clinical validation of relevant molecular targets remains challenging. In such situations, there is a high likelihood that tumor cell heterogeneity and the dysregulation of numerous pathways will limit the activity of any single molecularly targeted therapeutic intervention. Nevertheless, numerous rational strategies have been devised and tested in clinical trials for patients with SCLC.

4 Targeted Therapy for SCLC

For over four decades, clinical research in SCLC has focused on various combinations of cytotoxic chemotherapy drugs and radiotherapy. We have now entered the era of targeted therapy in oncology with the identification of agents that are more 'tumor-focused'. Theoretically, such treatment should improve anti-cancer efficacy and minimize the myriad toxicities that commonly occur with cytotoxic chemotherapy. A wide variety of molecularly targeted approaches have been explored in patients with SCLC, but, thus far, none of them have demonstrated convincing clinical utility.

4.1 Angiogenesis Inhibitors

Several lines of evidence support a major role for angiogenic pathways in SCLC, making them an attractive therapeutic target. SCLC is a highly vascular tumor with a high micro-vessel density, and most patients with SCLC have elevated serum levels of vascular endothelial growth factor (VEGF), a key mediator of angiogenesis [32]. In addition, many SCLC cells express the functional VEGFR receptors, VEGFR-2 and VEGFR-3, suggesting that this pathway may also serve as an autocrine growth regulator in SCLC [33, 34]. Elevated pre-treatment serum levels of VEGF and basic fibroblast growth factor (bFGF), another angiogenesis mediator, are associated with poor response to chemotherapy and reduced survival [35–37]. Although several anti-angiogenic agents have demonstrated benefit in other malignancies, clinically relevant predictive biomarkers have not yet been identified.

Three phase II studies investigated the role of bevacizumab, a humanized, anti-VEGF monoclonal antibody, in combination with standard chemotherapy. In the first trial, 63 patients with ES-SCLC received bevacizumab plus cisplatin and etoposide followed by maintenance bevacizumab [38]. The response rate (63.5 %), median progression-free survival (PFS) (4.7 months, 95 % CI, 4.3–5.5) and overall survival (OS) (median, 10.9 months, 95 % CI, 7.9–12.2; 1-year, 38 %) were similar to those achieved historically with chemotherapy alone. In addition, baseline, serum VEGF levels did not correlate with survival. The second trial randomized 102 patients with ES-SCLC to receive platinum/etoposide plus either bevacizumab or placebo concurrently and as maintenance therapy [39]. The bevacizumab arm demonstrated a superior response rate compared to placebo (58 %, 95 % CI, 43–71 % vs. 48 %, 95 % CI, 34–62 %), but no OS benefit was identified (median 9.4 vs. 10.9 months, HR, 1.16; 95 % CI 0.66–2.04). The third trial combined bevacizumab with cisplatin/irinotecan without maintenance therapy in 72 patients with ES-SCLC [40]. Although the survival results were encouraging with a median PFS of 7.0 months (95 % CI, 6.4–8.4) and a median OS of 11.6 months (95 % CI, 10.5–15.1), the trial did not meet its primary endpoint with a 1-year OS rate of only 44 % (95 % CI 33–58 %). Serum VEGF levels were not associated with PFS, but patients who developed grade ≥1 hypertension, a common side effect of bevacizumab, demonstrated a trend towards improved OS. Although bevacizumab plus chemotherapy has been well tolerated in ES-SCLC, the lack of an apparent improvement in survival has tempered enthusiasm for this approach. However, the development of hypertension may be an indicator of effective inhibition of the VEGF pathway and is being evaluated as a surrogate biomarker for benefit from bevacizumab [41, 42]. In LS-SCLC, the use of anti-angiogenic therapy has been more problematic. A phase II study of irinotecan, carboplatin, and bevacizumab with concurrent radiotherapy followed by maintenance bevacizumab was terminated early due to an unacceptable incidence of tracheoesophageal fistulae [43].

A randomized, phase II, placebo-controlled trial evaluated topotecan plus either aflibercept, a recombinant fusion protein that binds circulating VEGF, or placebo in 98 patients with recurrent ES-SCLC after platinum-based chemotherapy [44].

Although 3-month PFS favored aflibercept over placebo (26 % vs. 9 %; p=0.01), only one partial response was identified and median OS was similar between the two arms (4.6 vs. 3.9 months; p=0.25).

Several oral multi-kinase inhibitors that target VEGFR have been investigated as maintenance or second-line therapy in SCLC, but poor tolerability has been limiting. Sunitinib is a small-molecule inhibitor of receptor tyrosine kinases, including VEGFR, c-kit, FLT3, RET, and PDGFR. Two small trials utilized 50 mg/day for 4 weeks of a 6-week cycle as either maintenance therapy after platinum-based chemotherapy or as monotherapy following relapse [45, 46]. In both studies, no improvement in survival was noted and the majority of patients were unable to tolerate sunitinib due to profound fatigue. Interestingly, a continuous, lower dose schedule of sunitinib has shown promise as maintenance therapy in two other trials. The first phase II trial utilized sunitinib 25 mg/day without interruption in 34 patients after they had received six cycles of carboplatin and irinotecan [47]. The 1-year OS of 54 % and median PFS of 7.6 months were superior to historical controls, and the severe toxicity rate was relatively low. Similarly, trial CALGB 30504 randomized 85 patients to receive platinum/etoposide followed by either sunitinib 37.5 mg/day or placebo. The primary endpoint was met with an improvement in median PFS (3.8 vs. 2.3 months; HR=1.53, 95 % CI, 1.03–2.27; p=0.037). However, median OS was similar between the two arms and tolerability was a concern, with 46 % of patients having grade 3/4 toxicity and 20 % grade 3 fatigue.

Sorafenib is another multi-targeted, small-molecule inhibitor that targets B-RAF, VEGFR-1,-2,-3, PDGFR-β, c-kit, FLT3 and RET. The primary mechanism of anti-tumor activity is believed to be inhibition of VEGFR-2 [48]. A phase II trial of sorafenib 400 mg twice daily in 89 patients with recurrent, platinum-treated SCLC reported a response rate of 11 % (95 % CI, 3–25 %) with median OS of 6.7 months (95 % CI, 6.1–9.1 months) in patients deemed platinum-sensitive. Not surprisingly, the response rate (2 %, 95 % CI, 0–12 %) and median OS (5.3 months) were lower in platinum-resistant patients. Unfortunately, 23 % of patients stopped sorafenib because of toxicity. Serial serum VEGF levels did not correlate with clinical benefit and further investigation with this agent in SCLC was not recommended. Vandetanib targets VEGFR-2 and, to a lesser extent, EGFR. A randomized phase II study of vandetanib 300 mg/day vs. placebo in patients who responded to induction chemotherapy did not improve median PFS (2.7 vs. 2.8 months; HR, 1.01; 80 % CI, 0.75–1.36) or median OS (10.6 vs. 11.9 months; HR, 1.43; 80 % CI 1.00–2.05) [49]. Vandetanib was also poorly tolerated with frequent dose-reductions for rash and gastrointestinal toxicity. A phase II trial of cediranib, a selective inhibitor of VEGFR-1,-2,-3, in the second-line setting also failed to demonstrate any promising clinical activity [50]. The initial dose of cediranib 45 mg/day was intolerable due to grade 3/4 fatigue, diarrhea and elevated liver enzymes. In summary, these trials indicate that tyrosine kinase inhibitors (TKIs) targeting VEGFR are not suited for single-agent therapy in patients with SCLC.

Thalidomide inhibits angiogenesis by repressing key angiogenic genes and down-regulating the secretion of VEGF and bFGF [51]. Two phase III trials randomized patients with ES-SCLC to platinum-based chemotherapy plus either thalidomide or placebo. The first trial utilized an induction regimen of etoposide, cisplatin, cyclophosphamide and 4′-epidoxorubicin (PCDE) for 6 cycles plus thalidomide 400 mg/day or placebo in patients who had a response to the first two cycles of chemotherapy [52]. Ninety-two patients were enrolled and although a trend towards improved survival with thalidomide was identified, it was not statistically significant (median OS 11.7 vs. 8.7 months; HR, 0.74; 95 % CI, 0.49–1.12; p=0.16). Paradoxically, patients with a performance status (PS) of 1 or 2 had better survival than those with PS 0 (HR, 0.59; 95 % CI, 0.37–0.92; p=.02). Toxicity was generally manageable, but there were four toxic deaths as a result of myelosuppression in the thalidomide arm. A larger phase III trial combined thalidomide 100–200 mg/day or placebo with 6 cycles of carboplatin/etoposide followed by maintenance thalidomide or placebo [53]. Over 700 patients with both LS- and ES-SCLC were randomized. The addition of thalidomide did not improve median OS compared to placebo (10.1 vs. 10.5 months; HR, 1.09; 95 % CI, 0.93–1.27). An exploratory subgroup analysis suggested increased risk of death in patients with ES-SCLC (HR, 1.36; 95 % CI, 1.10–1.68). In addition, patients treated with thalidomide had twice the risk of thromboembolic events, but this did not appear to contribute to increased mortality. The authors suggested that the lower dose of thalidomide used in this trial may have contributed to the lack of therapeutic benefit, but a dose–response relationship has not been identified for this agent in other malignancies.

Several trials of other agents targeting angiogenic pathways, such as pazopanib and nintedanib which both inhibit VEGFR, are on-going in patients with SCLC. However, given the lack of clinical benefit and significant toxicity associated with anti-angiogenic agents in SCLC thus far, it appears unlikely that such studies in unselected patients will lead to improvements in survival. The identification of effective predictive biomarkers should help guide more rational use of these agents, but this has proven elusive given the heterogeneity of angiogenic signaling within tumors.

4.2 Growth Factor Inhibitors

A wide variety of growth factor receptors are overexpressed in SCLC and have been investigated as therapeutic targets. Epidermal growth factor receptor (EGFR) is over-expressed in 60 % of NSCLCs and EGFR TKIs have shown dramatic clinical benefits in patients whose tumors harbor activating EGFR mutations [54, 55]. In contrast, such mutations are extremely rare in SCLC, occurring primarily in combined SCLC/NSCLC tumors [56]. Despite this, preclinical data suggested that SCLC cells with low EGFR expression may respond to EGFR-TKIs though inhibition of the downstream mediators, ERK-1/2 [57]. However, a phase II trial of the EGFR-TKI, gefitinib, in 19 patients with relapsed SCLC failed to demonstrate any objective responses, likely due to the paucity of activating EGFR mutations in these tumors [58].

C-kit is a transmembrane, tyrosine kinase receptor that is detectable by immunohistochemistry (IHC) in 30–70 % of SCLCs [59, 60]. Imatinib, an oral inhibitor of both BCR–ABL and c-kit, has been investigated as both maintenance and second-line therapy for SCLC. In a small phase II trial, 14 patients with c-kit-IHC positive SCLC received maintenance imatinib 400 mg twice daily after induction cisplatin/irinotecan [61]. No improvement in median PFS (4.3 months) was identified relative to historical controls. Similarly, two phase II trials evaluated imatinib in patients with relapsed SCLC whose tumors expressed c-kit by IHC [62, 63]. There were no objective responses and median OS was only 2.0–5.3 months. Of note, these three trials are the only SCLC studies reported to date in which a predictive biomarker was utilized in an attempt to enrich the enrolled patient population for improved response to a targeted drug. A larger phase II study combined imatinib with carboplatin/irinotecan as initial therapy for in 68 patients with ES-SCLC who were not selected for c-kit expression [64]. Median PFS and OS were a disappointing 5.4 and 8.4 months, respectively. Retrospectively, 70 % of patients had tumors that expressed c-kit by IHC, but expression of c-kit had no impact on overall survival. Dasatinib is an oral TKIs with activity against c-kit and c-src, both of which are commonly expressed in SCLC. A phase II trial of dasatinib 70 mg twice daily in 45 patients with chemo-sensitive, relapsed SCLC reported no objective responses and survival appeared lower than that of historical controls (median PFS 1.4 months, median OS 3.9 months) [65]. A recurring theme in oncology is that the benefit of TKIs is largely limited to patients with tumors that harbor activating mutations in the target gene, as evidenced by the profound activity of imatinib in gastrointestinal stromal tumors harboring c-kit mutations. Unfortunately, c-kit-activating mutations have not been consistently identified in SCLC, highlighting the point that mere expression does not define the biological relevance of a potential therapeutic target.

The insulin-like growth factor (IGF) signaling pathway is under investigation as a potential therapeutic target in several malignancies, including SCLC. The type-1 IGF receptor (IGF-1R) is commonly over-expressed in lung cancer cell lines and tumors, and preclinical studies in SCLC have demonstrated that inhibition of IGF-1R disrupts cell proliferation and survival [66, 67]. Cixutumumab (IMC-A12) is a monoclonal antibody that targets IGF-1R. A randomized, phase II trial in patients with untreated ES-SCLC compared cisplatin/etoposide plus concurrent and maintenance cixutumumab to cisplatin/etoposide alone [68]. There was no evidence of improvement in efficacy with cixutumumab with response rate, PFS and OS being nearly identical in the two arms. A randomized, phase II study of the IGF-1R inhibitor linsitinib (OSI-906) vs. topotecan in patients with relapsed SCLC is currently enrolling patients. However, IGF-1R inhibition has not demonstrated substantial clinical benefit in several tumor types, and it appears that further studies are needed to identify predictive biomarkers that can define the optimal patient subgroups most likely to benefit from these agents.

Temsirolimus is a novel inhibitor of the mammalian target of rapamycin (mTOR) which has demonstrated cytostatic properties in other tumors, including renal cell carcinoma and mantle cell lymphoma. A randomized, phase II trial of temsirolimus at either 25 mg/week or 250 mg/week as consolidation therapy following initial chemotherapy enrolled 87 patients with ES-SCLC [69]. Only one patient had a partial response, and both median PFS (2.2 months, 95 % CI, 1.8–2.9) and OS (8.0 months; 95 % CI, 6.5–9.5) were unimpressive, suggested that temsirolimus does not warrant further study in SCLC.

Tipifarnib is an oral farnesyl transferase inhibitor that blocks the membrane-localization, and thus the activity, of the *RAS*-family of proto-oncogenes that are critical for signal transduction. Even though *RAS* mutations are not found in SCLC, tipifarnib was evaluated in a phase II study of 22 patients with relapsed SCLC. Somewhat unsurprisingly, there was no evidence of clinical activity [70].

Clinical trials of agents targeting other proliferative signaling pathways in SCLC are on-going. Targets under evaluation include: c-met (tivantinib); c-abl (ponatinib); Fyn3 (the antibody-drug conjugate SC16LD6.5); cyclin dependent kinases (BAY-100394); and somatostatin receptor SSTR2 (pasireotide; the radio-immunoconjugate Rh^{188}-P2045).

4.3 Matrix Metalloproteinase Inhibitors (MMPI)

Inhibition of matrix metalloproteinases (MMPs) has been investigated as a treatment strategy for SCLC. MMPs are produced and secreted by many cancers and are frequently detected in both malignant and stromal cells within tumors. MMPs digest basement membrane and extracellular matrix to facilitate local tumor invasion. Several MMPs have been found to be over-expressed in SCLC and this over-expression predicts for poorer survival [71, 72]. Marimastat is an orally administered MMP inhibitor. Based on preclinical data suggesting a tumoristatic effect, a randomized clinical trial was designed evaluating marimastat 10 mg twice daily vs. placebo as adjuvant therapy following induction chemotherapy in over 400 patients with either LS- or ES-SCLC [73]. Both median PFS (4.3 vs. 4.4 months; HR, 0.977; 95 % CI, 0.807–1.184; $p=0.81$) and median OS (9.3 vs. 9.7 months; HR = 1.013; 95 % CI, 0.831–1.235; $p=0.90$) were nearly identical in the marimastat and placebo arms, respectively. In addition, the drug was poorly tolerated with over 50 % of patients requiring dose-reductions and 32 % stopping therapy prematurely due to toxicity. Quality-of-life favored the placebo arm with increased pain and reduced global quality-of-life noted with marimastat. Another MMP inhibitor, BAY 12-9566, was also compared to placebo as adjuvant therapy for SCLC, but after enrollment of only 327 patients, an interim analysis noted a PFS advantage favoring the placebo arm (5.3 vs. 3.2 months; $p=0.05$), and the study was discontinued [74].

4.4 Pro-Apoptotic Agents

Suppression of the apoptotic inhibitor Bcl-2 has been extensively investigated as a therapeutic strategy in SCLC. *Bcl-2* is an oncogene that produces an inhibitor of programmed cell death that acts through binding to the BH3 domain of pro-apoptotic family members to suppress cell death. Over-expression of Bcl-2 is associated with resistance to chemotherapy and has been reported in up to 90 % of SCLC. Xenograft models suggest that suppression of Bcl-2 enhances the cytotoxic effects of cisplatin and etoposide [75]. Oblimersen is an antisense oligonucleotide that is complementary to *Bcl-2* mRNA. Upon entering the cell, oblimersen hybridizes to *Bcl-2* mRNA and facilitates its degradation by RNaseH, thus decreasing Bcl-2 protein production [76, 77]. Given its chemotherapy sensitizing properties, oblimersen plus carboplatin/etoposide was compared to chemotherapy alone in a randomized, phase II study of 63 patients with ES-SCLC [78]. However, both median OS (8.6 vs. 10.6 months) and 1-year OS (24 % vs. 47 %) favored the control arm. Toxicity was similar between the two arms, and it was postulated that oblimersen may not have adequately penetrated SCLC cells to suppress Bcl-2.

Three other Bcl-2 antagonists, obatoclax, navitoclax (ABT-263), and AT-101 are small-molecule BH3 mimetics that act by inhibiting the interaction of Bcl-2 with BH3-containing pro-apoptotic proteins, such as Bax and Bak [79]. An encouraging phase I trial of obatoclax in combination with carboplatin/etoposide enrolled 25 patients with untreated SCLC and reported a favorable response rate of 68 % and median OS of 12.5 months at the recommended phase II schedule [80]. However, a phase II trial of obatoclax plus topotecan in patients with recurrent SCLC was stopped early due to lack of responses and dismal PFS after the first stage of enrollment [81]. Neurologic toxicity was also problematic with somnolence in 89 % of patients and ataxia in 56 %. Navitoclax also demonstrated promising activity in a phase I study in heavily pretreated patients with SCLC or atypical bronchial carcinoid with a 35 % stable disease rate and one durable partial response lasting over 35 months [82]. However, the phase II study of single-agent navitoclax in 39 patients with relapsed SCLC yielded a response rate of only 2.6 % with stable disease in 23 % and median OS of only 3.2 months [83]. AT-101 is an oral BH3 mimetic that has been shown to increase concentrations of the pro-apoptotic proteins NOXA and PUMA [84], and has synergistic activity with topotecan in a SCLC xenograft model [85]. A phase II trial of AT-101 in 15 patients with chemotherapy-sensitive, recurrent SCLC reported no responses, and a correlative analysis of peripheral blood mononuclear cells demonstrated a paradoxical reduction of pro-apoptotic caspase activity with treatment [86]. Similarly, a phase I/II study of AT-101 plus topotecan in 30 patients with relapsed/refractory SCLC yielded only three partial responses in the chemo-sensitive, relapsed cohort with a median time to progression (TTP) of 4 months, and no responses in the refractory cohort with a median TTP of only 2.7 months [87]. Once again, the trial did not meet its endpoint of improved response rate and was stopped after the first stage of accrual. Recently, a phase I study of AT-101 plus cisplatin/etoposide in seven patients with SCLC reported a favorable response rate of 83 %, suggesting that further studies of this combination are warranted in the first-line setting [88]. Overall, however, despite solid biological rationale and promising preclinical data, efforts to target apoptotic pathways in patients with SCLC have thus far been disappointing.

4.5 Cancer Stem Cell-Targeted Therapy

SCLC responds extremely well to first-line chemotherapy or chemoradiotherapy. However, most patients with LS-SCLC and all patients with ES-SCLC relapse with relatively resistant disease, suggesting that there is a sub-population of tumor cells in the initial tumor that are profoundly resistant to current standard therapy. It has been postulated that a small population of cancer stem cells (CSCs) could be responsible for this clinical phenomenon, and that SCLC may represent the best solid tumor model in which to test the CSC hypothesis. Treatment strategies targeting chemo-resistant CSCs are based on the elucidation of the pathways that regulate CSC traits, such as self-renewal. Thus far, interest has focused mainly on the inhibition of the Hedgehog, Notch and Wnt signaling pathways that are critical for stem cell development and self-renewal [89, 90].

Recent data suggest that the inhibition of Hedgehog signaling has an antitumor effect in SCLC [91]. Several Hedgehog pathway inhibitors are under clinical investigation in SCLC, including vismodegib (GDC-0449), erismodegib (LDE-225), LY2940680 and BMS-833923. In a primary SCLC xenograft model, LDE225 enhanced tumor cell kill after initial treatment with chemotherapy [92]. Vismodegib is an orally administered, small-molecule that binds to and inhibits Smoothened (SMO), a membrane protein that facilitates signaling through the Hedgehog pathway. A randomized, phase II study in 103 patients with ES-SCLC evaluated first-line cisplatin/etoposide with or without concurrent and maintenance vismodegib, and reported no significant differences in response rate, PFS or OS between the two arms [68].

Inhibition of the Notch and Wnt signaling pathways involved in CSC regulation is also undergoing active investigation. The Notch pathway is a primary regulator of normal adult stem cell differentiation and proliferation that is frequently dysregulated in SCLC [93]. Notch pathway inhibitors, such as the anti-Notch 2/3 monoclonal antibody OMP-59R5, are currently in clinical development in SCLC and other cancers [94]. Similarly, the Wnt pathway plays a critical role in adult stem cell regulation through control of cell differentiation and proliferation [95]. Aberrations of the Wnt pathway have been identified in lung cancer, and monoclonal antibodies targeting Wnt-1 and Wnt-2 are in early development [96, 97]. Hopefully, further investigations of the CSC hypothesis will open the door to new targets and subsequent therapies for SCLC in the near future.

4.6 Histone Deacetylase Inhibitors/Aurora Kinase Inhibitors

Histone deacetylases (HDACs) are a family of enzymes that regulate gene transcription, and the dysregulation of HDACs has been implicated in cancer proliferation, survival and apoptosis [98]. In light of this central role in malignant transformation,

HDACs have emerged as therapeutic targets in a variety of malignancies. In preclinical models of SCLC, HDAC inhibitors have altered histone acetylation, enhanced apoptosis, and reduced cell viability [99]. The CALGB conducted a phase II study of the HDAC inhibitor, romidepsin, in 16 patients with chemo-sensitive, relapsed SCLC [100]. No objective responses were identified, and both median PFS (1.8 months, 95 % CI, 1.54–3.52) and OS (5.9 months, 95 % CI, 4.63–16.5) were relatively low. The authors concluded that romidepsin did not warrant further study in SCLC. Vorinostat and belinostat, two newer HDAC inhibitors, are currently undergoing clinical evaluation in SCLC.

Aurora A kinase (AAK) is a protein kinase that facilitates chromosomal segregation during mitotic cell division, a process vital for tumor progression [101]. AAK is commonly amplified and over-expressed in many tumor types, including lung cancer, and preclinical studies have demonstrated mitotic arrest and cell death in tumor cells after AAK inhibition, making AAK an appealing therapeutic target [102, 103]. A phase I/II study of the AAK inhibitor, alisertib (MLN8237), enrolled patients with solid tumors, including 47 with SCLC, refractory to standard therapy [104]. Partial response was reported in 21 % of SCLC patients with a median PFS of 2.8 months and manageable toxicity, including neutropenia, anemia and stomatitis. In light of this clinically relevant response rate, further studies of alisertib in SCLC are underway.

Several other agents that affect DNA integrity are also being studied in clinical trials in patients with SCLC. Defects in DNA repair are commonly found in nearly all types of cancer. Poly-ADP ribose polymerase 1 (PARP1) is involved in DNA repair and inhibition of PARP1 results in irreparable double-strand breaks and cell death. Veliparib is currently being evaluated in patients with SCLC. Another trial is assessing the potential anti-SCLC activity of KML001, an anti-telomerase that induces cytotoxicity through DNA damage at the telomere in cancer cells.

4.7 Immunotherapy

Immunotherapy is a novel therapeutic approach with the goal of augmenting the patient's innate immune cytotoxic response to cancer cells. In SCLC, vaccine therapy has primarily been investigated as consolidation treatment after initial chemotherapy in an attempt to prolong the duration of tumor response. Bec2 is an anti-idiotypic antibody that mimics GD3, a ganglioside antigen that is over-expressed in 60 % of SCLCs, and induces anti-GD3 antibodies [105]. A large, phase III trial evaluated adjuvant vaccination with Bec2 after chemoradiation in over 500 patients with LS-SCLC [106]. Patients were randomized to observation vs. five vaccinations of Bec2 plus bacillus Calmette-Guerin (BCG) to enhance an anti-GD3 response. Common side effects of the vaccine included flu-like symptoms, local skin reactions and lethargy. No statistically significant improvement in survival was identified with the Bec2 vaccine compared to observation alone, with median PFS of 5.7 vs. 6.3 months, median OS of 14.3 vs. 16.4 months, and 2-year survival rate of 36 % vs. 38 %, respectively. The authors surmised that these disappointing results may have been due to the induction of a humoral anti-GD3 response in only 1/3 of patients receiving the vaccine.

A similar, rational vaccine strategy targeted the p53 antigen. *P53* is mutated in over 90 % of SCLCs and mutant p53 has a longer half-life and higher concentrations than wild-type p53 [107], making it an ideal immunotherapeutic target. Twenty-nine patients receiving platinum-based chemotherapy underwent leukopheresis for collection of dendritic cells which were then infected with an adenoviral construct containing p53 [108]. This adenovirus-based p53 vaccine was injected intradermally every 2 weeks over a 6-week period followed by monthly injections. Sixteen patients had significant p53-specific T-cell responses to immunization, but this did not translate into a significant clinical benefit, with only one patient demonstrating a short-lived partial response and five patients having stable disease with tumor progression within 6 months. Median OS from the time of first vaccination was 11.8 months and 1-year OS was 38 %. The authors suggested that dendritic cell function was reduced in most of the patients, possibly due to induction chemotherapy, which may have reduced the efficacy of the vaccine. Chemotherapy may also directly blunt antigen-specific, T-cell responses. Interestingly, 75 % of the patients who developed a p53-specific immune response demonstrated an objective response to subsequent chemotherapy which is unexpected given that the response rate in relapsed/refractory SCLC is typically 20 % or less. The reason for this degree of chemo-sensitivity after vaccination is unclear, but warrants further investigation. Despite these predominantly negative results, other vaccine-based approaches are in clinical development in SCLC, including a novel peptide vaccine targeting HLA-A*24-positive SCLC cells.

Interferon-α (IFN-α) is a cytokine that promotes antigen presentation on tumor cells and stimulates immune response. IFN-α has been evaluated as maintenance therapy after chemoradiation for SCLC in two trials. The first study randomized 237 patients to three arms: maintenance IFN-α, maintenance chemotherapy, or observation, with no difference reported in OS between the arms [109]. A smaller, phase II study also treated patients with induction chemoradiation followed by randomization to one of three arms: maintenance IFN-α plus retinoic acid, maintenance trophosphamide, or observation [110]. Median OS was not statistically different among the three arms at 17, 12 and 14 months, respectively. These and other trials have failed to identify a significant clinical benefit with IFN-α in SCLC and further studies were not recommended.

Immune checkpoint inhibitors have shown promise in several tumor types, including NSCLC. CTLA-4 is an immune checkpoint protein expressed on activated T-cells whose main function is to down-regulate T-cell activation [111]. Cancers can hijack the CTLA-4 system in order to escape the host's natural immune response to the malignancy, suggesting that CTLA-4 inhibition may induce a clinically beneficial, immune, anti-tumor response [112]. Ipilimumab is a fully human, monoclonal antibody that binds to CTLA-4 and inhibits ligand binding, enhancing T-cell activation and infiltration into tumor tissue. Ipilimumab was combined with carboplatin and paclitaxel in a randomized, phase II trial in 164 patients with

ES-SCLC [113]. Patients were randomized to one of three arms: carboplatin/paclitaxel/ipilimumab×4 cycles followed by 2 cycles of carboplatin/paclitaxel (concurrent); carboplatin/paclitaxel×2 cycles followed by carboplatin/paclitaxel/ipilimumab×4 cycles (phased); or carboplatin/paclitaxel/placebo×6 cycles. Patients without tumor progression then received maintenance with ipilimumab or placebo. The primary endpoint was immune-related (ir) PFS based on newly proposed immune-related response criteria (irRC) that factor in the potential for initial tumor progression followed by delayed regression or stabilization. The median irPFS for the concurrent, phased and placebo arms were 5.7, 6.4 and 5.3 months, respectively (HR, 0.64; p=0.03). The median OS favored the phased ipilimumab arm over the concurrent and placebo arms; 12.9, 9.1 and 9.9 months, respectively (HR, 0.75; p=0.13). Tumor response rates also favored the phased arm over the concurrent arm, suggesting that chemotherapy may sensitize SCLC to ipilimumab. Treatment was generally well tolerated with more rash, pruritus, and diarrhea in patients receiving ipilimumab. Given these results, two phase III trials with ipilimumab in advanced lung cancer are currently underway.

PD-1 is another immune checkpoint receptor expressed by activated T-cells that modulates immunosuppression through binding of its ligand, PD-L1. Many cancer cells produce and secrete PD-L1, resulting in localized immunosuppression that protects the cancer from immune surveillance. A phase Ib trial of pembrolizumab, an anti-PD1 antibody, enrolled 20 patients with PDL1-positive SCLC with a response rate of 35% and disease-control rate of 55% [114]. Another phase I/II study of patients with relapsed SCLC evaluated both single-agent nivolumab, an anti-PD1 antibody, and the combination of nivolumab plus ipilumumab, an anti-CTLA4 antibody. Response rates and disease control rates were 18% and 38%, respectively, in 40 patients treated with single-agent nivolumab, and 17 % and 54 %, respectively, in 46 patients treated with the combination [115]. Further trials of PD-1/PD-L1 inhibitors in SCLC are currently under way.

4.8 Oncolytic Virus Therapy

Finally, oncolytic virus therapy is an area of active investigation in several tumor types. These efforts have faced many challenges that have limited efficacy, including low viral titers, pre-existing host immunity, and lack of viral tropism for cancer cells. However, promising results from a phase I study of the oncolytic picornavirus, Seneca Valley Virus (SVV-001), in neuroendocrine tumors, including SCLC, generated renewed interest in this approach [116]. Thirty patients with neuroendocrine tumors, including 6 with SCLC, were treated with SVV-001and no dose-limiting toxicity was identified. Intratumoral viral replication was noted in vivo with increased blood viral titers several days after the initial administration and viral clearance several months later. Interestingly, one patient with SCLC resistant to several lines of chemotherapy demonstrated a progression-free interval of over 10 months. The reason for the apparent affinity of SVV-001 to neuroendocrine tumors remains unknown. Despite these promising findings, a randomized, phase II trial of 58 patients with ES-SCLC treated with induction chemotherapy followed by either the Seneca Valley virus (NTX-010) or placebo was prematurely closed after an interim analysis demonstrated no survival benefit [117]. The median PFS for both NTX-010 and placebo was only 1.7 months and the 3-month OS was also nearly identical at 83 % for NTX-010 and 85 % for placebo. Surprisingly, patients with detectable viral RNA 7 and 14 days post-treatment had a worse PFS compared to those with undetectable viral loads.

5 Conclusion

The development of molecular targeted strategies in SCLC has followed a common theme: identification of a putative target; development of an associated therapeutic approach; promising activity in preclinical models; suggestion of clinical activity in phase I studies; and abjectly disappointing results in phase II/III clinical trials. Thus far, no biologically rational or personalized treatments have demonstrated clinical utility in patients with SCLC. Nevertheless, clinical investigators continue to develop and evaluate new, molecularly targeted agents and combinations of agents in an attempt to overcome the molecular heterogeneity and resistance inherent in SCLC. Table 1 lists many such agents that have already been evaluated or are under investigation for the treatment of SCLC.

SCLC offers many unique barriers to the design and development of successful therapy. Adequate banks of ample tumor samples are relatively hard to come by since few patients are eligible for surgical resection and most diagnoses are made by fine needle aspiration or a small bronchoscopic biopsy. Although numerous cell lines have been established, the clinical failure of so many rational strategies suggests that the existing preclinical models do not adequately reflect the broad molecular heterogeneity of the actual disease in humans. The virtually universal link between SCLC and heavy tobacco smoking results in a very high mutational burden that severely challenges the ability to isolate relevant driver mutations and will undoubtedly limit the clinical activity of any single targeted therapy. Clinically, patients with SCLC tend to be quite ill at presentation due to the aggressive nature of the disease and the multitude of comorbid conditions brought on by years of tobacco use. In addition, despite robust tumor responses during initial standard treatment, they usually decline rapidly upon disease recurrence, hampering attempts for enrollment on investigational clinical trials.

Most of the strategies discussed in this chapter were designed in a rational manner with preclinical studies demonstrating interference with a specific biological target, pathway or process. However, nearly all of them were then clinically evaluated in an empiric manner, enrolling patients who were not selected for any specific biological characteristic aside from having SCLC. Of all of the completed trials described in this chapter, only three of them, all evaluating anti-c-kit therapy, selected patients based on the presence of the putative target, and even those trials

Table 1 Selected molecularly targeted agents evaluated in clinical trials in small cell lung cancer

Mechanism of action	Agent	Targets	Phase	Line of therapy
VEGF inhibitors	Bevacizumab	VEGF	II	1st line/maintenance
	Aflibercept	VEGF	II	relapsed
Multi-kinase inhibitors	Sunitinib	VEGFR, c-kit, FLT3, RET, PDGFR	II	maintenance/relapsed
	Sorafenib	B-raf, VEGFR, RET, PDGFR, c-kit, FLT3,	II	relapsed
	Vandetanib	VEGFR-2, EGFR	II	relapsed
	Cediranib	VEGFR-1,-2,-3	II	relapsed
	Nintedanib[a]	VEGFR, FGFR, PDGFR	II	relapsed
	Pazopanib[a]	VEGFR, FGFR, PDGFR, c-kit	II	maintenance/relapsed
Angiogenesis inhibitors	Thalidomide	angiogenic genes	III	1st line/maintenance
Growth factor pathway inhibitors	Imatinib	c-kit	II	maintenance/relapsed
	Dasatinib	c-kit, c-src	II	relapsed
	Temsirolimus	mTOR	II	maintenance
	Tipifarnib	farnesyl transferase	II	relapsed
	Cixitumumab	IGF-1R	II	1st line/maintenance
	Linsitinib[a]	IGF-1R	II	relapsed
	Ponatinib[a]	c-abl		relapsed
	Tivantinib	c-met	I	relapsed
	SC16LD6.5[a]	Fyn3	II	relapsed
	Pasireotide[a]	SSTR2	II	relapsed
	Rh^{188}-P2045[a]	SSTR2	I/II	relapsed
	BAY-1000394[a]	CDKs	I/II	1st line/maintenance
MMP inhibitors	Marimastat	MMPs	III	maintenance
	BAY 12-9566	MMPs	II	maintenance

Pro-apoptotic agents	Oblimersen	Bcl-2 mRNA	II	1st line
	Obatoclax mesylate	Bcl-2	II	relapsed
	Navitoclax	Bcl-2	II	relapsed
	AT-101	Bcl-2, Bcl-xL, Mcl-1	II	relapsed
Cancer stem cell-targeting agents	Vismodegib	SMO	III	1st line/maintenance
	Erismodegib[a]	SMO	I	1st line
	LY2940680[a]	SMO	II	1st line/maintenance
	BMS-833923[a]	SMO	I	1st line/maintenance
	OMP-59R5[a]	Notch 2/3	I/II	1st line
HDAC inhibitors	Romidepsin	HDAC	II	relapsed
	Vorinostat	HDAC	I/II	1st line/relapsed
	Belinostat[a]	HDAC	I	1st line
Aurora kinase inhibitor	Alisertib	Aurora kinase	I/II	relapsed
PARP inhibitor	Veliparib[a]	PARP 1/2	I/II	1st line
HSP inhibitor	Ganetespib[a]	HSP 90	II	relapsed
Therapeutic vaccine	Bec2	GD3 ganglioside	III	adjuvant
	INGN-225	p53	II	relapsed
Immune checkpoint inhibitor	Ipilimumab[a]	anti-CTLA-4	III	1st line
Oncolytic tumor virus	SVV-001	neuroendocrine cells	I	relapsed
	NTX-010	neuroendocrine cells	II	adjuvant
Surface antigen-targeting agents	Lorvotuzumab[a]	CD56 (NCAM)	I/II	1st line/maintenance
	BIW-8962	GM2 ganglioside	I/II	relapsed
	TF2/Lu^{177}- IMP-288[a]	CEA	I/II	adjuvant/relapsed

[a]On-going clinical trials

Abbreviations: *VEGFR* vascular endothelial growth factor receptor, *PDGFR* platelet derived growth factor receptor, *EGFR* epidermal growth factor receptor, *FGFR* fibroblast growth factor receptor, *mTOR* mammalian target of rapamycin, *IGF-1R* insulin-like growth factor receptor 1, *SSTR2* somatostatin receptor 2, *CDK* cyclin-dependent kinase, *MMP* matrix metalloproteinase, *SMO* smoothened, *HDAC* histone deacetylase, *PARP* poly-ADP ribose polymerase, *HSP* heat shock protein, *CTLA-4* cytotoxic T-lymphocyte antigen 4, *NCAM* neural cell adhesion molecule, *CEA* carcinoembryonic antigen failed to demonstrate promising clinical activity [61–63]. A recent review of clinical trial databases revealed 31 on-going therapeutic studies of molecularly targeted agents in SCLC. Of these, only six are utilizing predictive biomarkers to select a patient population that might be more apt to respond to the study drug, and only seven are incorporating correlative studies aimed at defining predictive biomarkers for future studies. The optimal development of personalized therapy requires the identification and utilization of predictive biomarkers so we can selectively treat those who will gain the most while avoiding treatment of those with little to no chance for benefit.

The age of personalized medicine in oncology has arrived, but it is still in its infancy. Advances in technology are rapidly expanding our ability to identify driver mutations across many tumor types and to design novel, biologically rational therapeutic strategies. Thus far, few of these strategies have been fully developed into clinical reality. The ultimate goal of personalized therapy in oncology is to improve the outcome for patients with cancer. This requires the analytical and clinical validation of predictive biomarkers followed by the demonstration that a therapeutic strategy based on these biomarkers has favorable clinical utility. The tools to accomplish these goals are already at hand. For patients with SCLC, little has changed over the past 30 years. It is hoped that our expanding understanding of the biology of SCLC will yield new, personalized interventions that will dramatically improve the prognosis and quality-of-life of patients with this dreaded disease.

References

1. Pesch B, Kendzia B, Gustavsson P et al (2012) Cigarette smoking and lung cancer: relative risk estimates for the major histological types from a pooled analysis of case-control studies. Int J Cancer 131:1210–1219
2. Churg A (1994) Lung cancer cell type and occupational exposure. In: Samet JM (ed) Epidemiology of lung cancer. Marcel Dekker, New York, pp 413–436
3. Navada S, Lai P, Schwartz AG, Kalemkerian GP (2006) Temporal trends in small cell lung cancer: analysis of the national surveillance, epidemiology, and end-results database. J Clin Oncol 24(18S):384s
4. Govindan R, Page N, Morgensztern D et al (2006) Changing epidemiology of small-cell lung cancer in the United States over the last 30 years: analysis of the surveillance, epidemiologic, and end-results database. J Clin Oncol 24:4539–4544
5. Siegel R, Ma J, Zou Z, Jemal A (2014) Cancer statistics, 2014. CA Cancer J Clin 64:9–19
6. Zelen M (1973) Keynote address on biostatistics and data retrieval. Cancer Chemother Rep 3 4:31–42
7. Goldstraw P, Crowley JJ, Chansky K et al (2007) The IASLC lung cancer staging project: proposals for the revision of the TNM stage groupings in the forthcoming (seventh) edition of the TNM classification for malignant tumors. J Thorac Oncol 2:706–714
8. Shepherd FA, Crowley J, Van Houtte P et al (2007) The IASLC lung cancer staging project: proposals regarding the clinical staging of smallcell lung cancer in the forthcoming (seventh) edition of the tumor, node, metastasis classification for lung cancer. J Thorac Oncol 2:1067–1077
9. Pignon JP, Arriagada R, Ihde DC et al (1992) A meta-analysis of thoracic radiotherapy for small-cell lung cancer. N Engl J Med 327:1618–1624

10. Warde P, Payne D (1992) Does thoracic irradiation improve survival and local control in limited-stage small-cell carcinoma of the lung? A meta-analysis. J Clin Oncol 10:890–895
11. Fried DB, Morris DE, Poole C et al (2004) Systematic review evaluating the timing of thoracic radiation therapy in combined modality therapy for limited-stage small cell lung cancer. J Clin Oncol 22:4785–4793
12. Turrisi AT, Kim K, Blum R et al (1999) Twice-daily compared with once-daily thoracic radiotherapy in limited small-cell lung cancer treated concurrently with cisplatin and etoposide. N Engl J Med 340:265–271
13. Auperin A, Arriagada R, Pignon JP et al (1999) Prophylactic cranial irradiation for patients with small-cell lung cancer in complete remission. N Engl J Med 341:476–484
14. Slotman B, Faivre-Finn C, Kramer G et al (2007) Prophylactic cranial irradiation in extensive small-cell lung cancer. N Engl J Med 357:664–672
15. Hanna NH, Einhorn LH (2002) Small-cell lung cancer: state of the art. Clin Lung Cancer 4:87–94
16. Von Pawel J, Schiller JH, Shepherd FA et al (1999) Topotecan versus cyclophosphamide, doxorubicin, and vincristine for the treatment of recurrent small-cell lung cancer. J Clin Oncol 17:658–667
17. O'Brien MER, Ciuleanu TE, Tsekov H et al (2006) Phase III trial comparing supportive care alone with supportive care with oral topotecan in patients with relapsed small-cell lung cancer. J Clin Oncol 24:5441–5447
18. Chute JP, Chen T, Feigal E et al (1999) Twenty years of phase III trials for patients with extensive-stage small-cell lung cancer: perceptible progress. J Clin Oncol 17:1794–1801
19. Gazdar AF, Minna JD (1996) NCI series of cell lines: an historical perspective. J Cell Biochem 24(suppl):1–11
20. Kalemkerian GP, Mabry M (1993) Cellular and molecular biology of small-cell lung cancer. In: Roth JA, Cox JD, Hong WK (eds) Lung cancer. Blackwell Scientific, Boston, pp 57–84
21. Naylor SL, Johnson BE, Minna JD, Sakaguchi AY (1987) Loss of heterozygosity of chromosome 3p markers in small-cell lung cancer. Nature 329:451–454
22. Hensel CH, Hsieh CL, Gazdar AF et al (1990) Altered structure and expression of the human retinoblastoma susceptibility gene in small cell lung cancer. Cancer Res 50:3067–3072
23. D'Amico D, Carbone D, Mitsudomi T et al (1992) High frequency of somatically acquired p53 mutations in small-cell lung cancer cell lines and tumors. Oncogene 7:339–346
24. Johnson BE, Ihde DC, Makuch RW et al (1987) myc family oncogene amplification in tumor cell lines established from small cell lung cancer patients and its relationship to clinical status and course. J Clin Invest 79:1629–1634
25. Kalemkerian GP (2000) Host-tumor interactions: growth factors. In: Pass HI, Mitchell JB, Johnson DH, Turrisi AT, Minna JD (eds) Lung cancer: principles and practice, 2nd edn. Lippincott Williams & Wilkins, Philadelphia, pp 181–198
26. Kelley MJ, Linnoila RI, Avis IL et al (1997) Antitumor activity of a monoclonal antibody directed against gastrin-releasing peptide in patients with small cell lung cancer. Chest 112:256–261
27. Peifer M, Fernandez-Cuesta L, Sos ML et al (2012) Integrative genome analyses identify key somatic driver mutations of small-cell lung cancer. Nature Genet 44:1104–1110
28. Rudin CM, Durnick S, Stawiski EW et al (2012) Comprehensive genomic analysis identifies SOX2 as a frequently amplified gene in small-cell lung cancer. Nature Genet 44:1111–1116
29. Byers LA, Wang J, Nilsson MB et al (2012) Proteomic profiling identifies dysregulated pathways in small cell lung cancer and novel therapeutic targets including PARP1. Cancer Discov 2:798–811
30. Sos ML, Dietlein F, Peifer M et al (2012) A framework for identification of actionable cancer genome dependencies in small cell lung cancer. Proc Natl Acad Sci U S A 109: 17034–17039

31. Hou JM, Krebs MG, Lancashire L et al (2012) Clinical significance and molecular characteristics of circulating tumor cells and circulating microemboli in patients with small-cell lung cancer. J Clin Oncol 30:525–532
32. Lucchi M, Mussi A, Fontanini G et al (2002) Small cell lung carcinoma (SCLC): the angiogenic phenomenon. Eur J Cardiothorac Surg 21:1105–1110
33. Tanno S, Ohsaki Y, Nakanishi K et al (2000) Human small cell lung cancer cells express functional VEGF receptors, VEGFR-2 and VEGFR-3. Lung Cancer 46:11–19
34. Tas F, Duranyildiz D, Oguz H et al (2006) Serum vascular endothelial growth factor (VEGF) and interlukin-8 (IL-8) levels in small cell lung cancer. Cancer Invest 24:492–495
35. Salven P, Ruotsalainen T, Mattson K et al (1998) High pre-treatment serum level of vascular endothelial growth factor (VEGF) is associated with poor outcome in small-cell lung cancer. Int J Cancer 79:144–146
36. Routsalainen T, Joensuu H, Mattson K et al (2002) High pretreatment serum concentration of basic fibroblast growth factor is a predictor of poor prognosis in small cell lung cancer. Cancer Epidemiol Biomarkers Prev 11:1492–1495
37. Ueno K, Inoue Y, Kawaguchi T et al (2001) Increased serum levels of basic fibroblast growth factor in lung cancer patients: relevance to response of therapy and prognosis. Lung Cancer 31:213–219
38. Horn L, Dahlberg SE, Sandler AB et al (2009) Phase II study of cisplatin plus etoposide and bevacizumab for previously untreated, extensive-stage small-cell lung cancer: Eastern Cooperative Oncology Group Study E3501. J Clin Oncol 27:6006–6011
39. Spigel DR, Townley PM, Waterhouse DM et al (2011) Randomized phase II study of bevacizumab in combination with chemotherapy in previously untreated extensive-stage small-cell lung cancer: results from the SALUTE trial. J Clin Oncol 29:2215–2222
40. Ready NE, Dudek AZ, Pang HH et al (2011) Cisplatin, irinotecan, and bevacizumab for untreated extensive-stage small-cell lung cancer: CALGB 30306, a phase II study. J Clin Oncol 29:4436–4441
41. Murukesh N, Dive C, Jayson GC (2010) Biomarkers of angiogenesis and their role in the development of VEGF inhibitors. Br J Cancer 102:8–18
42. Jubb AM, Harris AL (2010) Biomarkers to predict the clinical efficacy of bevacizumab in cancer. Lancet Oncol 11:1172–1183
43. Spigel DR, Hainsworth JD, Yardley DA et al (2009) Tracheoesophageal fistula formation in patients with lung cancer treated with chemoradiation and bevacizumab. J Clin Oncol 28:43–48
44. Allen JW, Moon J, Gadgeel SM et al (2012) SWOG 0802: A randomized phase II trial of weekly topotecan with and without AVE0005 (aflibercept) in patients with platinum-treated extensive-stage small cell lung cancer (E-SCLC). J Clin Oncol 30(15S):453s; abstract 7005
45. Schneider BJ, Gadgeel SM, Ramnath N et al (2011) Phase II trial of sunitinib maintenance therapy after platinum-based chemotherapy in patients with extensive-stage small cell lung cancer. J Thorac Oncol 6:1117–1120
46. Han JY, Kim HY, Lim KY et al (2013) A phase II study of sunitinib in patients with relapsed or refractory small cell lung cancer. Lung Cancer 79:137–142
47. Spigel DR, Greco FA, Rubin MS et al (2012) Phase II study of maintenance sunitinib following irinotecan and carboplatin as first-line treatment for patients with extensive-stage small-cell lung cancer. Lung Cancer 77:359–364
48. Gitlitz BJ, Moon J, Glisson BS et al (2010) Sorafenib in platinum-treated patients with extensive stage small cell lung cancer. J Thorac Oncol 5:1835–1840
49. Arnold AM, Seymour L, Smylie M et al (2007) Phase II study of vandetanib or placebo in small-cell lung cancer patients after complete or partial response to induction chemotherapy with or without radiation therapy: National Cancer Institute of Canada Clinical Trials Group Study BR.20. J Clin Oncol 25:4278–4284
50. Ramalingam SS, Belani CP, Mack PC et al (2010) Phase II study of Cediranib (AZD 2171), an inhibitor of the vascular endothelial growth factor receptor, for second-line therapy of small cell lung cancer (National Cancer Institute #7097). J Thorac Oncol 5:1279–1284

51. D'Amato RJ, Loughton MS, Flynn E et al (1994) Thalidomide is an inhibitor of angiogenesis. Proc Natl Acad Sci U S A 91:4082–4085
52. Pujol JL, Breton JL, Gervais R et al (2007) Phase III double-blind, placebo-controlled study of thalidomide in extensive-disease small-cell lung cancer after response to chemotherapy: an Intergroup Study FNCLCC cleo04-IFCT 00-01. J Clin Oncol 25:3945–3951
53. Lee SM, Woll PJ, Rudd R et al (2009) Anti-angiogenic therapy using thalidomide combined with chemotherapy in small cell lung cancer: a randomized, double-blind, placebo controlled trial. J Natl Cancer Inst 101:1049–1057
54. Mok TS, Wu YL, Thongprasert S et al (2009) Gefitinib or carboplatin-paclitaxel in pulmonary adenocarcinoma. N Engl J Med 361:1–11
55. Rosell R, Carcereny E, Gervais R et al (2012) Erlotinib versus standard chemotherapy as first-line treatment for European patients with advanced EGFR mutation-positive non-small-cell lung cancer (EURTAC): a multicentre, open-label, randomized phase 3 trial. Lancet Oncol 13:239–246
56. Lu HY, Sun WY, Chen B et al (2012) Epidermal growth factor mutations in small cell lung cancer patients who received surgical resection in China. Neoplasma 59:100–104
57. Tanno S, Ohsaki Y, Nakanishi K et al (2004) Small cell lung cancer cells express EGFR and tyrosine phosphorylation of EGFR is inhibited by gefitinib ("Iressa", ZD1839). Oncol Rep 12:1053–1057
58. Moore AM, Einhorn LH, Estes D et al (2006) Gefitinib in patients with chemo-sensitive and chemo-refractory relapsed small cell cancers: a Hoosier Oncology Group phase II trial. Lung Cancer 52:93–97
59. Hibi K, Takahashi T, Sekido Y et al (1991) Co-expression of the stem cell factor and the c-kit genes in small cell lung cancer. Oncogene 6:2291–2296
60. Plummer H, Catlett J, Leftwich J et al (1993) C-myc expression correlates with suppression of c-kit proto-oncogene expression in small cell lung cancer cell lines. Cancer 53:4337–4342
61. Schneider BJ, Kalemkerian GP, Ramnath N et al (2010) Phase II trial of imatinib maintenance therapy after irinotecan and cisplatin in patients with c-Kit-positive, extensive-stage small-cell lung cancer. Clin Lung Cancer 11:223–227
62. Dy GK, Miller AA, Mandrekar SJ et al (2005) A phase II trial of imatinib (ST1571) in patients with c-kit expressing relapsed small-cell lung cancer: a CALGB and NCCTG study. Ann Oncol 16:1811–1816
63. Krug LM, Crapanzano JP, Azzoli CG et al (2005) Imatinib mesylate lacks activity in small cell lung carcinoma expressing c-kit protein. Cancer 103:2128–2131
64. Spigel DR, Hainsworth JD, Simons L et al (2007) Irinotecan, carboplatin, and imatinib in untreated extensive-stage small-cell lung cancer: a phase II trial of the Minnie Pearl Cancer Research Network. J Thorac Oncol 2:854–861
65. Miller AA, Pang H, Hodgson L et al (2010) A phase II study of dasatinib in patients with chemosensitive relapsed small cell lung cancer (Cancer and Leukemia Group B 30602). J Thorac Oncol 5:380–384
66. Kaiser U, Schardt C, Brandscheidt D et al (1993) Expression of insulin-like growth factor receptors I and II in normal human lung and in lung cancer. J Cancer Res Clin Oncol 119:665–668
67. Warshamana-Greene GS, Litz J, Buchdunger E et al (2004) The insulin-like growth factor-1 (IGF-1) receptor kinase inhibitor NVP-ADW742, in combination with STI571 delineates a spectrum of dependence of small cell lung cancer on IGF-1 and stem cell factor signaling. Mol Cancer Ther 3:527–535
68. Belani CP, Dahlberg SE, Rudin CM et al (2013) Three-arm randomized phase II study of cisplatin and etoposide (CE) versus CE with either vismodegib (V) or cixitumumab (Cx) for patients with extensive-stage small cell lung cancer (ES-SCLC) (ECOG 1508). J Clin Oncol 31(15S):460s; abstract 7508

69. Pandya KJ, Dahlberg S, Hidalgo M et al (2007) A randomized, phase II trial of two dose levels of temsirolimus (CCI-779) in patients with extensive-stage small-cell lung cancer who have responding or stable disease after induction chemotherapy: a trial of the Eastern Cooperative Oncology Group (E1500). J Thorac Oncol 2:1036–1041
70. Heymach JV, Johnson DH, Khuri FR et al (2004) Phase II study of the farnesyl transferase inhibitor R115777 in patients with sensitive relapsed small-cell lung cancer. Ann Oncol 15:1187–1193
71. Kodate M, Kasai T, Ghashimoto H et al (1997) Expression of matrix metalloproteinase (gelatinase) in T1 adenocarcinoma of the lung. Pathol Int 47:461–469
72. Michael M, Babic B, Khokha R et al (1999) Expression and prognostic significance of metalloproteinases and their tissue inhibitors in patients with small-cell lung cancer. J Clin Oncol 17(6):1802–1808
73. Shepherd FA, Giaccone G, Seymour L et al (2002) Prospective, randomized, double-blind, placebo-controlled trial of marimastat after response to first-line chemotherapy in patients with small-cell lung cancer: a trial of the National Cancer Institute of Canada-Clinical Trials Group and the European Organization for Research and Treatment of Cancer. J Clin Oncol 20:4434–4439
74. Rigas JR, Denham CA, Rinaldi DA et al (2003) Randomized placebo-controlled trials of the matrix metalloproteinase inhibitor, BAY12-9566, as adjuvant therapy for patients with small cell and non-small cell lung cancer. Proc Am Soc Clin Oncol 22:628; abstract 2525
75. Zangemeister-Wittke U, Schenker T, Luedke GH et al (1998) Synergistic cytotoxicity of bcl-2 antisense oligodeoxynucleotides and etoposide, doxorubicin and cisplatin on small-cell lung cancer cell lines. Br J Cancer 78:1035–1042
76. Reed JC, Stein C, Subasinghe C et al (1990) Antisense-mediated inhibition of BCL2 protooncogene expression and leukemic cell growth and survival: comparisons of phosphodiester and phosphorothioate oligodeoxynucleotides. Cancer Res 50:6565–6570
77. Smith MR, Abubakr Y, Mohammad R et al (1994) Antisense oligodeoxyribonucleotide down-regulation of bcl-2 gene expression inhibits growth of the low-grade non-Hodgkin's lymphoma cell lines WSU-FSCCL. Cancer Gene Ther 2:207–212
78. Rudin CM, Salgia R, Wang X et al (2008) Randomized phase II study of carboplatin and etoposide with or without the bcl-2 antisense oligonucleotide oblimersen for extensive-stage small-cell lung cancer: CALGB 30103. J Clin Oncol 26:870–876
79. Li J, Viallet J, Haura E (2008) A small molecule pan-Bcl-2 family inhibitor, GX15-070, induces apoptosis and enhances cisplatin-induced apoptosis in non-small cell lung cancer cells. Cancer Chemother Pharmacol 61:525–534
80. Chiappori AA, Schreeder MT, Moezi MM et al (2012) A phase I trial of pan-Bcl-2 antagonist obatoclax administered as a 3-h or a 24-h infusion in combination with carboplatin and etoposide in patients with extensive-stage small cell lung cancer. Br J Cancer 106:839–845
81. Paik PK, Rudin CM, Pietanza MC et al (2011) A phase II study of obatoclax mesylate, a Bcl-2 antagonist, plus topotecan in relapsed small cell lung cancer. Lung Cancer 74:481–485
82. Gandhi L, Camidge R, Ribeiro de Oliveira M et al (2011) Phase I study of navitoclax (ABT-263), a novel Bcl-2 family inhibitor, in patients with small-cell lung cancer and other solid tumors. J Clin Oncol 29:909–916
83. Rudin CM, Hann CL, Garon EB et al (2012) Phase II study of single-agent navitoclax (ABT-263) and biomarker correlates in patients with relapsed small cell lung cancer. Clin Cancer Res 18:3163–3169
84. Tang XC, Zhu MK, Shi QX (1980) Comparative studies on the absorption, distribution and excretion of 14C-gossypol in four species of animals (author's transl). Yao Xue Xue Bao 15:212–217
85. Wang G, Min P, Zhang Y et al (2007) Preclinical studies of orally active, pan Bcl-2 small molecule inhibitor AT-101 in small cell lung cancer. In: AACR-NCI-EORTC International Conference on Molecular Targets and Cancer Therapeutics, abstract A:51

86. Baggstrom MQ, Qi Y, Koczywas M et al (2011) A phase II study of AT-101 (Gossypol) in chemotherapy-sensitive recurrent extensive-stage small cell lung cancer. J Thorac Oncol 6:1757–1760
87. Heist RS, Fain J, Chinnasami B et al (2010) Phase I/II study of AT-101 with topotecan in relapsed and refractory small cell lung cancer. J Thorac Oncol 5:1637–1643
88. Schelman WR, Mohammed TA, Traynor AM et al (2013) A phase I study of AT-101 with cisplatin and etoposide in patients with advanced solid tumors with an expanded cohort in extensive-stage small cell lung cancer. Invest New Drugs 32(2):295–302
89. Chari NS, McDonnell TJ (2008) The sonic hedgehog signaling network in development and neoplasia. Adv Anat Pathol 14:344–352
90. Fan X, Matsui W, Khaki L et al (2006) Notch pathway inhibition depletes stem-like cells and blocks engraftment in embryonal brain tumors. Cancer Res 66:7445–7452
91. Watkins DN, Berman DM, Burkholder SG et al (2003) Hedgehog signaling within airway epithelial progenitors and in small-cell lung cancer. Nature 422:313–317
92. Park KS, Martelotto LG, Peifer M et al (2011) A crucial requirement for Hedgehog signaling in small cell lung cancer. Nat Med 17:1504–1508
93. Androutsellis-Theotokis A, Leker RR, Soldner F et al (2006) Notch signaling regulates stem cell numbers in vitro and in vivo. Nature 442:823–826
94. Salcido CD, Larochelle A, Taylor BJ et al (2010) Molecular characterization of side population cells with cancer stem cell-like characteristics in small-cell lung cancer. Br J Cancer 102:1636–1644
95. Andrade AC, Nilsson O, Barnes KM et al (2007) Wnt gene expression in the post-natal growth plate: regulation with chondrocyte differentiation. Bone 40:1361–1369
96. Lemjabbar-Alaoui H, Dasari V, Sidhu SS et al (2006) Wnt and Hedgehog are critical mediators of cigarette smoke-induced lung cancer. PLoS One 1, e93
97. You L, He B, Xu Z et al (2004) Inhibition of Wnt-2 mediated signaling induces programmed cell death in non-small-cell lung cancer cells. Oncogene 23:6170–6174
98. Hess-Stump H (2005) Histone deacetylase inhibitors and cancer: from cell biology to the clinic. Eur J Cell Biol 84:109–121
99. Zhu WG, Lakshmanan RR, Beal MD et al (2001) DNA methyltransferase inhibition enhances apoptosis induced by histone deacetylase inhibitors. Cancer Res 61:1327–1333
100. Otterson GA, Hodgson L, Pang H et al (2010) Phase II study of the histone deacetylase inhibitor Romidepsin in relapsed small cell lung cancer (Cancer and Leukemia Group B 30304). J Thorac Oncol 5:1644–1648
101. Katayama H, Sen S (2010) Aurora kinase inhibitors are anticancer molecules. Biochim Biophys Acta 1799:829–839
102. Zhang XH, Rao M, Loprieato JA et al (2008) Aurora A, Aurora B and survivin are novel targets of transcriptional regulation by histone deacetylase inhibitors in non-small cell lung cancer. Cancer Biol Ther 7:1388–1397
103. Kaestner P, Stolz A, Bastians H (2009) Determinants for the efficiency of anticancer drugs targeting either Aurora-A or Aurora-B kinases in human colon carcinoma cells. Mol Cancer Ther 8:2046–2056
104. Melichar B, Adenis A, Libor H et al (2013) Phase I/II study of investigational Aurora A kinase inhibitor MLN8237 (alisertib): Updates ph II results in patients with small cell lung cancer, non-SCLC, breast cancer, head and neck squamous cell carcinoma, and gastroesophageal cancer. J Clin Oncol 31(15S):33s; abstract 605
105. Brezicka T, Bergman B, Olling S et al (2000) Reactivity of monoclonal antibodies with ganglioside antigens in human small cell lung cancer tissues. Lung Cancer 28:29–36
106. Giaccone G, Debruyne C, Felip E et al (2005) Phase III study of adjuvant vaccination with Bec2/Bacille Calmette-Guerin in responding patients with limited-disease small-cell lung cancer (European Organisation for Research and Treatment of Cancer 08971B; Silva Study). J Clin Oncol 23:6854–6864

107. Bodner SM, Minna J, Jensen SM et al (1992) Expression of mutant p53 proteins in lung cancer correlates with the class of p53 gene mutation. Oncogene 7:743–749
108. Antonia SJ, Mirza N, Fricke I et al (2006) Combination of p53 cancer vaccine with chemotherapy in patients with extensive stage small cell lung cancer. Clin Cancer Res 12:878–887
109. Mattson K, Niiranen A, Pyrhönen S et al (1992) Natural interferon alfa as maintenance therapy for small cell lung cancer. Eur J Cancer 28A:1387–1391
110. Ruotsalainen T, Halme M, Isokangas OP et al (2000) Interferon-alpha and 13-cis-retinoic acid as maintenance therapy after high-dose combination chemotherapy with growth factor support for small cell lung cancer-a feasibility study. Anticancer Drugs 11:101–108
111. Salama AK, Hodi FS (2011) Cytotoxic T-lymphocyte-associated antigen-4. Clin Cancer Res 17:4622–4628
112. Seliger B (2005) Strategies of tumor immune evasion. BioDrugs 19:347–354
113. Reck M, Bondarenko I, Luft A et al (2013) Ipilimumab in combination with paclitaxel and carboplatin as first-line therapy in extensive-disease-small-cell lung cancer: results from a randomized, double-blind, multicenter phase 2 trial. Ann Oncol 24:75–83
114. Ott PA, Fernandez MEE, Hiret S et al (2015) Pembrolizumab (MK-3475) in patients with extensive-stage small cell lung cancer: Preliminary safety and efficacy results from KEYNOTE-028. J Clin Oncol 33(15S):400s; abstract 7502
115. Antonia SJ, Bendell JC, Taylor MH et al. Phase I/II study of nivolumab with or without ipilumumab for treatment of recurrent small cell lung cancer: CA209-032. J Clin Oncol 33(15S):400s; abstract 7503
116. Rudin CM, Poirier JT, Senzer NN et al (2011) Phase I clinical study of Seneca Valley Virus (SVV-001), a replication-competent picornavirus, in advanced solid tumors with neuroendocrine features. Clin Cancer Res 17:888–895
117. Molina JR, Mandrekar SJ, Dy GK (2013) A randomized double-blind phase II study of the Seneca Valley virus (NTX-010) versus placebo for patients with extensive stage SCLC who were stable or responding after at least four cycles of platinum-based chemotherapy: Alliance (NCCTG) N0923 study. J Clin Oncol 31(15S):460s; abstract 7509

Personalized Radiation Therapy (PRT) for Lung Cancer

Jian-Yue Jin and Feng-Ming (Spring) Kong

Abstract This chapter reviews and discusses approaches and strategies of personalized radiation therapy (PRT) for lung cancers at four different levels: (1) clinically established PRT based on a patient's histology, stage, tumor volume and tumor locations; (2) personalized adaptive radiation therapy (RT) based on image response during treatment; (3) PRT based on biomarkers; (4) personalized fractionation schedule. The current RT practice for lung cancer is partially individualized according to tumor histology, stage, size/location, and combination with use of systemic therapy. During-RT PET-CT image guided adaptive treatment is being tested in a multicenter trial. Treatment response detected by the during-RT images may also provide a strategy to further personalize the remaining treatment. Research on biomarker-guided PRT is ongoing. The biomarkers include genomics, proteomics, microRNA, cytokines, metabolomics from tumor and blood samples, and radiomics from PET, CT, SPECT images. Finally, RT fractionation schedule may also be personalized to each individual patient to maximize therapeutic gain. Future PRT should be based on comprehensive considerations of knowledge acquired from all these levels, as well as consideration of the societal value such as cost and effectiveness.

Keywords Personalized radiation therapy • Biomarkers • Adaptive radiation therapy • Radiomics • Lung cancer

1 Introduction

Lung cancer is the leading cause of cancer death in the United States and worldwide [1, 2]. Radiation therapy (RT) plays an important role in the treatment of lung cancers, including both non-small cell lung cancer (NSCLC) and small cell lung cancers (SCLC). The majority of lung cancer patients require RT as a sole modality or an essential part of a multi-modality approach for cure or palliation. However, treatment outcome for lung cancer, primarily measured by tumor control and overall survival, remains suboptimal. Treatment toxicity can be remarkable for many patients. Personalized radiation therapy (PRT) tailors an RT regimen according to a patient's individual characteristics, and is one approach to

J.-Y. Jin, Ph.D. • F.-M. (Spring) Kong, M.D., Ph.D. (✉)
Cancer Center, Georgia Regents University, Augusta, GA, USA
e-mail: fkong@gru.edu

A. Ahmad, S.M. Gadgeel (eds.), *Lung Cancer and Personalized Medicine: Novel Therapies and Clinical Management*, Advances in Experimental Medicine and Biology 890, DOI 10.1007/978-3-319-24932-2_10

improving treatment outcome. Different patients may have very different tumor and normal tissue response to the same RT regimen due to patient heterogeneity. These different responses may be predicted by or correlated with patient factors, such as stage, tumor histology, patient performance, tumor (target) volume, tumor location, measured tumor response and critical organs response to treatment at the middle of RT, and various biomarkers. PRT may achieve maximal therapeutic gain for each individual patient according to these patient factors for an optimized balance of tumor control and treatment toxicity. The total RT dose is the most pivotal parameter in customization to improve treatment outcome, and the fractionation schedule of an RT regimen may be another important parameter to be personalized in the PRT.

The standard of care for RT has some components of PRT, such as individualization based on a patient's stage, histology and performance status. Standard RT regimens for NSCLC and SCLC, and for patients at different stages, are quite different. However, PRT has not been well implemented in treatment of patients with the same histology and stage with the exception of tumor volume based planning. The current standard of care for locally advanced stage NSCLC is still a "one dose fits all" uniform RT regimen with concurrent chemotherapy. Researches and some clinical trials have been carried out to explore PRT in this level. In this chapter, we will discuss PRT approaches and their progress including: (1) clinically established PRT based on a patient's histology, stage, tumor volume and tumor locations; (2) personalized adaptive RT based on image response during treatment; (3) personalized RT dose based on biomarkers; (4) Personalized fractionation schedule. Finally a summary of PRT approaches will be given.

2 PRT in Current Practice

PRT has been partially implemented in current practice, exemplified by (1) different RT regimens established as the standard of care according to a patient's histology (SCLC and NSCLC) and stage (limited stage versus extensive stage for SCLC, stage I, I/III, versus IV for NSCLC); (2) minor variation of dose prescription based on a patient's tumor volume, location, and estimated risk of RT toxicity.

2.1 PRT Based on Histology and Stage

The national comprehensive cancer network (NCCN) has provided detailed guidelines of RT regimens for lung cancers with various histology, stages and operational status [3]. Table 1 gives a brief summary of these regimens.

For Stage I and IIa non-operative patients (T1 and T2, <5 cm, N0) with peripherally located NSCLC, stereotactic body radiotherapy (SBRT) is the standard of care. Recent results from RTOG236 showed a 3-year primary tumor

Table 1 PRT regimens based on histology, stage and performance

Histology, stage, and performance	RT regimen
NSCLC	
Stage I, IIa (medical inoperable early stage disease)	
Stereotactic body radiotherapy (SBRT) is the standard care for peripheral diseases	34–60 Gy in 1–5 fx
Conventional RT is used for the centers without SBRT capability	70+ Gy in 30–35 fx
Stage I–III combined with surgery Postoperative radiation	
Positive or suspicious surgical margins	60 Gy in 30 fx
Mediastinal lymph nodes (N2 and above disease)	50–54 Gy in 25 fx
Chest wall invasion (T3 and T4)	50–60 Gy in 25–30 fx
Preoperative	
Radiation combined with chemotherapy	45–50 Gy in 20–25 fx
Marginally operable patients (stage IIIa or Ib)	60 Gy in 30–33 fx
Stage III Unresectable patients	60–70 Gy in 30–35 fx
Stage IV	
External beam radiation	16–17 Gy in 2 fx
	48 Gy in 12 fx
	30–45 Gy in 10–15 fx
	50 Gy in 20 fx
Intraluminal brachytherapy	10–16 Gy in 2 fx
SCLC	
	45 Gy in 15 twice daily
	54–60 Gy in 27–30 fx

control rate of 97.6 % (95 % CI, 84.3–99.7 %) in patients with medically inoperable stage I disease (<5 cm) [4, 5]. The RTOG trial used an RT regimen of 54–60 Gy/fx in 3 fractions [4]. Other fractionation regimens, such as 48 Gy in 4 fractions, 50–55 Gy in 5 fractions have also shown excellent results [6–8]. Studies suggest that a BED > 100 Gy is required to have a ~90 % tumor control rate [6–8]. For clinics without SBRT capability, the conventional fractionation may be still acceptable.

For Stage I-III NSCLC patients involving surgery, conventional fractionation is usually used, and RT dose depends on the stage and how surgery is implemented [3, 9]. A dose of 45–50 Gy in 1.8–2 Gy daily fractions is recommended for preoperative radiation. When postoperative RT is indicated, the mediastinum is commonly treated to 50 Gy in 25 fractions, and regions of extracapsular extension and/or bulky nodal disease boosted by an additional 10 Gy. Areas of gross residual disease may be treated to 66–70 Gy, if dose to normal structures can be limited. When T3N0 chest tumors with chest wall invasion are given postoperative RT, the regional nodal area does not require postoperative RT if mediastinal nodes were adequately staged surgically. However, patients with positive margin should be given 60 Gy postoperatively.

For unresectable stage III diseases, a dose of 60–70 Gy in 30–35 fractions is usually given, although several single institution and meta-analysis studies suggest that dose escalation might improve local control and thus potentially improve the survival [10–12]. In the results of RTOG 0617 a 74 Gy arm had worse survival than a 60 Gy arm [13]. A total dose of 60 Gy in 30 fractions is the current recommended dose for stage II/III receiving concurrent chemoradiation.

For stage IV NSCLC disease, a regimen of 30 Gy in 10 daily fractions is typically used for palliative treatment [14]. While using this dose regimen does initially relieve symptoms, it may not have a sustained effect. If patients continue to have good performance status and their symptoms improve, an additional 20 Gy in four fractions, or 30 Gy in 10 fractions may be delivered to sustain palliative benefit [9]. Other palliative regimens in use include 10 Gy × 1, 4 Gy daily × 5, 8.5 Gy weekly × 2, 3Gy daily × 13 or 15, 2.5 Gy daily × 20 or even 2 Gy daily × 30, based on a recent survey performed among ASTRO members [9]. Selection of regimen should be based on comprehensive consideration of age, performance status, tumor burden, and symptoms of each individual patient. Patients with poor performance status, and patients with large distant tumor burden regardless of their performance status, should be treated by a short course of relatively low dose radiotherapy. A definitive dose of radiation with combined chemotherapy may also be acceptable for patients with good performance and limited distant disease (such as solitary brain metastasis). There is limited evidence showing that higher dose thoracic radiation is associated with extension of survival in patients with good performance status [14].

For SCLC patients, RT is delivered early and concurrently with cisplatin-based chemotherapy. The standard of care RT regimen is 45 Gy in 1.5 Gy twice-daily fractions [9]. If hyperfractionation is not possible, a dose of at least 54–60 Gy in 2 Gy daily fractions should be given. If chemotherapy has been given prior to thoracic RT, 50–54 Gy in 1.8–2.0 Gy fractions should be given to complete responders and 60 Gy to partial responders. Daily fractionation with higher dose (60–70 Gy in 2 Gy fractions) is also an acceptable alternative [9].

2.2 *Variation of Dose Prescription Based on Estimated Toxicity*

A simple and clinically feasible PRT approach for stage III patients is to modify the standard dose prescription to the tolerance of organs at risk (OAR) with the aim of serious toxicity rate <5 %, and/or other iso-toxicity criteria. A patient's potential toxicity from the standard prescription dose (60 Gy in 30 fractions) can be estimated by clinically-derived normal tissue complication probability (NTCP) models. The prescription dose of the patient can be increased or decreased based on estimated toxicities. For patients with relatively small tumor volumes, tumors in a peripheral location, or tumors relatively far away from OARs, OARs usually receive less dose resulting from target prescription optimization. Thus, estimated toxicities will be relatively lower than "the safe limit", so that a higher prescription dose (usually 66–74 Gy) can be given to these patients. On the other hand, patients with large tumor volumes, or a tumor in a disadvantageous location may require a lower prescription dose (<60 Gy) due to concerns of toxicity. Therefore, PRT is based on patients' tumor volume and location and is often unconsciously practiced by many clinicians in a single case-based setting.

Reliable clinical data based-NTCP models for various OARs are often required to implement PRT. Many studies have been performed to derive NTCP models and setup radiation dose tolerance criteria for OARs [15–18]. During 2008–2010, the American Society of Therapeutic Radiology and Oncology (ASTRO) and American Association of Medical Physicists (AAPM) sponsored a Quantitative Analyses of Normal Tissue Effects in the Clinic (QUANTEC) to determine the best NTCP models for each organ [15]. The radiation therapy and oncology group (RTOG) has also set up their own radiation dose tolerance criterion for each organ for their multi-center clinical trials. For treatment of lung cancer, the three major OARs are the lung, esophagus and heart. The lung NTCP model has been well studied. The mean lung dose was found to be a very reliable estimation for NTCP [18]. Table 2 shows the NTCP dosimetric limits for lung, heart and esophagus used in the RTOG 1106 trial.

3 Personalized Adaptive RT Based on Image Response during RT

Radiation treatment of locally advanced NSCLC usually takes 6 weeks or more. Tumor and normal tissue response to radiation can be detected by nuclear medicine imaging during the course of the typical 6-week treatment regimen (such as after 2–4 weeks of starting RT). The RT regimen may be individually tailored according to the response measured in a particular patient. For patients with great tumor response (significant tumor shrinkage), the radiation field can be shrunk accordingly to reduce the volume of the normal tissue irradiated. Two potential strategies may be used for adaptive RT according to the tumor response based on different assumptions: (1) Dose escalation is applied to the residual tumor volume for all

Table 2 Dose tolerance limits for lung, heart and esophagus used in the RTOH 1106

Structure name	Description	Metric	Tolerance per protocol
Lungs	Lungs minus Pre-RT GTV	Max dose (Gy, 0.03 cm^3)	≤110 % Rx dose
		Mean dose (Gy)	≤20 Gy
		Volume >20 Gy (%)	≤35 %
		Volume>5 Gy (%)	≤65 %
Heart	Heart/Pericardium (see Atlas in RTOG)	Max dose (Gy, 0.03 cm^3)	≤70 Gy
		Mean dose (Gy)	≤30 Gy
		Volume>30 Gy (%)	≤50 %
		Volume>40 Gy (%)	≤35 %
Esophagus	Esophagus	Max Dose (Gy, 0.03 cm^3)	≤74 Gy
		Mean Dose (Gy)	≤34 Gy

patients according to an iso-toxicity criterion at a save level, assuming that low radiation dose is the major factor for the poor local control and overall survival; (2) Dose escalation is applied only to poor responders, while dose de-escalation may be applied to good responders, assuming good responders have more radiosensitive tumors, and the standard dose (such as 60 Gy in 30 fractions) is sufficient for tumor control. In addition, treatment regimen may also been adapted according to normal organ response observed during the course of treatment.

3.1 Imaging Tumor Response

An image modality that can accurately measure tumor response during RT is the key for personalized adaptive RT. Both computed tomography (CT) and positron emission tomography (PET) have been reported to measure the tumor response after partial treatment of RT [19–25]. Kupelian et al. studied the tumor volume change in 10 patients with daily MV CT in a Helical Tomotherapy HiArt machine, and found an average of 1.2 % reduction in tumor volume per day [19]. These 10 patients exhibited large heterogeneity in tumor volume reduction. Kong et al. demonstrated that when FDG-PET is performed during-RT at appropriate times, treatment related inflammation causes confounding effects only negligibly [23]. It was found that FDG uptake and metabolic tumor volume (MTV) decreased significantly after 40–50 Gy of fractionated RT, and significantly correlated with findings of PET images 3–4 months after treatment. Thus, during-RT FDG-PET can potentially be used for prediction of treatment outcome, evaluation of response in the middle of treatment, and adaptation of remaining treatment [23]. These findings were confirmed later by other researchers [24–26]. An advantage of FDG-PET over CT in personalized adaptive RT is that reduction of CT tumor volume during RT does not reflect tumor killing (the dead cells were not immediately dissolved). It was reported that reduction in MTV was 20 % greater than reduction of the CT-gross tumor volume (GTV) during RT, and MTV can be defined more reproducibly [27]. It was also found that adapting the planned target volume to the reduced MTV with a fixed composite NTCP of 15 % allows escalation of the total dose by 30–102 Gy (mean: 58 Gy) or a reduction in NTCP if the dose remained unchanged [28]. Using the MTV during RT, tumor dose can be escalated above 74 Gy while keeping lung NTCP unchanged in a majority of patients with stage III NSCLC [29].

3.2 Personalized Adaptive RT Strategies According to Tumor Response

A prospective phase 2 single institution clinical trial of the personalized adaptive RT using the first strategy mentioned above to escalate radiation dose to the resistant part of tumors was conducted at the University of Michigan in patients with locally advanced NSCLC [29]. During-RT FDG-PET image was used as the imaging modality to measure the tumor response after 18–19 fractions of treatment, and the RT regimen for the final 9 fractions were adapted to cover the residual MTV. The total number of fractions was fixed to 30, therefore the dose per fraction varied from 2.2 to 3.8 Gy. An iso-toxicity of 17 % chance of grade 2 and above PILT estimated from a mean lung dose NTCP model, and strict limitations of esophageal and heart doses as listed in Table 2, were used as the criteria to limit the RT dose. Figure 1 shows the schematics of the design. The adaptive plan was generated so that not only the dose to the residual MTV was escalated; the doses to the pre-RT PTV, CTV were also designed to reach at least 50 and 60 Gy, respectively. Figure 2 shows the initial plan and the adaptive plan for the first patient. Preliminary results demonstrated overall survival at 1 and 2 years follow up significantly better than conventional RT of patients with stage III NSCLC treated with concurrent and adjuvant carboplatin and paclitaxel (Fig. 3). This concept has also been developed into a multicenter phase II clinical trial. RTOG 1106 was opened in 2012 and over 85 patients have been treated under the protocol.

The other strategy of personalized adaptive RT would be a very attractive approach if during-RT images can be used as a biomarker to predict a patient's radiosensitivity. Patients with greater tumor response may be more radiosensitive, thus a lower radiation dose may be required to control the tumor. RTOG 0617, a randomized phase 3 multicenter clinical trial, showed a surprised result that a 60 Gy arm had better overall survival than a 74 Gy arm [13]. This suggests that a good portion of patients may achieve complete tumor control after a radiation dose of 60 Gy, and this group of patients may suffer from treatment complications if radiation dose is escalated. During-RT PET may be used to identify this group of patients. Chui et al. studied 106 patients with during-RT (10–12 days after starting RT) and found that maximum standard uptake value (SUV) significantly correlated with tumor control [26]. This result is consistent with the results of Kong et al. [23], and suggests that maximum SUV of during-RT PET may be used as a biomarker to predict tumor radiosensitivity.

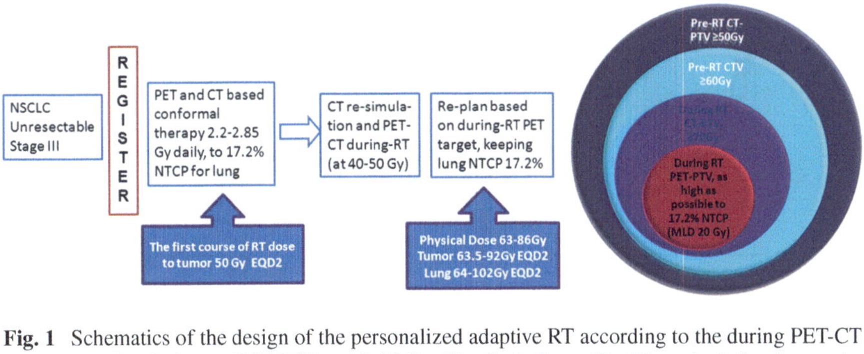

Fig. 1 Schematics of the design of the personalized adaptive RT according to the during PET-CT images. Re-simulation and PET-CT at 45–50 Gy. The final plan will achieve the following goals: During-RT PET-PTV: as high as possible dose limited by 17.2 % NTCP of lung (mean lung dose of 20 Gy); During-RT CT-PTV $\geq$ 70 Gy; Pre-RT CTV $\geq$ 60 Gy; Pre-RT PTV $\geq$ 50 Gy

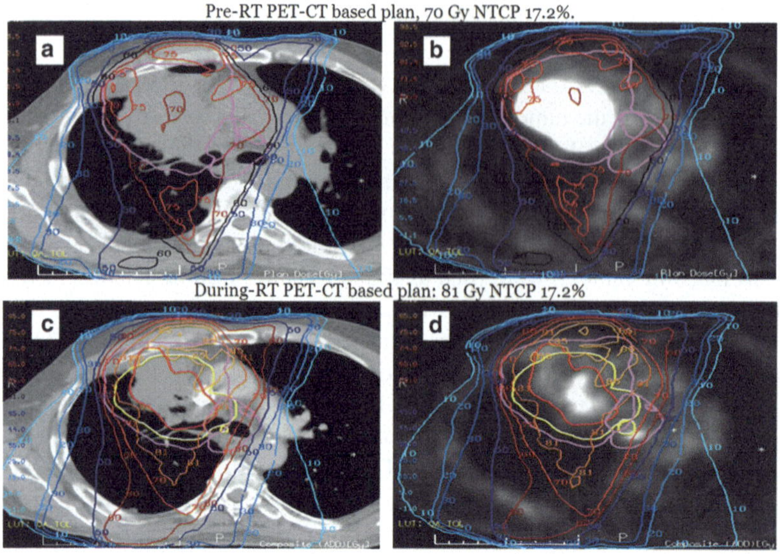

Fig. 2 Initial plan and the adaptive plan for the first patient using the during PET-CT image for re-planning. (**a**) Pre-RT plan in CT image: 17.2 % lung NTCP ~ 70 Gy; (**b**) The same pre-RT plan in PET image; (**c**) During-RT personalized adapted composite plan in During CT image: 17.2 % lung NTCP ~ 81 Gy to during-RT PET-MTV; (**d**) The same during-RT personalized adapted plan in PET image. Note the tumor response in the during RT PET. This patient had futile thoracotomy before, is currently doing well at 2 years with no evidence of tumor progression

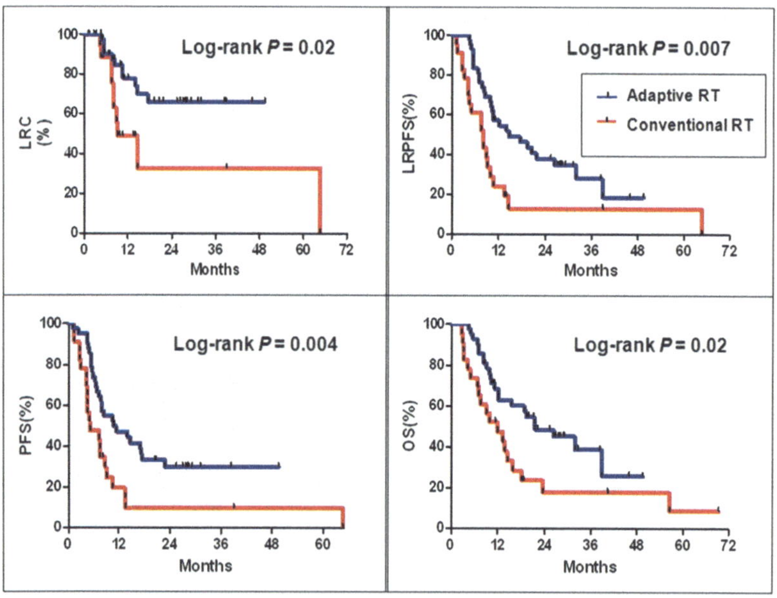

Fig. 3 preliminary results of comparison of local reginal control (LRC), local regional progression-free survival (LRPFS), progression-free survival (PFS), and overall survival between patients treated with personalized adaptive RT and patietns treated with conventional RT

3.3 Imaging Normal Tissue Response

OARs also change during the course of radiation therapy. Many image modalities, including, CT, magnetic resonance image (MRI), PET, and single photon emission computed tomography (SPECT), have been used to detect normal tissue response to radiation [30–49]. CT has been used to measure the change of radiopacity after radiation of lung tissue, and it was found that the change of radiopacity correlated with the radiation dose and the lung toxicity (such as radiation pneumonitis, cough and dyspnea) [31, 32]. MRI was used to measure lung density [33] and asymmetric enhancement on dynamic perfusion [34], which was shown to correlate with radiation pneumonitis. Increased FDG uptake was found in lung and esophagus on PET imaging, and correlated to lung and esophageal toxicities [35–41]. SPECT is an imaging modality that can directly measure the lung and heart function for their perfusion and ventilation, and it has been used to measure the radiation-induced changes in lung and heart function [31, 42, 43]. It was reported recently that lung ventilation can be derived from the patient's 4-dimensional CT [44–46]. However, most of these studies were performed after RT was completed. Therefore, there was no opportunity to alter the RT regimen.

Kong et al. observed increased FDG uptake on during-RT PET in the lung after 40–45 Gy of RT [23]. However, a correlation between FDG uptake and radiation induced lung toxicity (RILT) was not established. De Ruysscher et al. reported that in 18 patients, FDG uptake in the irradiated area of the lung outside GTV 7 and 14 days after initiating RT significantly correlated with the grade 2 or higher Dyspnea [47]. Li et al. reported in an abstract that in 84 patients, during-RT FDG uptake significantly correlated with RILT ($p=0.002$) [48]. Yuan et al. studied during-RT ventilation/perfusion (V/Q) SPECT in 56 stage I-III NSCLC patients [49]. Both studies found that both V and Q SPECT indicated improved lung function after ~45 Gy of radiation treatment, especially in the ipsilateral side of lung. This data suggests that some poor lung function regions measured by SPECT before RT resulted from tumor-based impairment of functional structure. Radiation treatment shrank the tumor and thus opened some of the functional structures and improved lung function. During-RT SPECT may identify which non-functional regions are due to intrinsic lung tissue damage, and which regions are due to tumor blockage and can be recovered after tumor to be controlled. Such information may be used for personalized adaptive RT plan to direct radiation beams to regions with intrinsically damaged lung tissue.

4 Individualized RT Based on Biomarkers Before RT

A patient's response to RT, including both tumor and normal structure responses, may differ remarkably from others, and may depend on the person's genomic characteristics, and thus may been predicted by biomarkers before the treatment starts.

Many studies have been performed to search for biomarkers to predict prognostics factors, tumor response and treatment toxicities in NSCLC [50–52]. These biomarkers have a broad spectrum and the concept is still evolving. The National Institutes of Health Biomarkers Definitions Working Group defined a biomarker as "a characteristic that is objectively measured and evaluated as an indicator of normal biological processes, pathogenic processes, or pharmacologic responses to a therapeutic intervention" [53, 54]. A joint venture on chemical safety, the International Program on Chemical Safety, has defined a biomarker as "any substance, structure, or process that can be measured in the body or its products and influence or predict the incidence of outcome or disease" [53]. For lung cancer, these biomarkers mainly include genomics, proteomics, microRNA, cytokines, metabolomics from tumor and blood samples, and radiomics from PET, CT, SPECT images. The biomarkers from tumor tissue have been widely studied for personalized medicine in chemotherapy and target therapy based treatment in lung cancer, which are discussed in detail in other chapters and are often not available for radiation oncology patients. This section will focus on the blood sample-based biomarkers, image biomarkers and their applications in PRT.

4.1 Genomic Biomarkers in Blood

Single nucleotide polymorphism (SNP) is a genomic biomarker which can be determined from a patient's blood sample and be used to predict a patient's response to RT, in either tumor and normal tissue. A SNP is a DNA sequence variation occurring when a Single Nucleotide (A, T, C or G) in the genome (or other shared sequence) differs between members of a biological species or paired chromosomes. SNPs usually occur more often in the non-coding area in the genome sequence. These genetic variations may underlie differences in the way our body responds to treatments. When a patient is under RT treatment, many cells, including tumor and normal tissue cells, suffer from radiation induced DNA damage in terms of single or double DNA strands break. The repair of DNA may differ between patients due to the difference in SNP genotypes, thus the patient may have different radiation sensitivities.

Yuan X et al. studied the association of SNPs in the transforming growth factor beta 1 (TGFβ 1) gene and risk of radiation pneumonitis (RP) in 164 NSCLC patients treated with RT [55]. They found CT/CC genotypes of TGFbeta1 rs1982073:T869C to be associated with a statistically significantly lower risk of RP grades ≥2 (hazard ratio [HR]=0.489; 95 % CI, 0.227–0.861; P=.013) and grades ≥3 (HR=0.390; 95 % CI, 0.197–0.774; P=0.007), respectively, compared with the TT genotype, after adjustment for Karnofsky performance status, smoking status, pulmonary function, and dosimetric parameters. Kelsey CR et al. also reported an association between SNP genotype and increasing slope of the dose–response curves (DRC) in SPECT lung [56]. The correlation of DRC with G(1301) A in XRCC1 (rs25487) was P=0.01 and to G(3748) A in BRCA1 (rs16942) was P=0.03. These results suggest that the SNPs may predict the radiation sensitivity of the lung tissue.

Tucker et al. have incorporated SNPs into a normal-tissue complication probability (NTCP) model to predict radiation pneumonitis (RP) risk [57]. Five SNPs (in genes for TGFβ, VEGF, TNFα, XRCC1 and APEX1) were selected from 16 SNPs from 10 different genes (XRCC1, XRCC3, APEX1, MDM2, TGFβ, TNFα, TNFR, MTHFR, MTRR, and VEGF) to incorporate into a mean lung dose based NTCP model from 141 NSCLC patients. As shown in Fig. 4, patients with 0, 1, and 2+ adverse SNPs showed 3 different NTCP dose response curves. The study also shows that with smoking status included in the multivariate model, the SNPs significantly associated with increased risk of RP in genes for TGFβ, VEGF, and XRCC3. The same research group used this SNP-incorporated NTCP model to test the potential benefits of PRT in a virtual clinic trial for 139 NSCLC patients treated with RT with radiation doses varying from 60 to 72 Gy [58]. They found that there were 82 patients (59 %) who would had a change in prescription of 5 Gy or more (either dose escalation or de-escalation), and 26 patients (19 %) would have had changes of 20 Gy or more. For 96 % of patients who developed radiation pneumonitis the model predicted that the prescription would have been lowered.

Kong et al. studied SNPs in blood samples of 119 NSCLC patients treated with RT with or without chemotherapy [59]. Twenty four SNPs in 11 genes were focused in the study. These SNPs were selected because they are located in one of the DNA repair pathways and have a minor allele frequency of at least 10 %, or they were previously reported association with toxicity, tumor response, outcome or cancer

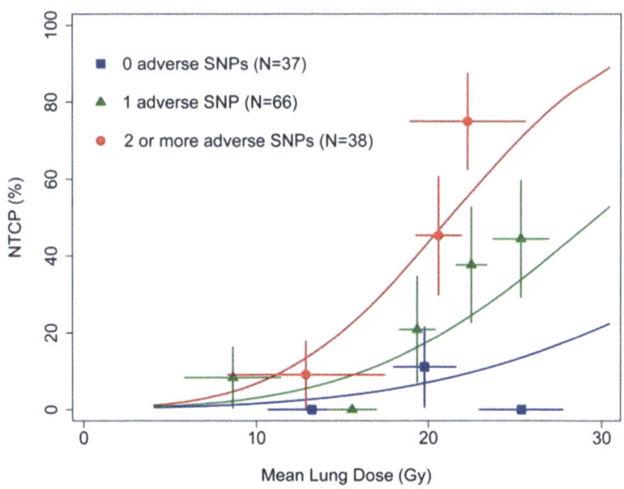

Fig. 4 Normal tissue complication probability (NTCP) dose response curves for patients with 0, 1, and 2+ adverse SNPs. The NTCP curve for patients with 0 adverse SNPs is least radiosensitive (Data from Tucker SL et al., Int J Radiat Oncol Biol Phys. 85:251–7.)

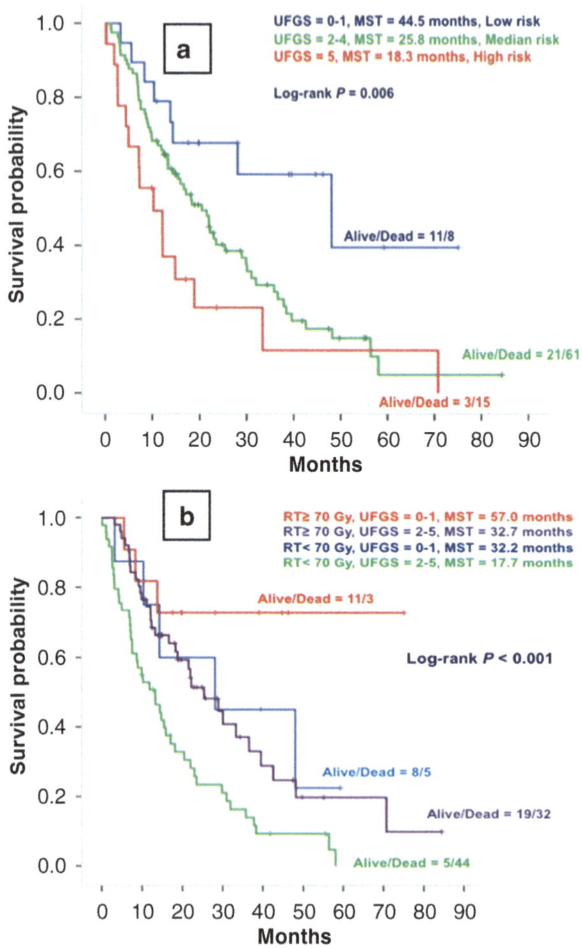

Fig. 5 SNPs in DNA repair genes on overall survival and their interaction with radiation doses. (**a**) Overall survival curves for three different groups according to the number of unfavorable genotypes (UFGS) in the 5 SNPs: (1) UFGS = 0–1, (2) UFGS = 2–4, and (3) UFGS = 5. (**b**) The OS of two different genotypes of patients (high risk: UFGS = 2–5, and low risk: UFGS = 0–1) were compared for different radiation doses (high dose: ≥70 Gy, and low dose: <70 Gy). Patients in both genotype groups showed survival benefit with higher radiation dose

risk. Five SNPs (ERCC2_rs238406, ERCC1_rs11615, ERCC1_rs3212948, XRCC4_rs9293329, XRCC4: rs2075685) were found to be independently associated with overall survival (OS) [59]. Figure 5a shows OS curves for three different groups according to the number of unfavorable genotypes (UFGS) in the 5 SNPs: (1) UFGS = 0–1, (2) UFGS = 2–4, and (3) UFGS = 5. These three groups of patients had significantly different survival. The OS of two different genotypes of patients (high risk: UFGS = 2–5, and low risk: UFGS = 0–1) were also compared for different radiation doses (high dose: ≥70 Gy, and low dose: <70 Gy) Fig. 5b. Patients in both genotype groups showed survival benefit with higher radiation dose.

4.2 micro-RNA Biomarkers in Blood

Micro-RNAs (miRNAs), a class of noncoding RNA about 18–25 nucleotides in length, are important post-transcriptional regulators of gene expression and are implicated in central biological processes such as development, cell proliferation, differentiation and apoptosis. It was reported that they were promising biomarkers for early cancer detection and prognosis [60–62]. Several miRNAs, including miR-15b, miR-34a; miR-221 and miR-130b, have been identified as associated with treatment response or prognosis for various cancers [63–66]. The expression of miRNAs can be measured in both tumor tissue and blood circulation. Detection in blood circulation is the preferred choice because the availability of blood samples. Many studies have demonstrated that miRNA can be stably, repeatable and reliably measured in serum/plasma [60–66]. While the miRNAs are potential biomarkers for prediction of treatment response, few study have demonstrated their potential to predict the response for RT.

Our group studied a panel of 84 detectable miRNAs in the circulating serum of 100 NSCLC patients from University of Michigan (UM) [67]. An miRNA signature consisting of 5 miRNA markers, which is expressed as 0.53*log(hsa-miR-15b) + 0.21*log(hsa-miR-34a)–0.27*log(hsa-miR-221)–0.27*log(hsa-miR-224)–0.07*log(hsa-miR-130b), was found and validated to be associated with the OS. The 100 patients were first randomized into a training group (47 patients) and a validation group (53 patients). Using only the training set, the signature was defined and patients were separated into high-risk and low-risk groups according to their signature values (> or < median value in the training group). Figure 6a, b show the comparison of survival curves for the high risk and low risk groups in training group and validation group, respectively. The result showed that there is a significant difference in OS between the high risk and low risk groups.

The high and low risk patients were also compared for different radiation doses (Fig. 7). The equivalent dose at 2 Gy/fraction (EQD2) of 70 Gy (median dose for these patients) was used to separate the high and low dose groups (Fig. 7a), and EQD2 = 83 Gy (BED = 100 Gy), a cut-off dose reported by many series for optimal tumor control for stereotactic body radiotherapy (SBRT) of lung cancers, was used as another stratification (Fig. 7b). It is interesting to note that low-risk patients (marker group 1) have, and the high-risk patients (marker group 2) do not have, the survival gain if dose is escalated to >70 Gy (Fig. 7a). On the other hand, while the high risk patients have survival gain if dose is escalated to >83 Gy (EQD2), low risk patients do not (Fig. 7b). These results suggest that this biomarker signature can differentiate between patients who will benefit from dose escalation at different dose levels and those who will not. At 70 Gy (EQD2) level, the high risk patients have limited gain of dose escalation, possibly, because the patients are in the beginning region of the sigmoid dose–response curve. On the other hand, at 83 Gy (EQD2) level, the low risk patients have

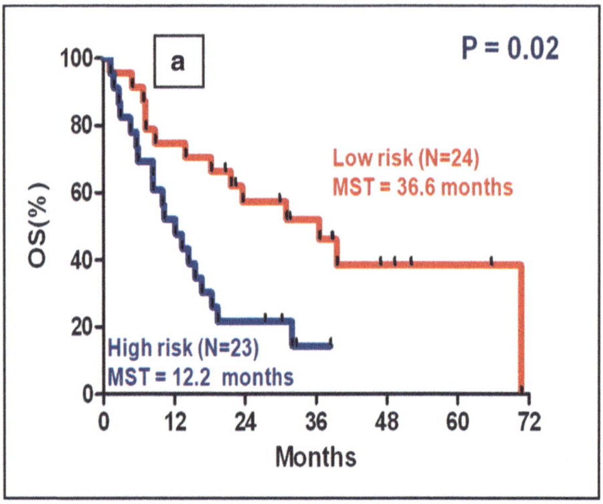

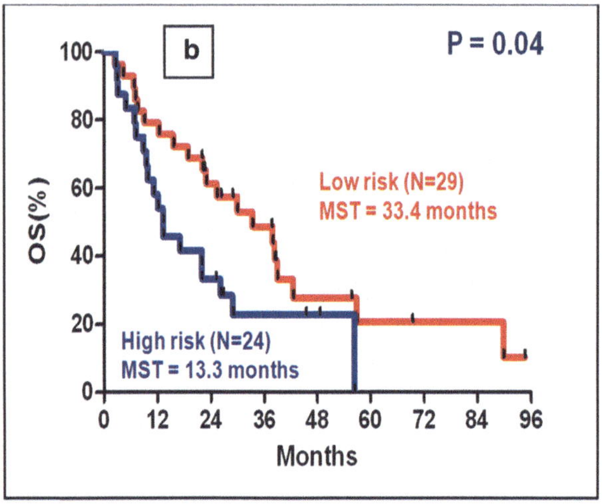

Fig. 6 MicroRNA signature on overall survival (OS) for the training and validation dataset. (**a**) Comparison of OS between the high and low risks miRNA signature for the training dataset and (**b**) for the validation set

limited gain of dose escalation because they may be at the plateau region of the sigmoid dose–response curve.

We also investigated the relationship between 84 miRNA markers and grade 2+ radiation pneumonitis (RP) [68]. Seventeen out of 100 NSCLC patients treated with RT developed grade 2+ RP. Nine miRNA markers showed significance in independent-*t* test and univariate logistic regression. However, only one marker, the hsa-miR-191, showed a significant correlation (P=0.01) using multivariate logistic regression. Figure 8 shows the incidence of cumulative RP over time for patients with low, median and high miR-191 levels. These results suggest miR-191 level may predict the incidence of RP.

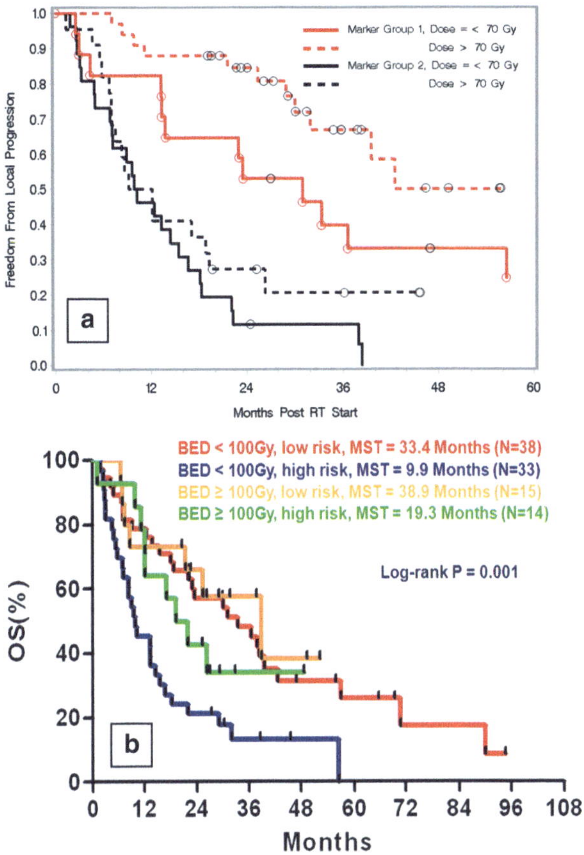

Fig. 7 MicroRNA on overall survival and dose response relationship at different dose levels. (**a**) comparison of the two groups of patients with low risk microRNA biomarker signature (marker group 1) and high risk microRNA biomarker signature (marker group 2) for two dose groups separated at 70 Gy; (**b**) comparison of the same two groups of patients with low and high risk biomarkers for 2 dose groups separated at 83 Gy (BED 100 Gy). We noted that the low-risk patients had, and the high-risk patients did not have, the survival gain when dose was escalated to >70 Gy. On the other hand, the low risk patients did not have, while the high risk patients had, the survival gain when dose was escalated to >83 Gy. These suggest that the low risk patients should have the dose at ≥70 Gy, while the high risk patients should have the dose at ≥83 Gy

4.3 *Cytokine Biomarkers in Blood*

Cytokines are a broad and loose category of small proteins that are important in cell signaling. They are released by cells and affect the behavior of other cells, and sometimes the behavior of the cell itself. One important function of cytokines is mediation of intercellular signaling to regulate homeostasis of the immune system. The effects of individual cytokines on immune response depend on several factors, including the local cytokine concentration, the pattern of cytokine receptor

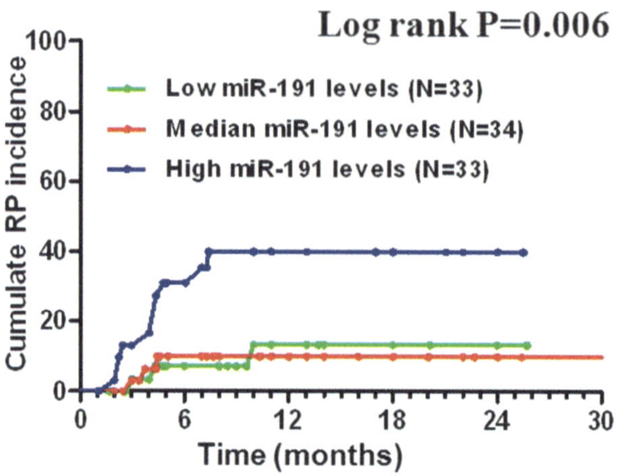

Fig. 8 Comparison of cumulated RP incidence with time for patients with low, median and high miR-191 levels

expression and the integration of multiple signaling pathways in responding immune cells. Recently, it was reported that the immune system plays an important role in RT of cancers, and immunotherapy and RT may act synergistically in cancer treatment [69, 70]. The levels of cytokines in the plasma may represent a status of interaction balance between the immune system and the tumor microenvironment, and thus may be associated with the outcome of RT treatment. Radiation treatment may break this balance, and the response of the treatment, including both tumor and normal tissue responses, may be reflected by the cytokine expression in the plasma. Common cytokines studied in the field of RT include granulocyte-macrophage colony stimulating factor (GM-CSF), interleukin (IL), interferon (IFN); tumor necrosis factor (TNF); transforming growth factor (TGF).

As early as 1999, Kong et al. reported that in 59 lung cancer patients, the patients without evidence of disease after RT or ChemoRT had significantly lower pretreatment TGFß1 level (6.0 ± 1.0 ng/mL) than those patients with diseases after treatment (12.5 ± 1.7 ng/mL) [71], suggesting that patients with low initial TGFß1 level have better outcome. Plasma TGFß1 level was 4.9 ± 0.7 ng/mL in 104 non cancer patients, and was 4.4 ± 0.2 ng/mL in normal volunteers. Zhao et al. reported that in 65 Stage III NSCLC patients TGF-ß1 ratio (during-RT/pre-RT TGF-ß1 level) was significantly correlated with OS [72]. The median OS was 30.7 months for patients with TGF-ß1 ratio ≤1 versus 13.3 months for those with TGF-ß1 ratio >1 ($p = 0.0029$). Other cytokines, such as hepatocyte growth factor (HGF), interleukin-6 (IL-6), and nicotinamide N-methyltransferase (NNMT), have also be reported to correlate with the prognostics of lung cancers [73, 74]. However, because these mechanisms are not well understood, the roles of these biomarkers in PRT are limited.

Many studies have reported that levels of inflammatory cytokines such as TNF-α, IL-1β, IL-6 and TGF-β1in plasma during RT predict radiation pneumonitis [75–78].

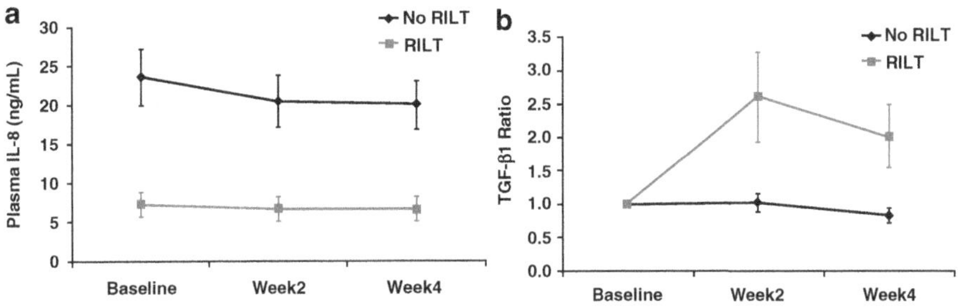

Fig. 9 Correlation of Cytokine levels and radiation induced lung toxicity (RILT). Comparison of IL-8 level (**a**) and the TGF-ß1 ratio (**b**) for patients with and without RILT at baseline, week-2 and week-4

Table 3 Personalized Radiation-induced lung toxicity (RILT) model combining 3 biophysical risk factors: 1) mean lung dose (MLD), 2) IL-8, and 3) TGF-β1

Risk groups	No RILT	With RILT	%RILT
0 risk factors	5	0	0
1 risk factor	18	1	5
2 risk factors	23	3	12
3 risk factors	2	6	75

Radiation-induced lung toxicity (RILT) risk factors are:
1st factor: MLD ≥14 GY
2nd factor: Interleukin8 (IL-8) <7.6 pg/ml
3rd factor: 2-week transforming growth factor beta1 (TGF-ß1)/baseline ≥0.5

Stenmark et al. found that the IL-8 level and TGF-ß1 ratio (between week-2 to baseline) may be predictive factors for RP [79]. Figure 9 compares IL-8 level (A) and the TGF-ß1 ratio (B) for patients with and without RILT at baseline, week-2 and week-4. The patients with RP had significantly higher levels of IL-8 at baseline, week-2 and week-4, and significantly higher TGF-ß1 ratios at week-2 and week-4.

A personalized toxicity model combining IL-8 and TGF-ß1 with mean lung dose (MLD) yielded an improved predictive ability (AUC 0.80, 95 % CI 0.66–0.94, $p<0.001$) as compared to MLD or any one variable individually [79]. Table 3 shows RILT risk grouping based on MLD, TGF-ß1, and IL-8. MLD ≥ 14 Gy, pre-treatment IL-8 < 7.6 pg/mL, and 2-week TGF-ß1 ratio ≥0.5 are the 3 risk factors. A validation study with 58 cases has been completed and it showed that for patient with 3 risk factors, the possibility of RILT reaches 75 % (Table 3).

However, cytokines are produced not only in normal lung tissue after irradiation, but are also over-expressed in tumor cells of NSCLC patients. The confounding effects of tumor-derived cytokine production may greatly influence the predictive value of RILT. A comprehensive model incorporating both effects may be needed in order to use cytokine information for PRT.

4.4 Image Biomarkers

As discussed in Sect. 2, images can be used to directly measure treatment response and thus for personalized adaptive radiotherapy. Images can also be used as biomarkers to predict a patient's tumor and normal tissue response to treatment before starting treatment, because some features of the images may reflect the intrinsic characteristics of a tumor and normal structures and their responses to the treatment. Recently, the term "radiomics" has been used to describe an approach of high-throughput extraction of large amounts of quantitative image features from radiographic images [80, 81]. The hypothesis is that quantitative analysis of medical image data through automatic or semi-automatic software of a given imaging modality can provide more and better information. This is supported by the fact that patients exhibit differences in tumor shape and texture measurable by different imaging modalities [80, 81]. In addition, advanced image analysis on conventional and novel medical imaging may capture additional information not currently used, and more specifically, that genomic and proteomics patterns can be expressed in terms of macroscopic image-based features.

Tumor shape and texture are important features in radiomics. Several texture analysis mathematical methods, including statistical-, model-, and transform-based methods, can be used to evaluate 'texture features' that provide a measure of intralesional heterogeneity for a patient [80–85]. The simplest approach is to use a statistical-based methodology with the pixel intensity histogram [80–84]. Parameters such as mean intensity, maximum intensity, minimum intensity, uniformity (uniformity of gray-level distribution), standard deviation of the gray-level histogram distribution, skewness (asymmetry of the histogram), and kurtosis (flatness of the histogram) can be quickly calculated using this approach. Other more complicated parameters, such as entropy (randomness of the matrix), energy/angular second moment (pixel repetition/orderliness and measures the homogeneity of an image), homogeneity (uniformity of concurrence matrix), dissimilarity (measurement of how different each element in the matrix is), and correlation (measurement of gray-tone linear dependencies) can be determined using a second-order statistics approach [80–84]. The fractal dimension is another measure to characterize the surface roughness of an image object, and can be determined using a model-based fractal analysis method [85].

Texture uniformity of the tumor in CT images was found to be a poor prognostic factor for NSCLC patients [83, 84]. Uniformity, entropy and fractal dimension in CT images have also been reported to correlate with the mean SUV of FDG PET image in NSCLC and esophageal cancer patients [86]. Kuo et al. reported the association of CT-derived imaging features with histo-pathologic markers, and several pre-defined gene expression modules on liver cancer [87]. For PET imaging, the maximum and median FDG uptake has been reported to have strong prognostic power [88]. Shape and texture features of FDG PET images have also been investigated for correlation with treatment response. El Naqa et al. demonstrated that several first- and second-order statistical textural features (energy, contrast, local homogeneity, and entropy) are useful in predicting outcome in head and neck (n=9) and cervical cancer (n=14) [89]. These methods achieved an area under curve (AUC) of 0.76 and 1.0 for the cervix and head and neck cohorts, respectively [89]. Tixier et al. have investigated its clinical application in 41 patients with esophageal cancer treated with chemoradiation and shown that baseline FDG PET texture is a sensitive predictive marker [90]. They found that local (i.e., entropy and homogeneity) and regional (i.e., size and intensity variabilities) texture parameters performed better than standard SUV measurements in differentiation of responders from non-responders following chemoradiation. The sensitivity, specificity, and AUC for SUVmax were 53 %, 73 %, and 0.59 compared to 73 %, 88 %, and 0.89 for local homogeneity in identifying responders [90].

In NSCLC, SUV measures of FDG uptake on the PET image before RT may also be used as a biomarker to predict radiation induced lung toxicity [91, 92]. The hypothesis is that pretreatment inflammation in the lung makes pulmonary tissue more susceptible to radiation damage. Petit SF et al. retrospectively studied 101 NSCLC patients treated with Chemo-RT [91]. FDG uptake in the lung volume, excluding clinical target volumes in the Pre-RT PET was related to RILT after RT in univariable logistic regression [91]. The 95th percentile of the FDG uptake in the lungs remained significant in multivariable logistic regression (p=0.016; odds ratio [OR]=4.3). Castillo R et al. performed similar work and confirmed that FDG uptake in pre-RT PET predict RILT [92], another potential tool to guide PRT.

5 Personalized Fractionation Schedule in PRT

Fractionation schedule could be an important part in PRT. However, there have been few studies on this topic. The conventional fractionation schedule of 1.8–2 Gy/fraction was based on clinical experiences in the 2-dimensional (2D) radiotherapy era. The dose delivered to the tumor was usually similar as the dose to the normal tissue in the 2D era. Because the α/β ratio is usually much lower for the normal tissue than for the tumor, a fractionation schedule with smaller dose/fraction would benefit a patient based on the therapeutic ratio calculated from the linear-quadratic (LQ) model. However, reducing the dose/fraction prolongs the treatment duration, and thus greatly reduces the power of radiation killing due to the tumor cell repopulation effect. The conventional 1.8–2 Gy/fraction was a balance of these 2 factors. With the rapid development of RT technology, such as 3D conformal RT, intensity modulated RT, and image-guided RT, radiation dose to the normal tissue has been greatly reduced. A dose-volume histogram (DVH) is usually used to represent the dose received by an organ at risk (OAR) and the tumor. The doses for the OARs are usually much lower than that of the tumor, and may depend largely on the tumor volume and location. Thus, a different fractionation schedule may need to be established for treatment with current technology.

Jin et al. demonstrated that hypo-fractionation (large dose/fraction) offers a higher therapeutic ratio than conventional fractionation for relatively small tumors, while conventional fractionation generally offers a therapeutic advantage for patients with large tumors for lung cancers in a theoretic study [93]. The therapeutic ratio was calculated based on the LQ model with the α/β ratio being 10 Gy for the tumor, and 3 Gy for the lung. The underlying principle of this fractionation effect on the therapeutic ratio was well illustrated by Gay et al. using a simple isodose line based approach [94]. As shown in Fig. 10, the 30 % isodose line divides the lung tissue into two regions (the number 30 % is calculated as the ratio of α/β ratio of normal lung tissue and the tumor, which are 3 and 10 Gy, respectively). For the region >30 %, the lung BED decreases with increasing fraction number, suggesting a benefit for conventional fractionation. On the other hand, for the region <30 %, the lung BED increases with increasing fraction number, suggesting a benefit for hypo-fractionation. For a relatively small tumor, the 30 % isodose line will encompass only small part of lung volume so that overall, hypo-fractionation is usually preferred. On the other hand, for large tumor, the isodose will encompass a large volume of lung, and thus conventional fractionation is preferred. Myerson also independently derived a hypo-fractionation sufficiency condition and a hyper-fractionation sufficiency condition to determine whether hypo- or hyper-fractionation may have the therapeutic advantage [95].

However, these studies used a simple LQ model without considering the tumor cell repopulation effect. Consequently, the calculated optimal fractionation regimen was either a single fraction, or one with infinite fraction (hypo-fractionation was considered as the choice if the optimal fractionation corresponding to a single fraction, and conventional fractionation was considered to be the choice if the optimal fractionation corresponding to infinite fractions). Xiao et al. have used a potential

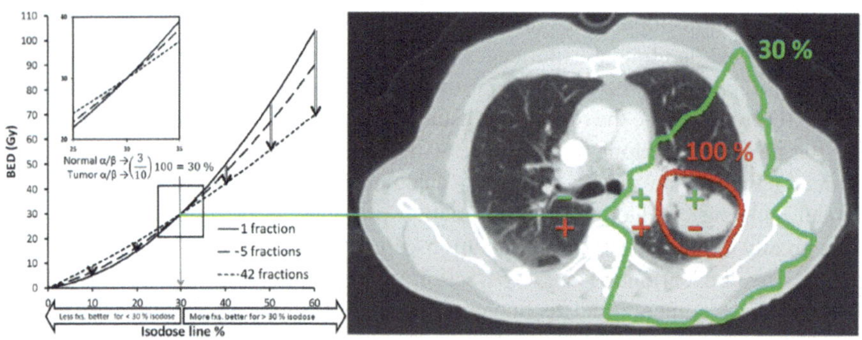

Fig. 10 A simple isodose line based approach to illustrate the fractionation effect. The left figure shows the how BED varies with the isodose line for different fractionation schedule. The 30 % isodose line divides the lung tissue into two regions (the number 30 % is calculated as the ratio of α/β ratio of normal lung tissue and the tumor, which are 3 and 10 Gy, respectively). For the region >30 %, the lung BED decreases with increasing fraction number, suggesting a benefit for conventional fractionation. On the other hand, for the region <30 %, the lung BED increases with increasing fraction number, suggesting a benefit for hypo-fractionation (Data from Gay HA, Jin JY, Chang AJ, et al. *Int J Radiat Oncol Biol Phys* 85:e81–87)

doubling time (T_{pot}) correction to account for the tumor cell repopulation effect for the LQ model [96]. The corrected LQ model is expressed below,

$$BED = n \cdot d\left(1 + \frac{d}{\alpha / \beta}\right) - \frac{0.693 \cdot t}{\alpha \cdot T_{pot}} \tag{1}$$

where n is the number of treatment fractions, d is the dose per fraction, and t is the number of treatment days for a specific radiotherapy treatment regimen. An α/β ratio of 10 Gy and α value of 0.30 Gy^{-1} were used for the tumor. Similar to the approach by Jin et al. [93], an iso-biologic equivalent dose (iso-BED) was given to the tumor to simplify the comparisons of therapeutic ratios among various fractionation schedules, so that the therapeutic ratio depended only on the modeled lung toxicity. A simple logistic model was used to determine the local effective damage and calculate the total damaged lung volume to represent the lung toxicity. The simple logistic model is expressed as

$$E(D) = 1 / \left(1 + \left(D_{50} / D\right)^2\right) \tag{2}$$

where $E(D)$ is the local effective damage at the dose D, and D_{50} is the dose causing 50 % of local damage and a parameter determining the radiosensitivity of the lung. Figure 11 shows changes of the relative lung damage volume (RDV) with number of fractions for different T_{pot} values at a fixed D_{50} value (D_{50} = 30 Gy). We noted that there was a minimal RDV, or maximal therapeutic ratio for each curve. The fraction number corresponding to the minimal RDV was the optimal fraction number. It was ~5 for T_{pot} = 5 days, and ~8 for T_{pot} = 10 days, and varied from 15 to 30 when T_{pot} further increased. The optimal fraction number also depended on the D_{50} and tumor size and location. This study demonstrated that the RT fractionation schedule should also be personalized according to the patient's factors to improve the therapeutic ratio. However, further studies, such as determining accuracy of the T_{pot}, D_{50}, α and β values for individual patients, are required to implement this strategy clinically.

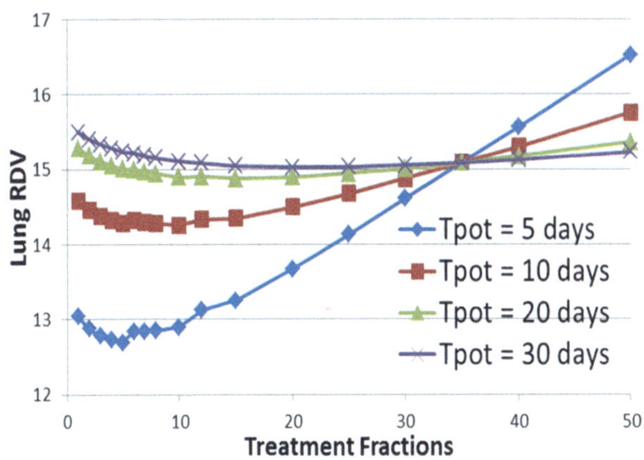

Fig. 11 Dependency of relative damaged volume (RDV) of lung on the numbers of treatment fractions for various T_{pot} with fixed D_{L50}

6 Summary

The current practice of radiation treatment for lung cancer is partially individualized to tumor histology (small cell versus non-small cell), stage, size/location, and combination with use of systemic therapy. During-RT image guided adaptive treatment is a promising individualization approach. During-RT PET-CT image guided adaptive treatment is currently being tested in multicenter trials such as RTOG1106. During-RT imaging may also measure an individual's response to treatment for both tumor and normal tissue, and thus empower us to further personalize the remaining treatment by either escalating or deescalating the total dose to the tumor according to the measured response. Research on biomarker guided PRT is ongoing, interesting clinical trials are proposed. In addition, RT fractionation schedule (radiation dose per fraction) may also be personalized to each individual patient to maximize therapeutic gain. Future PRT should be knowledge based to maximize the therapeutic gain in each individual patient by comprehensive considerations of knowledge acquired from patients in the clinic, imaging assessment, tumor pathology, testing of patient biologic features, radiation dosimetric analysis, responses of tumor and normal tissues to the treatment and combination of systemic therapy (Fig. 12). The future of PRT may also consider the societal value such as cost and effectiveness.

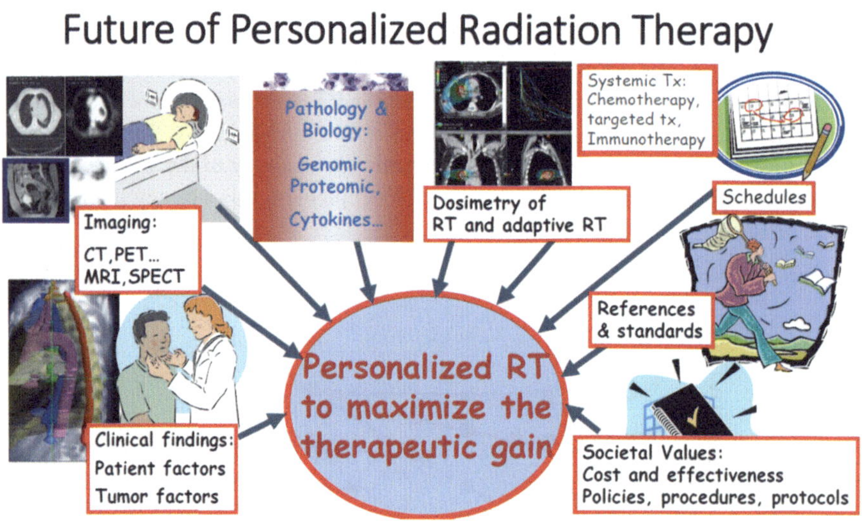

Fig. 12 Future of personalized radiation therapy. Personalized radiation therapy (PRT) will maximize the therapeutic gain in each individual patient by comprehensive considerations of knowledge acquired from patients in the clinic, imaging assessment, tumor pathology, testing of patient biologic features, radiation dosimetric analysis, responses of tumor and normal tissues to the treatment and combination of systemic therapy. The future of PRT should also consider the societal value such as cost and effective analysis

References

1. Jemal A, Siegel R et al (2009) Cancer statistics, 2009. Cancer J Clin 59(4):225–249
2. Ferlay JSH, Bray F, Forman D, Mathers C, Parkin DM (2010) "GLOBOCAN 2008." Cancer incidence and mortality worldwide: IARC CancerBase. International Agency for Research on Cancer; 2010 No. 10
3. Ettinger DS, Akerley W, Borghaei H et al (2013) National comprehensive cancer network. Non-small cell lung cancer, version 2.2013. J Natl Compr Canc Netw 11(6):645–653
4. Timmerman R, Paulus R et al (2010) Stereotactic body radiation therapy for inoperable early stage lung cancer. JAMA 303(11):1070–1076
5. Timmerman R, Bastasch M et al (2007) Optimizing dose and fractionation for stereotactic body radiation therapy. Normal tissue and tumor control effects with large dose per fraction. Front Radiat Ther Oncol 40:352–365
6. Onishi H, Araki T et al (2004) Stereotactic hypofractionated high-dose irradiation for stage I nonsmall cell lung carcinoma: clinical outcomes in 245 subjects in a Japanese multiinstitutional study. Cancer 101(7):1623–1631
7. Hiraoka M, Matsuo Y et al (2007) Stereotactic body radiation therapy (SBRT) for early-stage lung cancer. Cancer Radiother 11(1-2):32–35
8. Guckenberger M, Wulf J et al (2009) Dose-response relationship for image-guided stereotactic body radiotherapy of pulmonary tumors: relevance of 4D dose calculation. Int J Radiat Oncol Biol Phys 74(1):47–54
9. Kong F-M, Jin J-Y, Bradley J, Martel M (2011) *Cancers of the thorax* in treatment planning In: Faiz M. Khan (ed) Radiation Oncology. Williams & Wilkins
10. Kong FM, Ten Haken RK et al (2005) High-dose radiation improved local tumor control and overall survival in patients with inoperable/unresectable non-small-cell lung cancer: long-term results of a radiation dose escalation study. Int J Radiat Oncol Biol Phys 63(2):324–333
11. Rengan R, Rosenzweig KE et al (2004) Improved local control with higher doses of radiation in large-volume stage III non-small-cell lung cancer. Int J Radiat Oncol Biol Phys 60(3):741–747
12. Machtay M, Bae K et al (2010) Higher biologically effective dose of radiotherapy is associated with improved outcomes for locally advanced Non-small cell lung carcinoma treated with chemoradiation: an analysis of the Radiation Therapy Oncology Group. Int J Radiat Oncol Biol Phys 82(1):425–434
13. Cox JD (2012) Are the results of RTOG 0617 mysterious? Int J Radiat Oncol Biol Phys 82(3):1042–1044
14. Budach W, Belka C (2004) Palliative percutaneous radiotherapy in non-small-cell lung cancer. Lung Cancer 45(Suppl 2):S239–S245
15. Marks LB, Yorke ED, Jackson A, Ten Haken RK, Constine LS, Eisbruch A, Bentzen SM, Nam J, Deasy JO (2010) Use of normal tissue complication probability models in the clinic. Int J Radiat Oncol Biol Phys 76(3 Suppl):S10–S19
16. Yorke ED, Jackson A, Rosenzweig KE, Merrick SA, Gabrys D, Venkatraman ES, Burman CM, Leibel SA, Ling CC (2002) Dose-volume factors contributing to the incidence of radiation pneumonitis in non-small-cell lung cancer patients treated with three-dimensional conformal radiation therapy. Int J Radiat Oncol Biol Phys 54(2):329–339
17. Marks LB, Bentzen SM, Deasy JO, Kong FM, Bradley JD, Vogelius IS, El Naqa I, Hubbs JL, Lebesque JV, Timmerman RD, Martel MK, Jackson A (2010) Radiation dose-volume effects in the lung. Int J Radiat Oncol Biol Phys 76(3 Suppl):S70–S76
18. Kong FM, Hayman JA, Griffith KA, Kalemkerian GP, Arenberg D, Lyons S, Turrisi A, Lichter A, Fraass B, Eisbruch A, Lawrence TS, Ten Haken RK (2006) Final toxicity results of a radiation-dose escalation study in patients with non-small-cell lung cancer (NSCLC): predictors for radiation pneumonitis and fibrosis. Int J Radiat Oncol Biol Phys 65(4):1075–1086
19. Kupelian PA, Ramsey C, Meeks SL et al (2005) Serial megavoltage CT imaging during external beam radiotherapy for non-small-cell lung cancer: observations on tumor regression during treatment. Int J Radiat Oncol Biol Phys 63(4):1024–1028

20. Bosmans G, van Baardwijk A, Dekker A et al (2006) Intra-patient variability of tumor volume and tumor motion during conventionally fractionated radiotherapy for locally advanced non-small-cell lung cancer: a prospective clinical study. Int J Radiat Oncol Biol Phys 66(3):748–753
21. Fox J, Ford E, Redmond K et al (2009) Quantification of tumor volume changes during radiotherapy for non-small-cell lung cancer. Int J Radiat Oncol Biol Phys 74(2):341–348
22. Gay HA, Taylor QQ, Kiriyama F, Dieck GT, Jenkins T, Walker P, Allison RR, Ubezio P (2013) Modeling of non-small cell lung cancer volume changes during CT-based image guided radiotherapy: patterns observed and clinical implications. Comput Math Methods Med 2013:1–13
23. Kong FM, Frey KA, Quint LE, Ten Haken RK, Hayman JA, Kessler M, Chetty IJ, Normolle D, Eisbruch A, Lawrence TS (2007) A pilot study of [18F]fluorodeoxyglucose positron emission tomography scans during and after radiation-based therapy in patients with non small-cell lung cancer. J Clin Oncol 25(21):3116–3123
24. van Baardwijk A et al (2007) Time trends in the maximal uptake of FDG on PET scan during thoracic radiotherapy. A prospective study in locally advanced non-small cell lung cancer (NSCLC) patients. Radiother Oncol 82(2):145–152
25. Gillham C, Zips D, Pönisch F, Evers C, Enghardt W, Abolmaali N, Zöphel K, Appold S, Hölscher T, Steinbach J, Kotzerke J, Herrmann T, Baumann M (2008) Additional PET/CT in week 5-6 of radiotherapy for patients with stage III non-small cell lung cancer as a means of dose escalation planning? Radiother Oncol 88(3):335–341
26. Choi NC, Chun TT, Niemierko A, Ancukiewicz M, Fidias PM, Kradin RL, Mathisen DJ, Lynch TJ, Fischman AJ (2013) Potential of 18F-FDG PET toward personalized radiotherapy or chemoradiotherapy in lung cancer. Eur J Nucl Med Mol Imaging 40(6):832–841
27. Mahasittiwat P, Yuan S, Xie C, Ritter T, Cao Y, Ten Haken RK, Kong FM (2013) Metabolic tumor volume on PET reduced more than gross tumor volume on CT during radiotherapy in patients with non-small cell lung cancer treated with 3DCRT or SBRT. J Radiat Oncol 2(2):191–20231
28. Feng M et al (2009) Using fluorodeoxyglucose positron emission tomography to assess tumor volume during radiotherapy for non-small-cell lung cancer and its potential impact on adaptive dose escalation and normal tissue sparing. Int J Radiat Oncol Biol Phys 73(4):1228–1234
29. Kong FM, Ten Haken R et al (2013) A phase II trial of mid-treatment FDG-PET adaptive, individualized radiation therapy plus concurrent chemotherapy in patients with non-small cell lung cancer (NSCLC). J Clin Oncol 31(suppl; abstr 7522)
30. Robbins ME, Brunso-Bechtold JK, Peiffer AM, Tsien CI, Bailey JE, Marks LB (2012) Imaging radiation-induced normal tissue injury. Radiat Res 177(4):449–466
31. Boersma LJ, Damen EM, de Boer RW, Muller SH, Valdés-Olmos RA, van Zandwijk N, Lebesque JV (1996) Recovery and overall and local lung function loss 18 months after irradiation for malignant lymphoma. J Clin Oncol 14:1431–1441
32. Mah K, Van Dyk J, Keane T, Poon PY (1987) Acute radiation-induced pulmonary damage: a clinical study on the response to fractionated radiation therapy. Int J Radiat Oncol Biol Phys 13:179–188
33. Yankelevitz DF, Henschke CI, Batata M, Kim YS, Chu F (1994) Lung cancer: evaluation with MR imaging during and after irradiation. J Thorac Imaging 9:41–46
34. Ogasawara N, Suga K, Karino Y, Matsunaga N (2002) Perfusion characteristics of radiation-induced lung on Gd-DTPA-enhanced dynamic magnetic resonance imaging. Invest Radiol 37:448–457
35. Hicks RJ, MacManus MP, Matthews JP, Hogg A, Binns D, Rischin D, Ball DL, Peters LJ (2004) Early FDG-PET imaging after radical radiotherapy for nonsmall-cell lung cancer: inflammatory changes in normal tissues correlate with tumor response and do not confound therapeutic response evaluation. Int J Radiat Oncol Biol Phys 60:412–418
36. Guerrero T, Johnson V, Hart J, Pan T, Khan M, Luo D, Liao Z, Alani J, Stevens C, Komaki R (2007) Radiation pneumonitis: local dose versus [18F]-fluorodeoxyglucose uptake response in irradiated lung. Int J Radiat Oncol Biol Phys 68:1030–1035

37. Hart JP, McCurdy MR, Ezhil M, Wei W, Khan M, Luo D, Munden RF, Johnson VE, Guerrero TM (2008) Radiation pneumonitis: correlation of toxicity with pulmonary metabolic radiation response. Int J Radiat Oncol Biol Phys 71:967–971
38. Abdulla S, Salavati A, Saboury B, Basu S, Torigian DA, Alavi A (2014) Quantitative assessment of global lung inflammation following radiation therapy using FDG PET/CT: a pilot study. Eur J Nucl Med Mol Imaging 41(2):350–356
39. McCurdy M, Bergsma DP, Hyun E, Kim T, Choi E, Castillo R, Castillo E, Guerrero T (2013) The role of lung lobes in radiation pneumonitis and radiation-induced inflammation in the lung: a retrospective study. J Radiat Oncol 2(2):203–208
40. McCurdy MR, Castillo R, Martinez J, Al Hallack MN, Lichter J, Zouain N, Guerrero T (2012) [18F]-FDG uptake dose-response correlates with radiation pneumonitis in lung cancer patients. Radiother Oncol 104(1):52–57
41. Mac Manus MP, Ding Z, Hogg A, Herschtal A, Binns D, Ball DL, Hicks RJ (2011) Association between pulmonary uptake of fluorodeoxyglucose detected by positron emission tomography scanning after radiation therapy for non-small-cell lung cancer and radiation pneumonitis. Int J Radiat Oncol Biol Phys 80(5):1365–1371
42. Seppenwoolde Y, De Jaeger K, Boersma LJ, Belderbos JS, Lebesque JV (2004) Regional differences in lung radiosensitivity after radiotherapy for nonsmall-cell lung cancer. Int J Radiat Oncol Biol Phys 60:748–758
43. Marks LB, Fan M, Clough R, Munley MT, Bentel G, Coleman RE, Jaszczak R, Hollis D, Anscher M (2000) Radiation-induced pulmonary injury: symptomatic versus subclinical endpoints. Int J Radiat Biol 76:469–475
44. Vinogradskiy Y, Castillo R, Castillo E, Tucker SL, Liao Z, Guerrero T, Martel MK (2013) Use of 4-dimensional computed tomography-based ventilation imaging to correlate lung dose and function with clinical outcomes. Int J Radiat Oncol Biol Phys 86(2):366–371
45. Zhong H, Jin JY, Ajlouni M, Movsas B, Chetty IJ (2011) Measurement of regional compliance using 4DCT images for assessment of radiation treatment. Med Phys 38(3):1567–1578
46. Ding K, Bayouth JE, Buatti JM, Christensen GE, Reinhardt JM (2010) 4DCT-based measurement of changes in pulmonary function following a course of radiation therapy. Med Phys 37(3):1261–1272
47. De Ruysscher D, Houben A, Aerts HJ, Dehing C, Wanders R, Ollers M, Dingemans AM, Hochstenbag M, Boersma L, Borger J, Dekker A, Lambin P (2009) Increased(18) F-deoxyglucose uptake in the lung during the first weeks of radiotherapy is correlated with subsequent radiation-induced lung toxicity (RILT): a prospective pilot study. Radiother Oncol 91(3):415–420
48. Li L, Wang W, Stanton P, Bi N, Kong FM (2013) FDG pulmonary uptake changes during and post-radiation therapy compared to pretreatment in predicting radiation-induced lung toxicity in non-small cell lung cancer. Int J Radiat Oncol Biol Phys 87(2):S77
49. Yuan ST, Frey KA, Gross MD, Hayman JA, Arenberg D, Cai XW, Ramnath N, Hassan K, Moran J, Eisbruch A, Ten Haken RK, Kong FM (2012) Changes in global function and regional ventilation and perfusion on SPECT during the course of radiotherapy in patients with non-small-cell lung cancer. Int J Radiat Oncol Biol Phys 15:82(4)
50. Kim DN, Nam TK, Choe KS, Choy H (2012) Personalized combined modality therapy for locally advanced non-small cell lung cancer. Cancer Res Treat 44(2):74–84
51. Ausborn NL, Le QT, Bradley JD, Choy H, Dicker AP, Saha D, Simko J, Story MD, Torossian A, Lu B (2012) Molecular profiling to optimize treatment in non-small cell lung cancer: a review of potential molecular targets for radiation therapy by the translational research program of the radiation therapy oncology group. Int J Radiat Oncol Biol Phys 83(4):e453–e464
52. Salgia R, Hensing T, Campbell N, Salama AK, Maitland M, Hoffman P, Villaflor V, Vokes EE (2011) Personalized treatment of lung cancer. Semin Oncol 38(2):274–283
53. Strimbu K, Tavel JA (2010) What are biomarkers? Curr Opin HIV AIDS 5(6):463–466
54. Biomarkers Definitions Working Group (2001) Biomarkers and surrogate endpoints: preferred definitions and conceptual framework. Clin Pharmacol Ther 69(3):89–95

55. Yuan X, Liao Z, Liu Z, Wang LE, Tucker SL, Mao L, Wang XS, Martel M, Komaki R, Cox JD, Milas L, Wei Q (2009) Single nucleotide polymorphism at rs1982073:T869C of the TGFbeta 1 gene is associated with the risk of radiation pneumonitis in patients with non-small-cell lung cancer treated with definitive radiotherapy. J Clin Oncol 27(20):3370–3378
56. Kelsey CR, Jackson IL, Langdon S, Owzar K, Hubbs J, Vujaskovic Z, Das S, Marks LB (2013) Analysis of single nucleotide polymorphisms and radiation sensitivity of the lung assessed with an objective radiologic endpoin. Clin Lung Cancer 14(3):267–274
57. Tucker SL, Li M, Xu T, Gomez D, Yuan X, Yu J, Liu Z, Yin M, Guan X, Wang LE, Wei Q, Mohan R, Vinogradskiy Y, Martel M, Liao Z (2013) Incorporating single-nucleotide polymorphisms into the Lyman model to improve prediction of radiation pneumonitis. Int J Radiat Oncol Biol Phys 85(1):251–257
58. Vinogradskiy Y, Tucker SL, Bluett JB, Wages CA, Liao Z, Martel MK (2012) Prescribing radiation dose to lung cancer patients based on personalized toxicity estimates. J Thorac Oncol 7(11):1676–1682
59. Wang W et al (2012) 11 Single nucleotide polymorphisms in dna repair genes may be associated with survival in patients with non-small cell lung cancer treated with definitive radiotherapy, oral abstract, Chicago Multidisciplinary Symposium in Thoracic Oncology, Chicago, 06 Sept 2012.
60. Landi MT et al (2010) MicroRNA expression differentiates histology and predicts survival of lung cancer. Clin Cancer Res 16(2):430–441
61. Yu SL et al (2008) MicroRNA signature predicts survival and relapse in lung cancer. Cancer Cell 13(1):48–57
62. Vosa U et al (2011) Identification of miR-374a as a prognostic marker for survival in patients with early-stage nonsmall cell lung cancer. Genes Chromosomes Cancer 50(10):812–822
63. Hermeking H (2010) The miR-34 family in cancer and apoptosis. Cell Death Differ 17(2):193–199
64. Sen CK et al (2009) Micromanaging vascular biology: tiny microRNAs play big band. J Vasc Res 46(6):527–540
65. Yang C et al (2012) Epigenetic silencing of miR-130b in ovarian cancer promotes the development of multidrug resistance by targeting colony-stimulating factor 1. Gynecol Oncol 124(2):325–334
66. Franchina T, Amodeo V, Bronte G, Savio G, Ricciardi GR, Picciotto M, Russo A, Giordano A, Adamo V (2014) Circulating miR-22, miR-24 and miR-34a as novel predictive biomarkers to pemetrexed-based chemotherapy in advanced non-small cell lung cancer. J Cell Physiol 229(1):97–99
67. Bi N, Schipper MJ, Stanton P, Wang W, Kong FM (2013) Serum miRNA signature to identify a patient's resistance to high-dose radiation therapy for unresectable non-small cell lung cancer. J Clin Oncol 31(suppl; abstr 7580)
68. Bi N, Stanton P, Wang W, Kong FM (2013) Serum MicroRNA as a predictive marker for radiation pneumonitis in patients with inoperable/unresectable non-small cell lung cancer (NSCLC). Int J Radiat Oncol Biol Phys 87(Issue 2):S93
69. Golden EB, Demaria S, Schiff PB, Chachoua A, Formenti SC (2013) An abscopal response to radiation and ipilimumab in a patient with metastatic non-small cell lung cancer. Cancer Immunol Res 1(6):365–372
70. Ludgate CM (2012) Optimizing cancer treatments to induce an acute immune response: radiation Abscopal effects, PAMPs, and DAMPs. Clin Cancer Res 18(17):4522–4525
71. Kong F, Jirtle RL, Huang DH, Clough RW, Anscher MS (1999) Plasma transforming growth factor-beta1 level before radiotherapy correlates with long term outcome of patients with lung carcinoma. Cancer 86(9):1712–1719
72. Zhao L, Ji W, Zhang L, Ou G, Feng Q, Zhou Z, Lei M, Yang W, Wang L (2010) Changes of circulating transforming growth factor-beta1 level during radiation therapy are correlated with the prognosis of locally advanced non-small cell lung cancer. J Thorac Oncol 5(4):521–525

73. Ujiie H, Tomida M, Akiyama H, Nakajima Y, Okada D, Yoshino N, Takiguchi Y, Tanzawa H (2012) Serum hepatocyte growth factor and interleukin-6 are effective prognostic markers for non-small cell lung cancer. Anticancer Res 32(8):3251–3258
74. Chang CH, Hsiao CF, Yeh YM, Chang GC, Tsai YH, Chen YM, Huang MS, Chen HL, Li YJ, Yang PC, Chen CJ, Hsiung CA, Su WC (2013) Circulating interleukin-6 level is a prognostic marker for survival in advanced nonsmall cell lung cancer patients treated with chemotherapy. Int J Cancer 132(9):1977–1985
75. Rube CE, Wilfert F, Uthe D, Konig J, Liu L et al (2004) Increased expression of pro-inflammatory cytokines as a cause of lung toxicity after combined treatment with gemcitabine and thoracic irradiation. Radiother Oncol 72:231–241
76. Anscher MS, Kong FM, Andrews K, Clough R, Marks LB et al (1998) Plasma transforming growth factor beta1 as a predictor of radiation pneumonitis. Int J Radiat Oncol Biol Phys 41:1029–1035
77. Arpin D, Perol D, Blay JY, Falchero L, Claude L et al (2005) Early variations of circulating interleukin-6 and interleukin-10 levels during thoracic radiotherapy are predictive for radiation pneumonitis. J Clin Oncol 23:8748–8875
78. Chen Y, Hyrien O, Williams J, Okunieff P, Smudzin T et al (2005) Interleukin (IL)-1A and IL-6: applications to the predictive diagnostic testing of radiation pneumonitis. Int J Radiat Oncol Biol Phys 62:260–266
79. Stenmark MH, Cai XW, Shedden K, Hayman JA, Yuan S, Ritter T, Ten Haken RK, Lawrence TS, Kong FM (2012) Combining physical and biologic parameters to predict radiation-induced lung toxicity in patients with non-small-cell lung cancer treated with definitive radiation therapy. Int J Radiat Oncol Biol Phys 84(2):e217–e222
80. Lambin P, Rios-Velazquez E, Leijenaar R, Carvalho S, van Stiphout RG, Granton P, Zegers CM, Gillies R, Boellard R, Dekker A, Aerts HJ (2012) Radiomics: extractingmore information from medical images using advanced feature analysis. Eur J Cancer 48(4):441–446
81. Davnall F, Yip CS, Ljungqvist G, Selmi M, Ng F, Sanghera B, Ganeshan B, Miles KA, Cook GJ, Goh V (2012) Assessment of tumor heterogeneity: an emerging imaging tool for clinical practice? Insights Imaging 3(6):573–589
82. Srinivasan GN, Shobha G (2008) Statistical texture analysis. Proc World Acad Sci Eng Technol 36:1264–1269
83. Ganeshan B, Abaleke S, Young RC, Chatwin CR, Miles KA (2010) Texture analysis of non-small cell lung cancer on unenhanced computed tomography: initial evidence for a relationship with tumor glucose metabolism and stage. Cancer Imaging 10:137–143
84. Al-Kadi OS (2010) Assessment of texture measures susceptibility to noise in conventional and contrast enhanced computed tomography lung tumour images. Comput Med Imaging Graph 34(6):494–503
85. Kido S, Kuriyama K, Higashiyama M, Kasugai T, Kuroda C (2003) Fractal analysis of internal and peripheral textures of small peripheral bronchogenic carcinomas in thin-section computed tomography: comparison of bronchioloalveolar cell carcinomas with nonbronchioloalveolar cell carcinomas. J Comput Assist Tomogr 27(1):56–61
86. Rutman AM, Kuo MD (2009) Radiogenomics: creating a link between molecular diagnostics and diagnostic imaging. Eur J Radiol 70:232–241
87. Kuo MD, Gollub J, Sirlin CB, Ooi C, Chen X (2007) Radiogenomic analysis to identify imaging phenotypes associated with drug response gene expression programs in hepatocellular carcinoma. J Vasc Interv Radiol 18:821–831
88. Paesmans M, Berghmans T, Dusart M, Garcia C, Hossein-Foucher C, Lafitte JJ, Mascaux C, Meert AP, Roelandts M, Scherpereel A, Terrones Munoz V, Sculier JP, European Lung Cancer Working Party, and on behalf of the IASLC Lung Cancer Staging Project (2010) Primary tumor standardized uptake value measured on fluorodeoxyglucose positron emission tomography is of prognostic value for survival in non-small cell lung cancer: update of a systematic review and meta-analysis by the European Lung Cancer Working Party for the International Association for the Study of Lung Cancer Staging Project. J Thorac Oncol 5(5):612–9

89. El Naqa I, Grigsby P, Apte A et al (2009) Exploring feature-based approaches in PET images for predicting cancer treatment outcomes. Pattern Recognit 42(6):1162–1171
90. Tixier F, Le Rest CC, Hatt M et al (2011) Intratumor heterogeneity characterized by textural features on baseline 18 F-FDG PET images predicts response to concomitant radiochemotherapy in esophageal cancer. J Nucl Med 52(3):369–378
91. Petit SF, van Elmpt WJ, Oberije CJ, Vegt E, Dingemans AM, Lambin P, Dekker AL, De Ruysscher D (2011) [^{18}F]fluorodeoxyglucose uptake patterns in lung before radiotherapy identify areas more susceptible to radiation-induced lung toxicity in non-small-cell lung cancer patients. Int J Radiat Oncol Biol Phys 81(3):698–705
92. Castillo R, Pham N, Ansari S, Meshkov D, Castillo S, Li M, Olanrewaju A, Hobbs B, Castillo E, Guerrero T (2014) Pre-radiotherapy FDG PET predicts radiation pneumonitis in lung cancer. Radiat Oncol 9(1):74
93. Jin JY, Kong FM, Chetty IJ et al (2010) Impact of fraction size on lung radiation toxicity—hypofractionation may be beneficial in dose escalation of radiotherapy for lung cancer. Int J Radiat Oncol Biol Phys 76:782–788
94. Gay HA, Jin JY, Chang AJ et al (2013) Utility of normal tissue-to-tumor a/b ratio when evaluating isodoses of isoeffective radiation therapy treatment plans. Int J Radiat Oncol Biol Phys 85:e81–e87
95. Myerson RJ (2011) Normal tissue dose conformality measures to guide radiotherapy fractionation decisions. Med Phys 38:1799–1805
96. Xiao N, Kong FM, Chetty IJ, Burmeister J, Joiner M, Jin JY (2013) Toward individualized fractionation schedule for lung cancer radiation therapy. Int J Radiat Oncol Biol Phys 87(2):S542

Personalized Therapy of Non-small Cell Lung Cancer (NSCLC)

Shirish M. Gadgeel

Abstract Lung cancer remains the most common cause of cancer related deaths in both men and women in the United States and non-small cell lung cancer (NSCLC) accounts for over 85 % of all lung cancers. Survival of these patients has not significantly altered in over 30 years. This chapter initially discusses the clinical presentation of lung cancer patients. Most patients diagnosed with lung cancer due to symptoms have advanced stage cancer. Once diagnosed, lung cancer patients need imaging studies to assess the stage of the disease before decisions regarding therapy are finalized. The most important prognostic factors are stage of the disease and performance status and these factors also determine therapy. The chapter subsequently discusses management of each stage of the disease and the impact of several pathologic, clinical factors in personalizing therapy for each individual patient. Transition from chemotherapy for every patient to a more personalized approach based on histology and molecular markers has occurred in the management of advanced stage NSCLC. It is expected that such a personalized approach will extend to all stages of NSCLC and will likely improve the outcomes of all NSCLC patients.

Keywords Clinical symptoms • Staging • NSCLC • Chemotherapy • Histology • EGFR • ALK • Molecular markers

1 Introduction

Management of lung cancer, specifically NSCLC has evolved over the last 10 years from a more general and empiric approach to a more personalized approach, based on an understanding of the biological features of the patient's cancer and the clinical characteristics of the patient. This chapter discusses clinical characteristics, staging of lung cancer and particulars of a personalized approach to the management of NSCLC in deciding systemic therapy for lung cancer. Personalized approach to

S.M. Gadgeel, M.D. (✉)
Karmanos Cancer Institute, Wayne State University,
4100 John R, 4, HWCRC, Detroit, MI 48201, USA
e-mail: gadgeels@karmanos.org

A. Ahmad, S.M. Gadgeel (eds.), *Lung Cancer and Personalized Medicine: Novel Therapies and Clinical Management*, Advances in Experimental Medicine and Biology 890, DOI 10.1007/978-3-319-24932-2_11

surgical management and radiation therapy are discussed in other chapters. This chapter will discuss personalized approach to NSCLC. Another chapter is focusing on Small Cell Lung Cancer.

2 Clinical Features of Lung Cancer

The median age at presentation in the United States is around 71 years [1]. However about 10 % of the cases occur in patients below the age of 50. The incidence of lung cancer in US males is 83 per 100,000 and in US females is 55 per 100,000.

Usually patients with early stage lung cancer don't have any symptoms related to the cancer (Table 1). Lack of symptoms in early stage lung cancer patients is related to the sparse pain fiber innervation of the lungs and the significant respiratory reserve that two lungs provide. The lack of symptoms is particularly true for lung cancers that originate in the periphery of the lungs. The most common symptoms at diagnosis are cough, dyspnea, weight loss and chest pain [2, 3]. However in most patients by the time they develop symptoms the cancer has metastasized to either the regional lymph nodes or to distant sites. Approximately 5–10 % of lung cancer patients are asymptomatic at presentation [2, 4]. These cancers are often detected during evaluation for an unrelated medical problem or on a chest radiograph performed for pre-operative evaluation.

Recently a large randomized clinical trial showed that CT scan screening for lung cancer in individuals with significant smoking history reduced lung cancer related and overall mortality [5]. Based on this data it is expected that CT scan screening will become more common and this may lead to an increase in the percentage of lung cancer patients who are asymptomatic at diagnosis.

3 Staging of NSCLC

One of the most important factors in deciding management of NSCLC is stage of patient's cancer. The first step in a newly diagnosed NSCLC patient is to conduct tests to define the stage of the patient's cancer. This includes history and physical

Table 1 Symptoms at diagnosis of non-small cell lung cancer

Symptoms	Present at diagnosis (%)
Cough	45–75
Dyspnea	40–60
Weight loss	20–70
Chest pain	30–45
Hemoptysis	25–35
Bone pain	6–25
Fatigue	0–20

Table 2 Simplified staging system

Stage	Sites involved	Management
'Localized'	Tumor restricted to the lung or is associated with hilar lymph node metastases	Surgery Tumor ≥4 cm or involvement of hilar lymph nodes adjuvant chemotherapy
'Regional'	Tumor extending to mediastinum or is associated with metastases to mediastinal lymph nodes	Concurrent Chemotherapy and Radiation Therapy
		Select cases patients may be considered for surgery following concurrent therapy
'Metastatic'	Metastases to other organs including other parts of the same lung or other lung, pleura	Systemic Therapy

examination, blood tests including complete blood count and complete metabolic profile, CT scans of the chest including the upper abdomen, PET scan and a brain scan.

Staging studies are based on an understanding of the common areas of metastases with lung cancer patients. Lung cancer can metastasize to almost any area of the body but the most common sites of metastases are regional lymph nodes, other areas of the lungs, pleura, adrenal glands, brain, liver and bones. Thus the planned scans should assess these common areas of metastases.

Based on the staging studies, patients are staged from stage I to IV. From a practical point of view patients can be considered to have following three stages-cancer that is limited to the lung with or without metastases to the hilar lymph nodes (localized disease), cancer with metastases to the mediastinal lymph nodes or extension of the cancer to the mediastinum (regional disease) and cancer with distant metastases (distant disease) (Table 2). In patients with localized cancer surgical resection is the primary consideration. NSCLC patients with metastases to mediastinal lymph nodes or direct extension to mediastinal structures are generally managed with chemotherapy and radiation. Finally patients with distant metastases are managed with systemic therapy. The goals of therapy in patients with localized cancer and cancer with regional metastases is to eradicate the cancer, whereas the goals of therapy in patients with metastatic disease are to shrink and control the cancer so as to improve symptoms and prolong survival.

4 Patient Characteristics and Treatment Decisions

Many other considerations are important in deciding therapy including patient's performance status and co-morbid illnesses. A common co-morbid illness in lung cancer patients is COPD (Chronic Obstructive Pulmonary Disease) since smoking is the most common causative factor for both conditions. COPD is associated with impaired respiratory reserve and therefore can impact the ability to perform surgery or radiation. Since the median age of patients is 71 years and many patients are current or former smokers many patients have other co-morbid illnesses, including heart disease, renal failure, diabetes and related complications. All these conditions may impact the ability to deliver appropriate care for the patients.

An important consideration in deciding therapy is the performance status of the patient [6]. Performance status is determined by the treating physician and reflects the patient's activity level. Performance status has been consistently shown to have both prognostic and predictive importance. Performance status could be impaired due to the lung cancer or the co-morbid illnesses or both together. Patients with impaired performance have an inferior outcome and don't tolerate therapy very well.

Age of the patients should also be considered while deciding therapy [7]. Most trials show that older patients who have a good performance status and have adequate organ function tolerate therapy well and have outcomes as good as younger patients. However, older patients are more likely to have co-morbid illnesses and aging related loss of organ function that can impact the ability to tolerate treatments. Appropriate assessment of elderly patients is imperative before therapy is initiated in these patients.

5 Adjuvant Therapy in Early Stage NSCLC

Systemic recurrence occurs in over 50 % of patients who undergo surgery for early stage lung cancer [8]. Thus, post-operative systemic therapy in lung cancer is clinically justified. However, for almost 40 years none of the trials showed a survival advantage in favor of adjuvant chemotherapy. A meta-analysis of the initial trials, published in 1995, suggested that adjuvant cisplatin-based chemotherapy can improve survival of NSCLC patients by 5 %, though this improvement was not statistically significant [9]. In the 1990s drugs such as vinorelbine, paclitaxel and gemcitabine were introduced and evaluated for the treatment of NSCLC patients. Each of these agents when combined with cisplatin demonstrated a survival advantage in patients with advanced stage NSCLC compared to older platinum based combinations. These data spurred interest in evaluating these newer platinum based combinations as adjuvant therapy. Two trials have evaluated the combination of cisplatin and vinorelbine and both showed a survival improvement of 8–10 %. Based on these data use of adjuvant platinum based chemotherapy in patients with stage IB (tumors greater than 4 cm)–III NSCLC has become standard of care [10, 11].

The LACE meta-analysis, which included all adjuvant trials conducted after 1995 that enrolled over 300 patients and evaluated cisplatin based chemotherapy, showed a more modest benefit of 5.4 % survival improvement at 5 years [1]. The meta-analysis did suggest that the use of the combination of cisplatin and vinorelbine, led to slightly greater improvement in overall survival compared to older cisplatin based combinations.

The LACE meta-analysis showed that the benefit from adjuvant chemotherapy varies with stage. Patients with stage IA had an inferior survival with adjuvant chemotherapy (HR: 1.4, 95 % CI: 0.95–2.06) [1]. These data have to be viewed with a level of caution since the number of patients with stage IA disease in this meta-analysis was small and the 95 % confidence intervals are fairly wide. The benefit from adjuvant chemotherapy was minimal in stage IB patients (HR: 0.93, 95 % CI: 0.78–1.10) and modest in stage II and stage IIIA patients (HR: 0.83, 95 % CI: 0.72–0.95). Thus, the benefit from adjuvant chemotherapy may be proportionally greater in patients with higher stage disease. Further analysis of stage IB patients has been conducted. Retrospective analyses of two trials suggest that the benefit from adjuvant chemotherapy in stage IB patients is dependent upon the size of the tumor [10, 12]. Adjuvant chemotherapy was found to improve survival in patients with tumors ≥4 cm. However, in stage IB patients with tumors <4 cm adjuvant chemotherapy was associated with a non-significant worse survival.

The consensus that has emerged from all of these trials is that adjuvant chemotherapy is recommended for patients with tumors that have metastasized to regional lymph nodes (hilar or mediastinal) and based on retrospective analyses, to patients with large (≥4 cm) tumors.

5.1 Personalized Adjuvant Chemotherapy

The benefit rate of 5–10 % with adjuvant therapy suggests that not all patients treated with adjuvant therapy benefit from it. In addition, survival rates of at least 25 % following surgery suggest that not all patients need chemotherapy. Therefore there is a need to develop markers that can identify the patients who need adjuvant chemotherapy and the patients who are likely to benefit from adjuvant chemotherapy.

5.1.1 Prognostic Markers

Tumor stage remains one of the most important prognostic factors. The risk of relapse is higher with higher stage of lung cancer [13]. Also as mentioned earlier the benefits of adjuvant chemotherapy are higher n higher stage lung cancer. Among the clinical variables female sex and younger age ≤70 years are associated with better prognosis [13].

Various factors have been evaluated for prognostic utility. Pathologic features of high grade or poorly differentiated tumors and angio-lymphatic invasion predict for high risk of relapse [14–16]. However, it is not clear that, patients with tumors that have these features necessarily benefit from adjuvant chemotherapy.

5.1.2 Predictive Markers

Markers Predictive of Chemotherapy

Many markers that predict for benefit from adjuvant chemotherapy have been evaluated. The marker that has received the most attention is ERCC1 (Excision Repair Cross Complementation Group 1). Platinum analogues are the most commonly used drugs in the treatment of NSCLC. Platinum analogues bind to DNA and form adducts that inhibit DNA replication. Since tumor cells divide more rapidly, formation of these adducts cause cell death in these cells. The nucleotide excision repair complex can repair platinum-damaged DNA. ERCC1 is the rate limiting enzyme of this repair complex [17]. In vitro studies and clinical studies suggest that tumoral ERCC1 levels may predict for resistance to platinum analogues. Retrospective analyses of the IALT adjuvant trial suggested that benefit from cisplatin based chemotherapy was restricted to patients with tumors that had low ERCC1 levels [18]. However, assessment of this marker from tumors of patients on other enrolled trials did not confirm the predictive utility of ERCC1 [19]. Therefore this marker is currently not utilized to select patients for adjuvant cisplatin based chemotherapy. Other markers such as RRM1 (ribonucleotide reductase messenger 1) to predict sensitivity to gemcitabine and βIII tubulin expression levels to predict sensitivity to taxanes have also been evaluated without conclusive data to support the use of these markers for making decisions regarding use of these chemotherapy agents as adjuvant therapy [20].

Genetic Markers

An important advance in oncology has been the identification of 'driver' genetic alterations. Targeting these genetic alterations has led to significant clinical benefit primarily in patients with advanced cancer. Very few examples of utilizing these agents targeting 'driver' genetic alterations as adjuvant therapy exist to date in oncology. Adjuvant trastuzumab has demonstrated improved survival in patients with Her2 positive breast cancer. Also imatinib mesylate has shown similar survival advantage in patients with GIST (gastro-intestinal stromal tumor).

EGFR (epidermal growth factor receptor) mutations were the first 'driver' genetic alteration identified in NSCLC. EGFR-TKIs have been evaluated as adjuvant therapy in NSCLC. These clinical trials have established that EGFR-TKIs are not beneficial as adjuvant therapy in unselected NSCLC patients [21, 22]. However, conclusive data regarding the utility of these drugs in EGFR mutation positive NSCLC patients as adjuvant therapy is not available as yet. Recently the results of the RADIANT trial were presented. In this study about 1000 NSCLC patients were randomized to erlotinib or placebo for 2 years following surgery and adjuvant chemotherapy. Of the patients enrolled, 161 patients had EGFR mutation positive NSCLC. In this sub group erlotinib did improve the progression free survival with a hazard ratio of 0.61 but this did not reach statistical significance [22]. Data on overall survival from this study is still not available. In this study only about 50 % of the patients received erlotinib for the planned 24 months, suggesting that a higher proportion of patients receiving the drug for a longer period may lead to an even greater benefit.

Similar data is lacking for other genetic alterations such as ALK gene rearrangement. The National Cancer Institute in collaboration with the co-operative groups is about to launch a clinical trial called the ALCHEMIST. In this trial over

8000 patients will be enrolled. Patients with EGFR mutation positive NSCLC will be randomized to erlotinib or placebo whereas patients with ALK positive NSCLC will be randomized to crizotinib or placebo following surgery and adjuvant chemotherapy, if required. A prospective study focused on patients with tumors that have the specific genetic alterations will establish the utility of these agents as adjuvant therapy.

Genomic Analyses

Lung cancer, like any cancer is the result of the genetic alterations that impact the phenotype and biologic behavior of the tumor tissue. Therefore, there is significant interest in developing markers based on genomic analyses that have prognostic and predictive utility. This strategy is now routinely being applied in the management of breast cancer. Various groups of investigators have developed genomic signatures as prognostic and/or predictive markers [23, 24]. However, none of these signatures to date have shown clinical utility in prospective trials limiting the clinical applicability of these markers.

6 Management of Locally Advanced Non-small Cell Lung Cancer (Stage III)

Patients are considered to have locally advanced NSCLC when the tumor has invaded the mediastinum or the tumor has metastasized to mediastinal lymph nodes. The principle that guides therapy in this clinical situation is that patients already have systemic micro-metastases. Thus the goal of therapy is not only to treat the clinically evident disease but also to treat systemic metastases that are too small to be detected on staging scans.

These patients are generally treated with concurrent chemotherapy and radiation [25]. The chemotherapy is supposed to treat the systemic micro-metastases and the radiation therapy targets the cancer in the chest. The two treatment modalities are administered together since there is data to suggest that chemotherapy sensitizes the tumor to the effects of radiation. The two commonly used chemotherapy regimens when administered with radiation are cisplatin and etoposide or carboplatin and paclitaxel administered on a weekly basis. Radiation therapy is generally administered to 60 Gy over about 6–7 weeks.

Concurrent therapy is associated with higher rates of toxicities, particularly esophagitis, compared to sequential therapy. Therefore, not all patients are candidates for such concurrent therapy. Appropriate selection of patients based on performance status, presence of co-morbidities, particularly lung function is crucial. The median survival with concurrent therapy in locally advanced NSCLC is 20–25 months, with a 5 year survival of about 25 %. Attempts to improve these outcomes with addition of targeted agents or delivering further chemotherapy following completion of concurrent therapy have not been successful [25].

Surgical resection of the tumor following concurrent chemotherapy and radiation has been evaluated in patients with locally advanced NSCLC [26]. Randomized trials have not conclusively shown that surgery in this clinical situation is beneficial. These trials have shown that patients who require a pneumonectomy following concurrent chemotherapy and radiation have a higher rate of mortality and it is possible that this higher rate of mortality may have precluded trials from demonstrating a benefit from surgery. Based on the available data the consensus is that patients who require only a lobectomy may benefit from surgery following concurrent chemotherapy and radiation [27]. Surgery following chemotherapy and radiation is performed only in select patients after a thorough assessment by a multi-disciplinary team with experience in management of such patients.

The predictive and prognostic markers relevant in adjuvant therapy also have relevance in patients with locally advanced NSCLC. It is expected that clinical trials in the future will show benefits of integrating targeted therapy such as EGFR-TKIs in patients with genetically defined tumors.

7 Management of Advanced Non-small Cell Lung Cancer

In recent years major advances in lung cancer have occurred primarily in the management of advanced NSCLC. The treatment paradigm has shifted from using platinum based two drug combination to a treatment paradigm that tailors therapy based on histology and molecular markers (Fig. 1).

7.1 Chemotherapy

For many years the standard therapy for advanced NSCLC was platinum based two drug combinations. Such chemotherapy regimens not only prolonged survival but also improved quality of life. The efficacy of each of these combinations was the same in each of the histologic subtypes of NSCLC. Pemetrexed is the first chemotherapy that has differential efficacy in patients with squamous cell lung cancer and in patients with non-squamous histology. In a randomized trial the combination of cisplatin and pemetrexed demonstrated superior survival to the combination of cisplatin and gemcitabine in patients with advanced non-squamous tumors whereas the reverse was true in patients with squamous cell tumors (Treatment by histology interaction analysis $p=0.0011$) [28]. The precise reason for this difference is unclear but maybe related to higher levels of thymidylate synthase, the enzyme targeted by pemetrexed, in squamous cell lung cancers compared to non-squamous tumors [29]. Based on these data pemetrexed now is only approved for patients with non-squamous cell lung cancers. It is therefore imperative that every effort is made to define the histologic subtype of NSCLC, specifically obtaining sufficient tumor material during diagnostic biopsies.

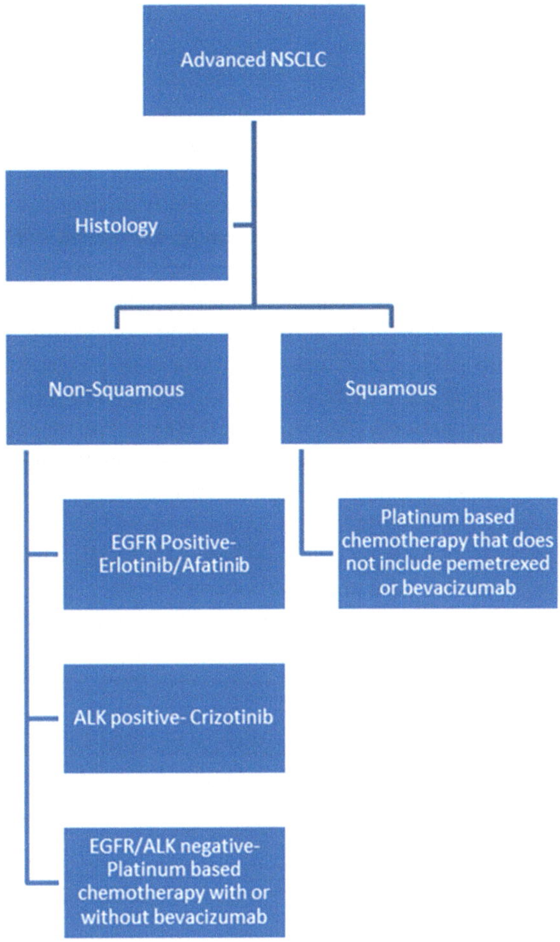

Fig. 1 Management of advanced non-small cell lung cancer

Another important aspect of chemotherapy is the survival advantage observed with maintenance therapy. For many years the standard of care was to deliver chemotherapy for 4–6 cycles. Over the last few years two drugs have been approved for maintenance therapy. In two separate randomized trials maintenance therapy with pemetrexed demonstrated a survival advantage. In the first trial Ciuleanu et al. randomized patients who had completed 4 cycles of a platinum based doublet chemotherapy and had stable or responding NSCLC to placebo or pemetrexed [30]. In non-squamous NSCLC patients the median survival in patients who received pemetrexed was 15.5 months versus 10.3 months (HR: 0.7, $p=0.002$). Similar survival advantage was not observed in squamous cell patients. Thus these results show that switching to maintenance pemetrexed therapy following completion of 4 cycles of platinum based doublet chemotherapy provides survival advantage.

In the Paramount trial Paez-Ares et al. enrolled 939 patients with advanced non-squamous NSCLC who were treated with 4 cycles of cisplatin and pemetrexed [31]. Subsequently 539 patients who had stable or responding disease and were eligible for maintenance portion of the trial were randomized to pemetrexed or placebo. The median survival with pemetrexed was 13.9 months and with placebo was 11 months (HR: 0.78, p=0.0195). Based on this data maintenance pemetrexed following a platinum and pemetrexed combination is accepted as standard therapy.

Erlotinib, the epidermal growth factor receptor (EGFR) tyrosine kinase inhibitor was also evaluated in advanced NSCLC patients as maintenance therapy [32]. Of the 1949 patients enrolled in the run in phase consisting of 4 cycles of chemotherapy, 889 patients with stable and responding cancers were randomized to erlotinib or placebo. Erlotinib improved progression free survival (PFS), the primary end point of the study, with a median PFS of 12.3 weeks versus 11.1 weeks in placebo patients (HE: 0.71, p<0.0001). The median survival was also improved (12 months versus 11 months, HR: 0.81, p=0.0088). These results have led to the approval of erlotinib as maintenance therapy. In subset analyses the benefit in patients with EGFR mutation positive NSCLC was greater (HR: 0.10, p<0.0001) compared to patients with wild type EGFR (HR: 0.78, p=0.0185), though this data has to be viewed with a level of caution since the total number of patients known to have EGFR mutations was only 49. In another subset analysis the relative benefit with erlotinib in squamous cell patients was modest. The PFS benefit in squamous cell patients was 0.76 (0.60–0.95) and the overall survival benefit was 0.86 (0.68–1.10).

Due to the greater acceptance of pemetrexed in non-squamous patients and due to the limited benefit of erlotinib in squamous cell patients use of erlotinib in the first line setting appears to be restricted to EGFR mutation positive NSCLC patients.

7.2 *Bevacizumab*

An important aspect of most cancer is the ability to induce angiogenesis. A major mediator of tumor angiogenesis is VEGF (vascular endothelial growth factor). Bevacizumab targets VEGF and in pre-clinical models inhibits tumor angiogenesis. In an exploratory study the addition of bevacizumab to chemotherapy demonstrated promising efficacy [33]. However, in the same study patients with squamous cell histology had increased rates of hemoptysis including fatal episodes. In the subsequent randomized phase III trial eligibility was restricted to patients with advanced non-squamous NSCLC [34]. In this trial bevacizumab in combination with carboplatin and paclitaxel demonstrated superior survival to carboplatin and paclitaxel alone (Median survival 12.3 months versus 10.3 months, Hazard ratio 0.79, p=0.003). Similar improvement in survival was not observed when bevacizumab was combined with cisplatin and gemcitabine, though the primary end point of this trial was progression free survival [35]. It is possible that addition of bevacizumab may improve outcomes only with specific chemotherapy combinations.

The POINTBREAK trial compared the combination of carboplatin, pemetrexed and bevacizumab to the combination of carboplatin, paclitaxel and bevacizumab, with the primary objective of demonstrating superior survival with the pemetrexed based combination in patients with advanced non-squamous NSCLC [36]. The study failed to show superior survival with the pemetrexed combination, though the progression free survival was superior with this combination.

Bevacizumab is associated with specific adverse events such as increased risk of bleeding, including hemoptysis and increased arterial thrombotic events such as myocardial infarction and cerebro-vascular accident. Therefore assessment of patients before initiating therapy with bevacizumab is very crucial.

7.3 Targeted Therapy Based on Genetic Alterations (Table 3)

An important consideration in initiating systemic therapy for advanced NSCLC is the assessment of 'driver' genetic alterations. The two genetic alterations for which we have data in the front line setting are EGFR mutations and ALK gene rearrangement. Clinical data regarding both these genetic alterations are discussed in other chapters in this book. Other genetic alterations for which clinical data exists will be discussed here.

Table 3 Driver genetic alterations other than EGFR and ALK

Gene/pathway	Smoking status	Histology	Genetic alteration
Kras	Primarily smokers	Predominantly adenocarcinomas	Kras mutations
ROS1	Primarily never smokers	Predominantly adenocarcinomas	ROS1 translocations
RET	Primarily never smokers	Predominantly adenocarcinomas	RET translocations
Her2	Primarily never smokers	Predominantly adenocarcinomas	Her2 mutations, Her2 amplification
Braf	Primarily smokers	Adenocarcinomas/ squamous cell carcinomas	Braf mutations
cMET	N/A	Adenocarcinomas/ squamous cell carcinomas	cMET overexpression, amplification and mutation
PI3K pathway	More in smokers	Squamous cell carcinomans/ adenocarcinomas	PTEN loss
			PI3K amplification
			PI3K mutations
			AKT mutations
FGFR1	Primarily smokers	Predominantly squamous cell carcinomas	FGFR1 amplification

7.3.1 Kras Mutations

Mutations in the Kras gene were identified in NSCLCs over 25 years ago [37]. Approximately 20 % of NSCLCs have Kras mutations [38]. Kras mutations occur more commonly in smokers than never smokers and occur much more commonly in adenocarcinomas than in squamous cell cancers. In addition the rate of these mutations is lower in Asian NSCLC patients compared to North American patients.

The protein encoded by the Kras gene functions as a guanosine diphosphate (GDP)/guanosine triphosphate (GTP) regulated on-off switch that can activate downstream signaling proteins [27]. Mutated Ras encodes for a protein that is insensitive to GTPase and therefore constantly bound to GTP and active. In NSCLC Kras mutations are restricted to codons 12 and 13. There are a variety of substitutions that can occur at these codons which result in mutated Kras.

Previous analyses suggested that presence of Kras mutations has a prognostic relevance but the data is inconsistent [39, 40]. This may be a result of different biologic behavior of the different Kras mutations; i.e., codon 12, 13, as well as different type of base substitutions encountered in these codons. In addition, some studies suggest that Kras mutations may predict for resistance to chemotherapy and EGFR-TKIs. Data in colon cancer also suggests that response to certain treatments may differ based on the type of Kras mutations [41].

Direct inhibition of Kras for therapeutic benefit has remained elusive. An alternative approach is to inhibit the downstream signaling proteins to effectively inhibit Kras signaling and thus its oncogenic consequences. Raf1 was the first effector protein of Ras to be identified. Raf1 signals through a pathway that involves the ERK-MEK signaling cascade [37]. The ERK-MEK signaling pathway is the primary mediator of the oncogenic effects of Ras mutations. Novel MEK inhibitors are in clinical trials and have been evaluated in NSCLC. The single agent activity of these drugs has been modest. Recently Janne et al. reported the results of a randomized phase II study that evaluated the addition of selumetinib (AZD6244), a MEK inhibitor, to docetaxel in patients with Kras mutation positive progressive NSCLC [42]. The addition of AZD6244 led to improved progression free survival (5.3 months vs. 2.1 month, $p=0.0138$) and response rate (37.2 % vs. 0 %, $p<0.0001$). The percentage of patients that were alive and progression free at 6 months was also superior in patients who received the combination, 37.1 %, compared to the patients who received docetaxel alone, 15.8 % ($p=0.0158$). The overall survival was numerically superior with the addition of AZD6244 (9.4 months vs. 5.2 months) but this did not reach statistical significance ($p=0.2069$). Data according to individual Kras mutations has not been reported and it is not clear if this combination will have differential efficacy in the different mutations. Adverse events were also higher among patients who received the combination of AZD6244 with docetaxel, primarily neutropenia, asthenia, diarrhea, edema, rashes and stomatitis. Based on the promising randomized phase II results there are plans to conduct a randomized phase III study to evaluate this combination in Kras mutation positive NSCLC patients.

Many other strategies are being evaluated to inhibit Kras in Kras mutation positive NSCLC including combination of MEK inhibitor with AKT inhibitor and hsp90 (heat shock protein 90) as discussed later. Ongoing clinical trials will define which of these strategies will lead to clinical benefit.

7.3.2 ROS1

ROS1 is a receptor tyrosine kinase (RTK), is related to the insulin receptor family and shares significant homology with ALK [43–45]. ROS1 can activate downstream signaling pathways such as PI3K, ERK/MEK and stat3 that result in increased cellular proliferation, invasion, and anti-apoptotic effects. ROS1 is detectable in many tissues including lung and skeletal muscle but its function is not clear. Recently ROS1 activation through gene rearrangements has been documented in NSCLC [39, 40]. ROS1 gene rearrangements form a chimeric protein which includes the tyrosine kinase domain of ROS1. The ROS1 tyrosine kinase in the chimeric protein is constitutively activated and oncogenic. There are many partner genes with which ROS1 can be rearranged in NSCLC. The rate of ROS1 gene rearrangements in NSCLC is about 2 % [46, 47]. It appears that clinical demographics and pathologic features of patients with ROS1 gene rearrangement are similar to ALK positive patients. Thus, they are younger, never smokers and predominantly have adenocarcinoma histology.

Since there is some homology between ROS1 and ALK, particularly in tyrosine kinase region, the ability of crizotinib to inhibit ROS1 was evaluated [41]. Ou et al. presented the results of 35 evaluable patients with ROS1 rearranged NSCLC treated with crizotinib [48]. The response rate was 60 % in these patients from crizotinib, activity that is similar to the drug's activity in ALK positive NSCLC patient. These results suggest that crizotinib is the preferred treatment in patients with ROS1 rearranged NSCLC.

7.3.3 MEt alterations

MET is a transmembrane tyrosine kinase receptor which is activated by its ligand Hepatocyte Growth Factor (HGF). Activated MET is involved in variety of cellular functions including motility, survival and proliferation [49]. Over expression of MET and HGF are well documented in NSCLC and is associated with worse prognosis [50]. In addition MET mutations and amplification occur in NSCLC [51, 52]. The oncogenic relevance of MET mutations in lung cancer is unclear. Recent data has shown that MET amplification is one of the mechanisms of resistance to EGFR-TKIs in EGFR mutation positive NSCLC [53, 54]. In addition, MET maybe amplified in about 7 % of NSCLCs.

Pre-clinical data has shown that the combination of a MET inhibitor and EGFR inhibitor provide greater anti-tumor efficacy than either agent alone [55, 56].

Two different randomized trials have evaluated met inhibitors in combination with erlotinib in patients with recurrent NSCLC. In one of the trials MetMAB, a humanized antibody targeting MET was evaluated in a randomized phase III study that enrolled 499 patients with progressive NSCLC following 1 or 2 prior treatments [57]. Patients were randomized to erlotinib alone or erlotinib with MetMAB. Based on a prior randomized phase II study results, only patients with tumors that were considered MET positive (at least 50 % of the tumor cells were moderately or strongly positive by IHC testing) were enrolled on the study. The study failed to show a survival advantage with the addition of metMAB to erlotinib.

Tivantinib is an oral MET tyrosine kinase inhibitor that has been evaluated in NSCLC patients [58]. In a phase II trial 167 patients were randomly assigned to the combination of erlotinib (150 mg daily) and tivantinib (360 mg twice daily) or to erlotinib alone. The proportional hazards model adjusting for known prognostic factors showed a hazard ratio of 0.68 in favor of the combination ($p=0.04$). There was no significant difference in overall survival between the 2 arms. A pre-planned analysis of efficacy according to histology showed that in non-squamous patients the combination resulted in significantly improved PFS and OS after adjusting for prognostic factors. These data were the basis for a phase III study evaluating the combination of tivantinib and erlotinib compared to erlotinib alone in patients with progressive non-squamous NSCLC. According to a recent press release this study has been discontinued after an interim analysis concluded that the study would not reach its primary end point of improved survival. Detailed results of the study are awaited.

Finally crizotinib which is also known to be a cMET inhibitor has been evaluated in MET positive NSCLC patients. Results of a small study were presented by Dr. Camidge and colleagues recently [59]. Tumors of patients were analyzed for MET amplification. Only patients with ratio of MET gene copy number to the number of centromere of chromosome 7 of ≥1.8 were enrolled on the trial. Patients were considered to have low (ratio of ≥1.8–≤2.2), intermediate (ratio of >2.2–<5.0) or high (≥5.0 copies) amplification in their tumors based on the ratios. Fourteen patients have been enrolled on the trial. Majority of these patients were current or former smokers. Among these 14 patients benefit from crizotinib was higher in patients with higher amplification of MET. The response rate in low amplified tumors was 0/2, in intermediate amplified 1/6 and in high amplified 4/6. The true rate of MET amplification or high MET amplification is unclear. Further study of the efficacy of MET inhibitors like crizotinib in patients with MET amplified tumors is required. However available data suggests that assessment of gene amplification maybe a better bio-marker to identify patients who respond to MET inhibitors compared to detection by immuno-histochemistry.

There are other MET inhibitors in development including cabozantinib, which has shown clinical activity in NSCLC patients in a single arm phase II trial, and foretinib [60]. Since MET amplification maybe a mechanism of acquired resistance to EGFR-TKIs in EGFR mutation positive NSCLC there is a significant interest in evaluating MET inhibitors in this patient population. Ongoing trials will determine the role of these drugs in the management of NSCLC patients in general and in patients with activation of the cMET pathway in their tumors.

RET translocations—RET is a receptor tyrosine kinase that is an established oncogenic target in medullary thyroid cancer and papillary thyroid cancers [61, 62]. Recently RET gene rearrangements leading to activation of the RET tyrosine kinase were identified in NSCLCs [46, 63]. The most common partner gene is the KIF5B with variable break points. An alternative partner gene CCDC6 has also been identified. The incidence of these rearrangements is rare, probably <1 % and appears to occur primarily in adenocarcinomas. There are many RET inhibitors currently approved for other tumor types such as cabozantinib, sunitinib, sorafenib. Recently Drilon et al. reported that cabozantinib, a known RET inhibitor approved for medullary thyroid carcinoma, demonstrated response in 2 RET positive NSCLC patients and stable disease in a third patient [64]. This study is ongoing and similar studies will define the activity of RET inhibitors in RET positive NSCLC patients.

Her2 gene alterations—Her 2 mutations that cause constitutive activation of Her2 tyrosine kinase were identified in about 2 % of NSCLC [65, 66]. They primarily occur in adenocarcinomas, never smokers and in female patients. Mazieres et al. reported a 50 % response rate and a disease control rate of 82 % in 16 patients treated with Her2 directed therapy [65]. Her2 amplification has also been reported to occur in 2–20 % of NSCLCs and there is at least one case report of clinical benefit from Her2 inhibitors in a patient with Her2 amplified NSCLC [67, 68]. Further data is necessary to define the role of Her2 inhibitors in patients with tumors that have Her2 mutations or amplification.

Braf mutations—Braf is a kinase downstream of Kras. Braf mutation occurs in about 50 % of melanomas and almost all the Braf mutations in melanoma are the V600E mutation in exon 15 of the gene [69]. Braf inhibitors have shown clinical benefit in melanoma patients with this mutation in their tumor [70]. Braf mutation occur in about 3–5 % of adenocarcinomas of the lung and <1 % of sqaumous cell carcinomas [71–73]. About 50 % of the Braf mutations detected in NSCLCs are V600E. Braf mutations occur more commonly in patients who are current or former smokers. At least one report suggests that the V600E mutation occurs more commonly in females and another reports states that Braf mutations occur more commonly in men [72, 73]. Dabrafenib a Braf inhibitor has shown activity in NSCLC patients with Braf V600E mutation positive tumors [74]. There are ongoing trials evaluating Braf inhibitors and MEK inhibitors in patients with Braf mutation positive NSCLC.

FGFR1 (fibroblast growth factor receptor) amplification—FGFR1 belongs to the FGFR family of membrane bound receptors and is involved in inflammation, wound healing and embryonic development. Weiss et al. first reported that this gene is amplified in sqaumous cell lung cancers and that this genetic alteration is oncogenic in these tumors [75]. The rate of FGFR1 amplification reported by various groups has varied from 7 to 20 % depending upon the test utilized to assess amplification [76–78]. FGFR1 amplification may occur also in adenocarcinomas but at a lower rate.

Pre-clinical studies have shown that FGFR inhibitors can induce apoptosis in NSCLC cell lines with FGFR1 amplification. Recently data on two separate FGFR inhibitors were presented at the annual meeting of the American Society of Clinical Oncology. BJ398 demonstrated a response rate of 15 % and another 35 % had stable disease among 26 squamous cell patients with FGFR1 amplified tumors [79]. Another FGFR inhibitor AZD4547 demonstrated response in 1 of 13 patients [80]. The activity observed with these drugs in limited number of patients is relatively modest compared to activity observed with targeted drugs in most other lung cancers with 'actionable' mutations. The reasons for this modest activity are unclear. It could be related to inability to identify the tumors that are truly dependent on this pathway.

8 Conclusion

Management of NSCLC has shifted from approaching it as a single disease to an entity consisting of several related disorders that are managed differently, taking into account histologic, molecular, and clinical characteristics.

References

1. http://www.cancer.org/research/cancerfactsstatistics/cancerfactsfigures2014/. Accessed 15 Sept 2014
2. Chute CG, Greenberg ER, Baron J et al (1985) Presenting conditions of 1539 population-based lung cancer patients by cell type and stage in New Hampshire and Vermont. Cancer 56: 2107–11
3. Koyi H, Hillerdal G, Brandén E (2002) A prospective study of a total material of lung cancer from a county in Sweden 1997–1999: gender, symptoms, type, stage, and smoking habits. Lung Cancer 36:9–14
4. Buccheri G, Ferrigno D (2004) Lung cancer: clinical presentation and specialist referral time. Eur Respir J 24:898
5. The National Lung Screening Trial Research Team (2011) Reduced lung-cancer mortality with low-dose computed tomographic screening. N Engl J Med 365:395–409
6. Langer C, Lilenbaum R (2004) Role of chemotherapy in patients with poor performance status and advanced non-small cell lung cancer. Semin Oncol 31(suppl 6):8–15
7. Aggarwal C, Langer CJ (2012) Older age, poor performance status and major comorbidities: how to treat high-risk patients with advanced nonsmall cell lung cancer. Curr Opin Oncol 24:130–6
8. Mountain CF (1997) Revisions in the international system for staging lung cancer. Chest 111:1710–1717
9. Non-small Cell Lung Cancer Collaborative Group (1995) Chemotherapy in non-small cell lung cancer: a meta-analysis using updated data on individual patients from 52 randomized clinical trials. BMJ 311:899–909
10. Butts CA, Ding K, Seymour L et al (2010) Randomized phase III trial of vinorelbine plus cisplatin compared with observation in completely resected stage IB and II non-small-cell lung cancer: updated survival analysis of JBR-10. J Clin Oncol 28:29–34

11. Douillard JY, Rosell R, De Lena M et al (2006) Adjuvant vinorelbine plus cisplatin versus observation in patients with completely resected stage IB–IIIA non-small cell lung cancer (Adjuvant Navelbine International Trialist Association [ANITA]): a randomised controlled trial. Lancet Oncology 7:719–727
12. Strauss GM, Herndon JE, Maddaus MA et al (2008) Adjuvant paclitaxel plus carboplatin compared with observation in stage IB non–small-cell lung cancer: CALGB 9633 with the Cancer and Leukemia Group B, Radiation Therapy Oncology Group, and North Central Cancer Treatment Group Study Groups. J Clin Oncol 26:5043–5051
13. Chansky K, Sculier JP, Crowley JJ et al (2009) The International Association for the Study of Lung Cancer Staging Project: prognostic factors and pathologic TNM stage in surgically managed non-small cell lung cancer. J Thorac Oncol 4(7):792–801
14. Fibla JJ, Cassivi SD, Brunelli A et al (2012) Re-evaluation of the prognostic value of visceral pleura invasion in stage IB non-small cell lung cancer using the prospective multicenter ACOSOG Z0030 trial data set. Lung Cancer 78(3):259–262
15. Schuchert MJ, Schumacher L, Kilic A et al (2011) Impact of angiolymphatic and pleural invasion on surgical outcomes for stage I non-small cell lung cancer. Ann Thorac Surg 91(4):1059–1065
16. Kato T, Ishikawa K, Aragaki M et al (2012) Angiolymphatic invasion exerts a strong impact on surgical outcomes for stage I lung adenocarcinoma, but not non-adenocarcinoma. Lung Cancer 77(2):394–400
17. Reed E (1998) Platinum-DNA adduct, nucleotide excision repair and platinum based anticancer chemotherapy. Cancer Treat Rev 24(5):331–344
18. Olaussen KA, Dunant A, Fouret P et al (2006) DNA repair by ERCC1 in non-small-cell lung cancer and cisplatin-based adjuvant chemotherapy. N Engl J Med 355(10):983–991
19. Friboulet L, Olaussen KA, Pignon JP et al (2013) ERCC1 isoform expression and DNA repair in non-small-cell lung cancer. N Engl J Med 368:1101–10
20. Gadgeel SM, Bepler G (2013) Prognostic and predictive markers for personalized adjuvant therapy for non-small-cell lung cancer patients. Future Oncol 9:1909–21
21. Goss GD, O'Callaghan C, Lorimer I et al (2013) Gefitinib versus placebo in completely resected non-small-cell lung cancer: results of the NCIC CTG BR19 study. J Clin Oncol 31:3320–6
22. Kelly K, Altorki N, Eberhart E et al (2014) A randomized, double-blind phase 3 trial of adjuvant erlotinib (E) versus placebo (P) following complete tumor resection with or without adjuvant chemotherapy in patients (pts) with stage IB-IIIA EGFR positive (IHC/FISH) non-small cell lung cancer (NSCLC): RADIANT results. J Clin Oncol 32: abstract 7501
23. Chen HY, Yu SL, Chen CH et al (2007) A five-gene signature and clinical outcome in non-small-cell lung cancer. N Engl J Med 356(1):11–20
24. Kratz JR, He J, Van Den Eeden SK et al (2012) A practical molecular assay to predict survival in resected non-squamous, non-small-cell lung cancer: development and international validation studies. Lancet 379(9818):823–832
25. Scarpaci A, Mitra P, Jarrar D et al (2013) Multimodality approach to management of stage III non-small cell lung cancer. Surg Oncol Clin N Am 22:319–28
26. Donington JS, Pass HI (2013) Surgical approach to locally advanced non-small cell lung cancer. Cancer J 19:217–21
27. Albain KS, Swann RS, Rusch VW et al (2009) Radiotherapy plus chemotherapy with or without surgical resection for stage III non-small-cell lung cancer: a phase III randomised controlled trial. Lancet 374:379–86
28. Scagliotti GV, Parikh P, von Pawel J et al (2008) Phase III study comparing cisplatin plus gemcitabine with cisplatin plus pemetrexed in chemotherapy-naive patients with advanced-stage non-small-cell lung cancer. J Clin Oncol 26:3543–51
29. Ceppi P, Volante M, Saviozzi S et al (2006) Squamous cell carcinoma of the lung compared with other histotypes shows higher messenger RNA and protein levels for thymidylate synthase. Cancer 107:1589–96
30. Ciuleanu T, Brodowicz T, Zielinski C et al (2009) Maintenance pemetrexed plus best supportive care versus placebo plus best supportive care for non-small-cell lung cancer: a randomised, double-blind, phase 3 study. Lancet 374:1432–40

31. Paz-Ares LG, de Marinis F, Dediu M et al (2013) PARAMOUNT: Final overall survival results of the phase III study of maintenance pemetrexed versus placebo immediately after induction treatment with pemetrexed plus cisplatin for advanced nonsquamous non-small-cell lung cancer. J Clin Oncol 31:2895–902
32. Cappuzzo F, Ciuleanu T, Stelmakh L et al (2010) Erlotinib as maintenance treatment in advanced non-small-cell lung cancer: a multicentre, randomised, placebo-controlled phase 3 study. Lancet Oncol 11:521–9
33. Johnson DH, Fehrenbacher L, Novotny WF et al (2004) Randomized phase II trial comparing bevacizumab plus carboplatin and paclitaxel with carboplatin and paclitaxel alone in previously untreated locally advanced or metastatic non-small-cell lung cancer. J Clin Oncol 22:2184–91
34. Sandler A, Gray R, Perry MC et al (2006) Paclitaxel-carboplatin alone or with bevacizumab for non-small-cell lung cancer. N Engl J Med 355:2542–50
35. Reck M, von Pawel J, Zatloukal P et al (2010) Overall survival with cisplatin-gemcitabine and bevacizumab or placebo as first-line therapy for nonsquamous non-small-cell lung cancer: results from a randomised phase III trial (AVAiL). Ann Oncol 21:1804–9
36. Patel JD, Socinski MA, Garon EB et al (2013) PointBreak: A randomized phase III study of pemetrexed plus carboplatin and bevacizumab followed by maintenance pemetrexed and bevacizumab versus paclitaxel plus carboplatin and bevacizumab followed by maintenance bevacizumab in patients with stage IIIB or IV nonsquamous non-small-cell lung cancer. J Clin Oncol 31:4349–57
37. Santos E, Martin-Zanca D, Reddy EP et al (1984) Malignant activation of a K-ras oncogene in lung carcinoma but not in normal tissue of the same patient. Science 223:661–4
38. Karnoub AE, Weinberg RA (2008) Ras oncogenes: split personalities. Nat Rev Mol Cell Biol 9:517–31
39. Mascaux C, Iannino N, Martin B et al (2005) The role of RAS oncogene in survival of patients with lung cancer: a systematic review of the literature with meta-analysis. Br J Cancer 92(1):131–139
40. Shepherd FA, Bourredjem A, Brambilla E et al (2012) Prognostic and predictive effects of KRAS mutation subtype in completely resected non-small cell lung cancer (NSCLC): A LACE-bio study. ASCO Meeting Abstracts; 30(15 suppl):7007
41. Tejpar S, Celik I, Schlichting M et al (2012) Association of KRAS G13D tumor mutations with outcome in patients with metastatic colorectal cancer treated with first-line chemotherapy with or without cetuximab. J Clin Oncol 30(29):3570–3577
42. Janne PA, Shaw AT, Pereira J et al (2013) Selumetinib plus docetaxel for KRAS-mutant advanced non-small-cell lung cancer: a randomised, multicentre, placebo-controlled, phase 2 study. Lancet Oncol 14:38–47
43. Nagarajan L, Louie E, Tsujimoto Y et al (1986) The human c-ros gene (ROS) is located at chromosome region 6q16----6q22. Proc Natl Acad Sci U S A 83:6568–72
44. Manning G, Whyte DB, Martinez R et al (2002) The protein kinase complement of the human genome. Science 298:1912–34
45. Acquaviva J, Wong R, Charest A (2009) The multifaceted roles of the receptor tyrosine kinase ROS in development and cancer. Biochim Biophys Acta 1795:37–52
46. Takeuchi K, Soda M, Togashi Y et al (2012) RET, ROS1 and ALK fusions in lung cancer. Nat Med 18:378–81
47. Bergethon A, Shaw AT, Ou SH et al (2012) ROS1 rearrangements define a unique molecular class of lung cancers. J Clin Oncol 30:863–70
48. Shaw AT, Camidge DR, Engelman JR et al (2012) Clinical activity of crizotinib in advanced non-small cell lung cancer (NSCLC) harboring ROS1 gene rearrangement. J Clin Oncol 30: abstract 7508
49. Gherardi E, Birchmeier W, Birchmeier C et al (2012) Targeting MET in cancer: rationale and progress. Nat Rev Cancer 12:89–103
50. Park S, Choi YL, Sung CO et al (2012) High MET copy number and MET overexpression: poor outcome in non-small cell lung cancer patients. Histol Histopathol 27:197–207

51. Ma PC, Jagadeeswaran R, Jagadeesh S et al (2005) Functional expression and mutations of c-Met and its therapeutic inhibition with SU11274 and small interfering RNA in non–small cell lung cancer. Cancer Res 65:1479–88
52. Cappuzzo F, Marchetti A, Skokan M et al (2009) Increased MET gene copy number negatively affects survival of surgically resected non–small-cell lung cancer patients. J Clin Oncol 27:1667–74
53. Engelman JA, Zejnullahu K, Mitsudomi T et al (2007) MET amplification leads to gefitinib resistance in lung cancer by activating ERBB3 signaling. Science 316:1039–43
54. Turke AB, Zejnullahu K, Wu YL et al (2010) Preexistence and clonal selection of MET amplification in EGFR mutant NSCLC. Cancer Cell 17:77–88
55. Zhang YW, Staal B, Essenburg C et al (2010) MET kinase inhibitor SGX523 synergizes with epidermal growth factor receptor inhibitor erlotinib in a hepatocyte growth factor–dependent fashion to suppress carcinoma growth. Cancer Res 70:6880–90
56. Liu L, Shi H, Liu Y et al (2011) Synergistic effects of foretinib with HER-targeted agents in MET and HER1- or HER2-coactivated tumor cells. Mol Cancer Ther 10:518–30
57. Spigel DR, Edelman MJ, O'Byrne K et al (2014) Onartuzumab plus erlotinib versus erlotinib in previously treated stage IIIb or IV NSCLC: Results from the pivotal phase III randomized, multicenter, placebo-controlled METLung (OAM4971g) global trial. J Clin Oncol 32: abstract 8000
58. Sequist LV, von Pawel J, Garmey EG et al (2011) Randomized phase II study of erlotinib plus tivantinib versus erlotinib plus placebo in previously treated non-small-cell lung cancer. J Clin Oncol 29:3307–15
59. Camidge DR, Ou, SH, Shapiro G et al (2014) Efficacy and safety of crizotinib in patients with advanced *c-MET*-amplified non-small cell lung cancer (NSCLC). J Clin Oncol 32: abstract 8001
60. Gordon MS, Vogelzang NJ, Schoffski P et al (2011) Activity of cabozantinib (XL184) in soft tissue and bone: Results of a phase II randomized phase II discontinuation trial in patients with advanced solid tumors. J Clin Oncol 29: abstract 3010
61. Alberti L, Carniti C, Miranda C, Roccato E, Pierotti MA (2003) RET and NTRK1 protooncogenes in human diseases. J Cell Physiol 195:168–86
62. Bongarzone I, Vigneri P, Mariani L, Collini P, Pilotti S, Pierotti MA (1998) RET/NTRK1 rearrangements in thyroid gland tumors of the papillary carcinoma family: correlation with clinicopathological features. Clin Cancer Res 4:223–8
63. Ju YS, Lee WC, Shin JY, Lee S, Bleazard T, Won JK et al (2012) A transforming KIF5B and RET gene fusion in lung adenocarcinoma revealed from whole-genome and transcriptome sequencing. Genome Res 22:436–45
64. Drilon A, Wang L, Hasanovic A et al (2013) Response to cabozantinib in patients with RET fusion-positive lung adenocarcinomas. Cancer Discov 3:630–5
65. Mazieres J, Peters S, Lepage B et al (2013) Lung cancer that harbors a HER2 mutation: epidemiologic characteristics and therapeutic perspectives. J Clin Oncol 31:1997–2003
66. Arcila ME, Chaft JE, Nafa K et al (2012) Prevalence, clinicopathologic associations, and molecular spectrum of ERBB2 (HER2) tyrosine kinase mutations in lung adenocarcinomas. Clin Cancer Res 18:4910–8
67. Pelligrini C, Falleni M, Marchetti A et al (2003) HER-2/Neu alterations in non-small cell lung cancer: a comprehensive evaluation by real time reverse transcription-PCR, fluorescence in situ hybridization, and immunohistochemistry. Clin Cancer Res 9:3645–52
68. Hirsch FR, Varella-Garcia M, Franklin WA et al (2002) Evaluation of HER-2/neu gene amplification and protein expression in non-small cell lung cancer. B J Cancer 86:1449–56
69. Davies H, Bignell GR, Cox C et al (2002) Mutations of the BRAF gene in human cancer. Nature 417:949–54
70. Chapman PB, Hauschild A, Robert C et al (2011) Improved survival with vemurafenib in melanoma with BRAF V600E mutation. N Engl J Med 364:2507–16
71. Paik PK, Arcila ME, Fara M et al (2011) Clinical characteristics of patients with lung adenocarcinomas harboring BRAF mutations. J Clin Oncol 29:2046–51

72. Marchetti A, Felicioni L, Malatesta S et al (2011) Clinical features and outcome of patients with non–small-cell lung cancer harboring BRAF mutations. J Clin Oncol 29:3574–3579
73. Kobayashi M, Sonobe M, Takahashi T et al (2011) Clinical significance of BRAF gene mutations in patients with non-small cell lung cancer. Anticancer Res 31:4619–23
74. Planchard D, Mazieres J, Riely GJ et al (2013) Interim results of phase II study BRF113928 of dabrafenib in *BRAF* V600E mutation–positive non-small cell lung cancer (NSCLC) patients. J Clin Oncol 31: abstract 8009
75. Weiss J, Sos ML, Seidel D et al (2010) Frequent and focal FGFR1 amplification associates with therapeutically tractable FGFR1 dependency in squamous cell lung cancer. Sci Transl Med 2(62):62ra93
76. Heist RS, Mino-Kenudson M, Sequist LV et al (2012) FGFR1 amplification in squamous cell carcinoma of the lung. J Thorac Oncol 7:1775–1780
77. Cancer Genome Atlas Research Network (2012) Comprehensive genomic characterization of sqaumous cell lung cancer. Nature 489:519–25
78. Gadgeel SM, Chen W, Cote ML et al (2013) Fibrobalst growth factor receptor 1 amplification in non-small cell lung cancer by quantitative real time PCR. PLoS One 8:e79820
79. Nogova L, Sequist L, Cassier PA et al (2014) Targeting FGFR-1 amplified lung squamous cell carcinoma with selective pan-FGFR inhibitor BGJ398. J Clin Oncol 32: abstract 8034
80. Paik PK, Shen R, Ferry D et al (2014) A phase Ib open label multicenter study of AZD4547 in patients with advanced squamous cell lung cancers: Preliminary antitumor activity and pharmacodynamic data. J Clin Oncol 32: abstract 8035

Index

A. Ahmad, S.M. Gadgeel (eds.), *Lung Cancer and Personalized Medicine: Novel Therapies and Clinical Management*, Advances in Experimental Medicine and Biology 890, DOI 10.1007/978-3-319-24932-2

V

W

X

Z

The manufacturer's authorised representative in the EU is Springer Nature Customer Service Centre GmbH, Europaplatz 3, 69115 Heidelberg, Germany. If you have any concerns regarding our products, please contact ProductSafety@springernature.com

Printed and bound by CPI Group (UK) Ltd, Croydon, CR0 4YY
29/07/2026
02180604-0001